Representing Ebola

The Fairleigh Dickinson University Press
Series in Law, Culture, and the Humanities

The Fairleigh Dickinson University Press Series in Law, Culture, and the Humanities publishes scholarly works in which the field of Law intersects with, among others, Film, Criminology, Sociology, Communication, Critical/Cultural Studies, Literature, History, Philosophy, and the Humanities.

General Editor: Caroline Joan "Kay" S. Picart,
MPhil (Cantab), PhD, JD, Esquire
Attorney at Law/Of Counsel, Tim Bower Rodriguez, P.A.

Publications

Marouf A. Hasian Jr., *Representing Ebola: Culture, Law, and Public Discourse about the 2013–2015 West African Ebola Outbreak* (2016)

Jacqueline O'Connor, *Law and Sexuality in Tennessee Williams's America* (2016)

Caroline Joan "Kay" S. Picart, Michael Hviid Jacobsen, and Cecil E. Greek, *Framing Law and Crime: An Interdisciplinary Anthology* (2016)

Caroline Joan "Kay" S. Picart, *Law In and As Culture: Intellectual Property, Minority Rights, and the Rights of Indigenous Peoples* (2016)

On the Web at http://www.fdu.edu/fdupress

Representing Ebola

Culture, Law, and Public Discourse about the 2013–2015 West African Ebola Outbreak

Marouf A. Hasian Jr.

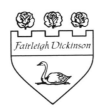

Fairleigh Dickinson

FAIRLEIGH DICKINSON UNIVERSITY PRESS
Madison • Teaneck

3 6 28 59 1

JUN 0 5 2017

Published by Fairleigh Dickinson University Press
Copublished by The Rowman & Littlefield Publishing Group, Inc.
4501 Forbes Boulevard, Suite 200, Lanham, Maryland 20706
www.rowman.com

Unit A, Whitacre Mews, 26-34 Stannary Street, London SE11 4AB

British Library Cataloguing in Publication Information Available

Library of Congress Cataloging-in-Publication Data

Names: Hasian, Marouf Arif, Jr., author.
Title: Representing ebola : culture, law, and public discourse about the
    2013–2015 West African ebola outbreak / Marouf A. Hasian Jr.
Description: Madison : Fairleigh Dickinson University Press ; Lanham,
    Maryland : The Rowman & Littlefield Publishing Group, Inc., [2016] |
    Series: The Fairleigh Dickinson University Press series in law, culture,
    and the humanities | Includes bibliographical references. | Description
    based on print version record and CIP data provided by publisher; resource
    not viewed.
Identifiers: LCCN 2016013710 (print) | LCCN 2016013354 (ebook) | ISBN
    9781611479577 (Electronic) | ISBN 9781611479560 (cloth : alk. paper)
Subjects: | MESH: Hemorrhagic Fever, Ebola | Disease Outbreaks |
Communicable
    Disease Control—legislation & jurisprudence | Human Rights | Social
    Responsibility | Colonialism | Africa, Western | United States
Classification: LCC RC140.5 (print) | LCC RC140.5 (ebook) | NLM WC 534 |
DDC 614.5/7—dc23   (RC 140.5. H27 2016)
LC record available at http://lccn.loc.gov/2016013710

∞™ The paper used in this publication meets the minimum requirements of
American National Standard for Information Sciences—Permanence of Paper
for Printed Library Materials, ANSI/NISO Z39.48-1992.

Printed in the United States of America

Contents

Acknowledgments   vii

1   Arguing about the Cultural and Legal Meanings of the 2013–2015 West African Ebola Outbreak   1

2   NGO Organizational Tales, the Discovery of "Patient Zero," and MSF's Stories about the Origins of the 2013–2015 West African Ebola Outbreak   23

3   The Legal and Ethical Duties That Are Owed to "Contact Tracers" and Other West African Volunteers   49

4   The Saga of Kaci Hickox and the Nature, Scope, and Limits of Human Rights Discourses in Ebola Contexts   77

5   The IMF, the World Bank, and Debates about the Role of Political Economy in Ebola Outbreak Contexts   107

6   Anticipating the Ebola Apocalypse and American Mediascapes   131

7   Liberia's 2014 Autoimmunization of the West Point Suburb and the Return of the Colonial *Cordon Sanitaire*   163

8   Belated Military Humanitarianism and American "Ebola Exceptionalism" during the West African Ebola Outbreak, 2014–2015   185

9 The Legal and Cultural Legacies of the 2013–2015 West
African Outbreak   209

Bibliography   235

Index   247

About the Author   253

Acknowledgments

I have incurred many debts along the way as I wrote this book on the latest Ebola outbreak in West Africa. I want to begin by thanking John, aka, the "bus guru," who sparked my initial interest in this topic when he explained to me some of the practices of health care workers at University of Utah's medical facilities. When we travel in on the bus to work every morning many of us engage in a lot of banter, some of it intellectual, and the more that John explained some of the challenges of these health care workers the more I realized that this raised all sorts of questions regarding Ebola transmission. This in turn led to many hundreds of days of research on various legal, cultural, medical, and military issues in Ebola contexts, and I can't thank John enough for sharing some of his ideas. His thirst for scientific knowledge was contagious. I am sure that he may not agree with much that I have to say about such topics as the West Point quarantines or the treatment of Kaci Hickox, but I thank him nevertheless.

I would also like to thank Jean Ho and Kijoung Na, and other members of the University of Utah Global Internship Program for allowing me to be a part of the 2015 summer internship program. Two delightful and hardworking students from South Korea, Kenneth Choi and Yubeen Kwon, spent several weeks in my office discussing Ebola situations or researching in the Marriott library as they learned about the trials and tribulations of Nina Pham or the "Africanization" of Ebola. These young high school students helped me immensely as I decided what to include in this particular book.

As usual there are many of my colleagues in the Department of Communication at the University of Utah who provided emotional support as

I worked on various chapters of this book. Professor Kent Ono, the chair of our department, listened patiently during many lunches as I explained some of the positions that I was taking in the book. All of the members of my Communication 7460 Social Movements class chimed in and offered suggestions when I commented on various topics that were covered in the book.

I could not have collected the books or stored the other research materials that I needed for this project if Dean Dianne Harris, our dean of College of Humanities, hadn't provided me with a research account. I have often told many colleagues that it is support like this that makes it a pleasure to study complex legal and cultural problems.

There are several people who work with Fairleigh Dickinson University Press, or Rowman & Littlefield, that I would like to thank. I want to thank the outside reviewers from communication studies that provided me with helpful suggestions on how to improve my biocriticism, as well as editors Brooke Bures, Zachary Nycum, and Hannah Fisher, and copyeditor Rae-Ann Goodwin. Caroline "Kay" Picart has supported my work from the very beginning, and this book would not have been written without her efforts and her endorsement. At the same time Harry Keyishian helped answer any questions that I had regarding the "unforgiving formatting" needed to get the manuscript ready for production. Both Kay and Harry helped me stay on task.

1

✚

Arguing about the Cultural and the Legal Meanings of the 2013–2015 West African Ebola Outbreak

It has become a truism among scholars, public health officials, scientists, and others that the fears associated with contracting "Zaire" Ebola, or Ebola virus disease (EVD), travel faster than Ebola itself. "The fear of being infected with Ebola and the desire to flee the area" noted Francesco Chiappelli and his colleagues, are "human universals."[1] This means that those who study the pathogenesis of EVD, or those who analyze the mass-mediated representations of Ebola transmission, are confronted with a number of difficult tasks as they try to track what many in communication studies would call the "rhetorical" or "argumentative" features of these outbreaks.[2]

Earlier Ebola outbreaks, that have killed hundreds of individuals since 1976, have occasionally garnered the attention of regional, national, and international audiences, but the massive loss of life, as well as the rampant anxieties that were caused by the most recent "Zaire" Ebola outbreak in Guinea, Sierra Leone, and Liberia appears to have catalyzed the efforts of those who seem to be convinced that somehow this outbreak was qualitatively different. By the spring of 2014 Ebola had "traveled" or "migrated" to urban areas in West Africa, and worries about mutations and lack of preparedness exacerbated the situation. Communities that were used to dealing with malaria, cholera, or other infectious diseases were now having to hear that they, or their neighbors, might have EVD.

Early misdiagnoses contributed to the early spread of EVD, but those in the West, or what is sometimes called "the North," who kept an eye on what was happening in West Africa also started to worry that Ebola could spread to places like Nigeria, Mali, or the Ivory Coast. The 2005 adoption of "The International Health Regulations" was supposed to help with the establishment of global surveillance triggers that would help with the prevention and containment of diseases,[3] but the poorer countries in the "South" simply did not have the type of surveillance equipment that was used by the wealthier nations. Moreover, cultural anthropologists, who recognized the importance of Ebola fears, complained that slashed World Health Organization (WHO) budgets hurt the efforts of those who tried to combat Ebola denialism, panic, and other anxieties. The anthropologists, and the other interdisciplinary scholars, started writing and talking about "neo-colonial" interventionism or the neglect of "the other" in Ebola contexts and more than a few openly questioned WHO's leadership. If WHO personnel were supposed to be in charge of this latest outbreak in West Africa, then why did *it take months* before WHO officials declared this to be an "international health" emergency?[4] At the same time, if WHO was in charge, did that mean that their employees and their supporters were the ones who were going to distribute the personal protective equipment (PPE), the gloves, the masks, the tents, and so on, that would be needed by the "Ebola fighters" in Sierra Leone, Liberia, and Guinea? If this was the case, then how did Doctors Without Borders, a moderately sized nongovernmental organization (NGO), end up treating one-third of all of the EVD patients in West Africa?[5]

Many scientists, administrators, or decision makers may have wanted to focus on epidemiological or clinical facets of these Ebola containment efforts, but J. Benton Heath has argued that the recent Ebola outbreak helped usher into the twenty-first century new transfers of *emergency power* at the international level that have helped with the legitimation of particular global institutions.[6] Heath was talking about the need for studies of hierarchical and horizontal power structures in the treatment of emerging diseases, and this raised questions about how organizations like WHO tried to recapture some legitimacy as their personnel tackled massive challenges during this latest Ebola outbreak.

CONTAMINATING DISCOURSES AND MASS MASS-MEDIATED TRANSMISSIONS: THE SIGNIFICANCE OF EBOLA STUDIES

The subject of this book is the discourse and argumentation patterns of politicians, NGOs, legal commentators and the media (in the United States/the "North" as well as West Africa) about the 2013–2015 outbreak of Ebola in West Africa. I will be arguing that the legal, medical, and political claims that are embedded in that Ebola discourse are inextricable shaped by existing cultural knowledges that are related to the cultural assumptions that we make regarding epidemiology, American exceptionalism, humanitarian intervention, and military action. All of this embeddedness has theoretical and pragmatic consequences for both the perceived resolution of the recent West African Ebola outbreak as well as the future of global public health practices. I hope that this and future critical scholarship will encourage awareness of the ways that the cultural knowledge of local communities in the "South" and humanitarian organizations in the "North" can impact, positively and negatively, humanitarian medical intervention and public health policies.

The 2013–2015 West African outbreak of Ebola was a major public health event involving a still little-understood disease, which in itself warrants extensive study. The critical analyses in this manuscript usefully apply emerging lines of scholarly inquiry into the reciprocal relationships that exist between cultural knowledge and public discourse (media, political, scientific) about any number of public policy issues. Concrete applications of this line of theoretical inquiry are necessary as they can extend the benefits of such theoretical awareness into the decisions of policy makers as well as the testing of the validity of these emerging theoretical frameworks.[7]

As I will explain in many chapters of this book, there were a host of personal, political, and technical reasons why so many Africans died from Ebola before the end of 2014, and for a long time many observers disagreed about the nature and the scope of the 2013–2015 West African outbreak. Both the reportage of failed regional attempts to contain EVD, as well as journalistic commentaries on community denialism, fear, and distrust only complicated matters for international organizations who found themselves being attacked for not taking charge during a major global pandemic. By the fall of 2014, after almost five thousand West Africans had died from Ebola, and medical humanitarians who usually scoffed at the very notion of "military humanitarianism" eventually pleaded that this "war" against EVD had to be fought by everyone who could join the lists. Fighting Ebola had become a global crusade, and later on medals would be handed out to some Anglo-American military leaders who helped those fighting on the frontlines of these EVD campaigns.[8]

As readers might imagine, talk of needed, but belated humanitarian as well as military interventionism raised a host of complex ideological questions as Ebola experts, virologists, public health administrators, and others started to realize that this was no longer just a "West African" problem. Writers in technical, public, and legal spheres started to debate about the theories and practices that would guide the war against Ebola. How, some asked, would those in the tri-state regions, who were living or working near the "epicenter" or the "center of gravity" of these Ebola battles, effectively "isolate" victims who needed to be segregated from healthier populations? Did the leaders of post-conflict societies in Liberia, Sierra Leone, or Guinea have the political will, or the economic resources, that were needed to pay contact tracers or volunteers who would need to locate EVD victims? Did regional militaries and police organizations have the trust of the people as they put in place restrictive cordons and quarantines at border crossings and in villages? Would the expatriate, foreign doctors and nurses who traveled to West Africa receive the same protection that was afforded African doctors? Would the military forces that were sent to help "Ebola hunters" respect the sovereign political and legal rights of West African governments?

These are just some of the questions that I will tackle in this book, and I will be extending the work of critical cultural scholars,[9] and critical legal writers,[10] as I try to underscore the contingent, partial, and ideological nature of the arguments that circulated in various transcontinental venues between December 2013 and the summer of 2015. Along the way, I will also be arguing that critical legal analyses of these situations reveals that at the very time that the thousands of West African contact tracers, public health workers, local ministers, and others got all of this under control, the foreign military powers arrived on the scene, just in time to claim credit for stopping the spread of EVD. In other words, I will be raising questions about whether organizations like Médecins Sans Frontières (MSF), or Doctors Without Borders, should have ever given up the hope that this could be contained by West Africans as they (reluctantly) joined those Westerners who called for the militarization of Ebola campaigns. If, as Paul Farmer has pointed out in *Infections and Inequalities*[11] "modern inequality" permeates the ways that we think about modern plagues, then it behooves us to highlight how those inequalities manifest themselves in Ebola contexts.

One heuristic way that both critical legal scholars and critical cultural scholars might accomplish some of the tasks that are needed to detect and to critique those inequities could involve the extension of the work of Michel Foucault, who once commented on the need to use methodologies that tracked the rhetorical and material formation of what were called *dispositifs*. In "The Confession of the Flesh" Foucault explains to Alain Grosrichard that a *dispositif,* or an apparatus, referred to the "thoroughly heterogeneous ensemble consisting of discourses, institutions, architectural forms, regulatory decisions, laws, administrative measures, scientific statements," and philosophical, moral and "philanthropic principles" that were elements of the apparatus that made up key "systems of relations."[12] Giorgio Agamben, who built on Foucault's usage of the term *dispositif,* emphasized how an apparatus of this kind could be used to position, manage, direct, or control particular forms of human agency.[13]

Although many representatives of WHO or NGOs who write or talk about the "lessons learned" from this latest outbreak often provide us with slivers of ideological commentary as they circulate what they often view as objectivist or neutral accounts of Ebola pathogenesis, prevention, containment, and preparedness, it will be one of my contentions that they often gloss over the more contradictory and chaotic features of these periods. For example, a few politicians and military leaders in West Africa who decided that emergencies dictated that they quarantine some of their suburbs in their own nations turned around and complained about how other foreign nations, during the fall of 2014, were stigmatizing them and hurting their economies by restricting air traffic to those same countries! These African decision makers did not seem to be bothered by the fact that their own stigmatization of the "other"—that was based on what they described as living in disease-ridden "slums"—looked much like the parallel national stereotyping that was taking place when other nations canceled flights in and out of West Africa. Supposedly real, evidence-based quarantining could be juxtaposed with supposedly unscientific rationales that were used by foreigners who canceled flights that might interfere with tourism or mining operations.

Debates about canceled flights or quarantines were not the only times where commentaries on ontological realities or epistemic beliefs became entangled with axiological claims regarding ethical behavior during medical humanitarian Ebola crises. Many chapters in this book underscore how contentious scientific theories about Ebola contagion were often linked to political, social, and military commentaries on cordon efficacy, legal discussions of quarantine infringements of human rights, stigmatization and identity politics.

Most journalists who traced West African outbreak seemed to write as if all Ebola patients deserved care and had the same access to medical facilities, but a more nuanced study of the material realities of the situations shows that throughout 2014 and 2015 there were publicized hints that countless complementary and contradictory logics were used to rationalize the differential treatment of African doctors and other public health care workers who got sick. Not everyone went through the same regimental procedures, and African intellectuals who cared about pan-African solutions to Ebola problems have reminded us that foreign doctors or health care workers who got sick were immediately flown out of the region. Authors of essays that appeared in scientific journals in the West often mentioned the need for "global health security," and this sounded like a noble goal, but when it came time to operationalize that notion, nationalist politics intruded and contributed to a dilution of that concept.

As I write this book, talk of new vaccines for EVD is in the air and transcontinental communities are writing and talking about how this could be the "game changer" that everyone was looking for. This search for vaccines is itself one manifestation of emergency-oriented ways of thinking about how to cope with catastrophic diseases, but we need to remember that the discovery of vaccines will not dispense with the need to tackle a host of legal and ethical issues that have to do with access to public health care treatments or infectious disease preparedness. Joseph Fins, writing in *The American Journal of Bioethics*, has argued that the recent West African Ebola outbreak provided the occasion for bioethicists and others to begin reevaluating how we are going to study the nexus that exists between ideology and microbiology, Ebola sciences and deliberative democracies.[14] He notes, for example, that after the first popularized cases of Ebola reached the Western Hemisphere, this led to a "media deluge, a good bit of hysteria, and predictable political posturing."[15]

I have written this book so that we can decode many of the textual and contextual features of this media deluge, and I will be extending the work of Fins, Heath, and others who worry about the ethical and legal conundrums that have been raised by the recent West Africa Ebola outbreak.[16]

My critical legal rhetorical approach is very different from traditional, formalistic, or positivist studies of the "rule of law" in that I view jurisprudential argumentation as a type of social act, an ideological performance, where the contingencies, the ambiguities, and the chaos of life are often papered over in order to produce coherent legal tales that appeal to those who want to see medical risk management and control. As a "child" of the legal realists,[17] the critical legal studies movement[18] and the recent critical security studies movement,[19] I am mainly interested in studying how empowered individuals and communities in West Africa or elsewhere actually interpreted and implemented legal guidelines during times of health emergencies. I am not that concerned with abstract, theoretical discussions of the "norms" that should be in place in global security contexts if those norms are not applied in concrete material situations. For example, I don't think that any legal tweaking of the 2005 "The International Health Regulations" is going to help anyone who might die during these outbreaks if the actions "on the ground" bear little relationship to metaphysical arguments that could be made about how Western powers should behave. If the work of scholars like Michel Foucault has taught us anything, it is that the ideologies and praxis that swirls around medical emergencies like the Ebola outbreaks, and the mediated representations of those situations, that garners our attention.[20] Those who defend the position that we need to improve or apply the International Health Regulations need to be able to demonstrate how that would have impacted the trajectories of the latest Ebola outbreak.

In Ebola contexts this is important, especially in rhetorical situations where some West Africans are accused of not understanding, or not appreciating, the legal histories and the governmental rationales that were used to justify the coercive imposition of quarantines. In situations like this we need to think of Western legal cultures as empowered groups who don't hesitate to shake their heads and complain about governmental corruptions, destroyed clinics, ineffective quarantines, and circumvented cordons. As Sung-Joon Park and René Umlauf explain, protecting "individuals from contracting Ebola is certainly necessary, but large-scale militarized interventions, cordoning off cities, districts, and whole regions raises the question of how far quarantine measures" can, or should be expanded.[21] At the same time, talk of West African "traditions" and burial habits by Western lawyers and journalists simply put on display the emotive and ideologically charged nature of some of the legal and ethical arguments that were used by some in the "North" to explain the difficulties they were having as they tried to make sure that Ebola did not travel to their shores. During periods when some public health officials were warning in medical journals that 1.4 million people could contract EVD if *West African behaviors* did not change,[22] legal scholars and Ebola experts were writing about the efficacy of historical quarantines that were used during colonial or postcolonial eras. Is it possible that some of this expressed not-so-veiled longings for earlier colonial or imperial times, before decolonization, when it was theoretically easier to control the spread of infectious diseases?

Another controversial argument that I will be making in this book, that extends the work of many other observers, involves the claim that Western media outlets significantly altered their coverage of this latest outbreak when EVD reached foreign shores. It is no coincidence that as soon as Western media outlets began carrying daily or weekly stores about the *failures of West African containment efforts* in July and August of 2014, legal interest in domestic discussions of quarantines of travelers spiked, as did coverage of the daily activities of individuals like Nina Pham (the nurse who treated a Liberian who traveled to Dallas) or Kaci Hickox (who would be quarantined in a tent by the state of New Jersey). The deaths of famed doctors in Africa who died before this did not often make front-page news, and these stories looked nothing like the personal interest stories that appeared in Anglo-American regional media venues.

In this book I will also underscore the idea that the adoption of a critical legal vantage point allows readers to see the contested nature of Ebola regulations and medical epistemologies. Conventional wisdom often assumes that there is some monolithic, objective collection of facts that are out there about Ebola that simply need to be circulated in order to help cut down on stereotyping of Ebola victims, but all of this *ignores of the power and cultural dimensions of epidemiological knowledge.* While organizations like the CDC or Doctors Without Borders liked to argue that it should be an uncontested "fact" that Ebola could only be spread by close contact with Ebola victims or their fluids, a number of anxious politicians, scientists, and others in the West started to contest the notion that EVD could only be transmitted through close "human-to-human" contact. Those who wanted to critique the CDC guidelines or WHO assumptions could talk about need for scientists and public health decision makers to apply the "precautionary principle"[23] as well as the need to protect American, Spanish, and British publics from possible "airborne" transmission. Some later chapters in the book illustrate how thousands of nurses often took the lead in asking for respirators and other protective measures that would help patients and health care workers in situations where "aerial" transmission of EVD threatened Western lives.

In these types of anxiety-producing situations legal rules or judicial principles were not going to be applied in any cultural vacuum, and talk of the rights of public health workers in West Africa or in other parts of the world were linked to how one argued about Ebola pathogenesis, disease transmission, "cultures," and the status of the health care infrastructures of nation-states. Complex ideological tapestries were fabricated by those who wove together cultural and legal threads that sometimes put on display contentious ways of talking about Ebola preparedness.

Before I supply some contextual material on the 2013–2015 West African Ebola outbreak that critiques some of these rhetorical tapestries let me provide readers with a few examples of the kind of questions that motivated me to write this book:

- What legal and cultural issues were raised during what Doctors Without Borders called the "first stage" of this outbreak (March 2014–July 2015)? This was the period of time when a few "Ebola hunters" from America and Europe joined public health officials from Guinea as they searched for the mysterious "patient zero."
- How did members of mainstream or alternative presses talk or write about the legal responsibilities and the ethical duties of local governments and foreign powers when they explained to their readers how thousands of West African "contact tracers" and volunteers were "tracking" down potential Ebola EVD victims?
- What are the *perceived* cultural and legal implications of having NGOs like Doctors Without Borders, or the U.S. military during "Operation United Assistance," intervene in the sovereign affairs of West African nations?
- What jurisprudential issues were said to have been raised when West African nations closed their borders and used colonial-style "*cordons sanitaires*" to keep out potential Ebola "carriers"?

- How do various regional or international communities debate about how economic institutions, like the World Bank or IMF, have any "responsibility to protect" when impoverished nations are suffering from the ravages of "emerging" infectious diseases?
- How do social agents argue about the nature, scope, and limits of U.S. legislative, executive, and judicial power during periods when returning doctors, nurses, and other "rescuers" come back to the "homeland" after "fighting" Ebola overseas?
- How do the "image events" (John Delicath and Kevin DeLuca)[24] that circulate in movies like *Outbreak* (1995) or *Contagion* (2011) influence the ways that communities interpret the core or "penumbral" legal lines that can be drawn between individual civil rights and public health interests?[25]
- Did the Ebola outbreak catalyze the efforts of bioethicists and others who might argue that West Africans and others deserve "global health security," or is that ideograph[26] simply a cultural sign that we have accepted the "militarization" of Ebola?

These are just a few of the types of research questions that I raise in this book, but this short list provides a summary of some of the key issues that I believe have been raised when we decode the various Ebola *dispositifs* that circulated in transatlantic public and legal spheres.

A CRITICAL LEGAL CONTEXTUALIZATION OF THE 2013–2015 EBOLA OUTBREAK

Elsewhere I have gone into much more detail explaining how critical legal rhetorical approaches differ from more formalistic and positivistic ways of viewing the "rule of law,"[27] and I will be applying this type of critical legal contextualization as I explore the contested nature of key Ebola rhetorics. Priscilla Wald has persuasively argued that there are contagion "outbreak" narratives that are made up of a "series of images, phrases, scenarios and story lines that unfold like so many movies,"[28] and I think of Ebola "*dispositifs*"[29] as those discursive formations that are made up of protean legal and bioethical fragments that circulated during the most recent Ebola outbreak in the same way. For example, those who debated about hospital duties or the rights of nurses, or those who wanted to make sure that contracts with "contact tracers" were enforced during the outbreak, were circulating ideologically loaded legal Ebola rhetorics that were providing specialized ways of advancing claims, providing evidence, and supplying argumentative warrants during heated judicial or bioethical debates.

The adoption of a critical legal rhetoric approach, that traces how these generic Ebola arguments drifted across, and between, legal and public spheres,[30] allows for a more nuanced critique of the claims that were advanced by many social actors, and not just jurists or lawyers, who had something to say about the legality or efficacy of particular Ebola prevention, containment, or preparedness policies. This "vernacular" way of viewing constellations of meaning, or *dispositifs*, invites us to see the ways that social actors, including lay persons, co-produce legal meanings as they deliberate about how to interpret public health regulations during epidemics.

As I write this book I join the growing community of rhetoricians and other interdisciplinary scholars who use a host of close-textual, contextual, or hybrid perspectives or methods as they study such topics as "viral rhetorics," "predatory" discourses, "contagion" stories, or post-apocalyptic narratives. For example, at times I will be drawing from the work of Jacques Derrida, Ann Stoler, and Roberto Esposito as I critique some of the cultural, social, political, economic, historical, and legal features of Ebola *dispositifs*.

Within my own discipline I am known as a critical legal rhetorician, and in this particular book I share Lisa Keränen's interest in biocriticism, a perspectival approach that she once described as "a mode of inquiry that analyzes the rhetorics of contagion across space and time."[31] She is the type of scholar who likes to review how these rhetorics circulate in technical and public spheres, and she tracks how some arguments about infectious diseases move across the porous boundaries that theoretically separate those fields or spheres. Keränen's analyses also draw from the work of Michel Foucault,[32] Priscilla Ward, and others who analyze the cultural, rhetorical, and biological features of these Ebola discourses that are geared toward making us feel less secure.

This type of a critical legal rhetorical approach has affinities with perspectival approaches that build on Michel Foucault's notion of the "truth effects" that go into our securitized governmental *epistemes*.[33] Given the fact that this book is concerned with Ebola politics it is noteworthy that Foucault once described his interventionist projects, filled with histories and counterhistories (later described as genealogies), as critical investigations of the power of victors and the powerless "vanquished." More specifically, he argued that his own critical approach to medical histories and vital sciences tried to "awaken" the discourse that existed "beneath the form of institutions and laws, the forgotten past of real struggles," that were often hidden behind the "masked victories of defeats" and the "blood that has dried in the codes."[34] Foucault's critiques thus combined commentaries on the politics of both life (biopolitics) and death (thanatopolitics).[35]

If those who died during the West Africa outbreak did so because of belated interventionism, ineffective quarantines, mismanaged cordons, sporadically enforced contracts, and so on, then there were a host of contestable legal and bioethical decisions that were made between 2013 and 2015 that need to be interrogated. This is one of the reasons readers will find that in the later sections of this book I will be constantly referring to the biopolitical as well as the thanatopolitical features of the circulation of Ebola texts and contexts.

The adoption of this critical legal rhetorical approach gives authors and readers the chance to review and critique the ways that national and international communities talked and wrote about global health security, public health leadership, and the stigmatization of Ebola victims and those who treated them. Instead of simply paying attention to a single, correct, or definitive interpretation of the "rule of law" during times of health emergencies, we would follow's Foucault's admonition and keep in mind the winners and losers in these heated historical, jurisprudential, or ethical Ebola contests.

Sadly, there are no shortage of discursive terrains that critics would need to keep track of as they study the *dispositifs* that circulated before, and after, the beginning of the latest Ebola outbreak. Talk of the "failed" states of West Africa, and discussion about the havoc that was wreaked by more than a dozen years of civil wars,[36] for example, formed antecedent rhetorics that circulated in Western circles before the latest EVD outbreak. These earlier figurations helped make sense of the ways that Ebola diverted precious resources away from the treatment of other diseases, like cholera, malaria, and Lassa fever. They could also be used to divert attention away from other functional or structural features of Ebola epidemics.

As I argue in more detail in later chapters of this book, some of the earliest discussion of duties in Ebola contexts had to do with the decisions that were made by the governments and public health authorities of Liberia, Guinea, and Sierra Leone before August of 2014. The six months that preceded this was a time when many in the West and other parts of the globe considered Ebola to be a localized, national, or regional outbreak situation, and they assumed that it could be controlled in the same way that previous Ebola outbreaks had been contained in places like "Zaire" (now the Democratic Republic of the Congo) or Uganda.

As noted above, mass-mediate discussions of legal and ethical liability were altered as soon as Spain, Nigeria, and the United States started to report that they were having to deal with Ebola patients, and the fact that regional or international travel restrictions were often involved signaled the revival of debates about state sovereignty and international health duties. This all heralded the appearance of permutations of the familiar jurisprudential balancing tests that considered the roles that legislatures or courts should play in the weighing of individual rights and collective interests during Ebola outbreaks. A critical legal rhetorical approach to all of this disputation would invite us to see how micro-commentaries about the treatment of individual patients like Thomas Eric Duncan, the Liberian who died from EVD in Dallas, could be linked to more macro debates about the propriety of restricting air travel, the duties of those who needed to put in place "mandatory" quarantines, and responsibilities of nation-states or WHO.

While some pundits in the blogosphere talked about the need for isolationism and the closing of the U.S.-Mexican borders to those who carried Ebola "contagion," others vociferously argued that this is exactly what we *should not do* if we wanted to be able to "contact trace" EVD victims. At the same time, the advocacy of travel restrictions and what were viewed by some as draconian quarantining were said to have an impact on the decisions that were made by doctors and nurses who wanted to travel overseas so that they could battle Ebola.

What might be called the securitization of Ebola rhetorics added even more ideological layers to these *dispositifs* as journalists and other pundits argued that those who believed in "military humanitarianism" needed to take serious their "responsibility to protect" (R2P) endangered populations that suffer from particular endemic or epidemic diseases. The victors and winners in these Ebola contests couldn't help using binary templates that invited readers to contrast the "speedy response" of Médecins Sans Frontières (MSF) or foreign militaries with the "late" interventions of WHO and the rest of the world.[37] This type of argumentation appealed to those who talked and wrote about "global health" needs or security "rights."

Legal performances, and public worries about scientific realities and jurisprudential issues, had everything to do with how one acted and behaved during this latest outbreak. For example, the hospitals in Dallas that treated some of the first Ebola patients had to worry about more than just their knowledge of epidemiology or virology. They were sued by one of the nurses who treated Thomas Duncan because concerns were raised about the privacy of public health caregivers, the lack of adequate training of nurses, and the lack of personnel protective equipment (PPE) in the hospital.[38] In other situations, newspapers—in West Africa and the United States—carried stories of how families of the dead were threatening lawsuits after they found out *that only some* of those who contracted Ebola were provided with experimental drug therapies.

Talk of the applicable law related to Ebola was not just a matter that concerned lawyers and judges. Rumors of how doctors in New York or nurses in Dallas were contracting Ebola meant that Western local clinics or hospitals now had to be aware of Centers for Disease Control (CDC) rules and protocols, and lay persons and journalists joined the ranks of those who talked about the rights and the duties of various parties in Ebola contexts.

It was one thing to think about Ebola threatening Africans overseas before August of 2014. It was quite another when your neighbor or family member also felt that they had to worry about contracting Ebola. Even though there were only a half dozen confirmed cases of Ebola throughout 2014, this did not stand in the way of the Anglo-American audiences who wanted to co-create their own Ebola *dispositifs*. No wonder that pundits in all sorts of media outlets talked and wrote about "state" versus "federal" interests during times of health emergencies, the legal responsibilities of governors, judges, and others who needed to "enforce" mandatory public measures.

As I explain in several chapters of this book, sometimes this led to a clash of political wills as the Obama administration and the CDC debated with local and regional communities about everything from the plausibility of "airborne" transmission of EVD to the wisdom of canceling flights from particular countries. The governors of New York and New Jersey, who wanted to show that they could get tough when it came to protecting the citizens in their states, used permutations of precautionary principle arguments as they demanded that doctors, nurses, and other volunteers returning from West Africa be quarantined for twenty-one days.

Would these heroines and heroes be allowed to practice individual acts of "self-surveillance," or would they be forced to undergo mandatory isolation in the name of protecting the collective interest in public health, safety, and welfare? A few journalists were fond of writing about the daily activities and movements of these returning volunteers as they supposedly went to subways, movie theaters, grocery stores, or even bowling alleys.

In these Western outbreak narratives, the personal became political, and even the riding of a bike by someone who traveled back from working with Ebola patients in West Africa could be symbolically coded as an act of defiance that threated the body politic. As I explain in more detail later on in this book, this involved a tension between what Roberto Esposito has called *communitas* and *immunitas*.[39]

Westerners often used theoretical models, risky scenarios, and hypothetical situations as they debated about what to do in the event that their populations had to experience life during full-scale epidemics, but in West Africa a type of situational awareness came when populations there dealt with different "phases" of foreign interventionism in West Africa.[40] As noted above the first phase lasted from March to July of 2014, while the second phase began in early September of 2014 and started to wind down by February of 2015. A few dozen foreign Ebola experts, doctors and other scientists traveled to Guinea, Liberia, and Sierra Leone during the first phase because they thought that they could treat this outbreak in the same way that they had treated dozens of others over the years, and they left when the number of "new" reported cases seemed to be going down. The second phase began after the World Health Organization, in August, finally declared this to be an international health emergency. This second phase came after months of listening to Doctors Without Borders complain about pathogenic, diagnostic, or treatment miscalculations and the underestimation of the scope of the EVD problem.

The importance of using legal and cultural frameworks for the study of Ebola debates comes from the recognition that there are diverse ways of framing how we make sense of both the world's inattentiveness to these problems during the initial phase, as well as their sudden rush to make up for lost time during the second phase. Was it some epidemiological conclusion, some "new" piece of scientific evidence, or some convincing graphic display of statistical information that led to a situation where West African populations suddenly witnessed the influx of Cuban and Chinese doctors, or the shipment of tons of personal protective equipment from warehouses in Belgium? Were the personnel working for MSF circulating poor arguments between June and August of 2014, and did that account for the relative lack of mainstream media coverage of EVD? If global communities had traveled to their cineplex to see movies like *Outbreak* (1995) or *Contagion* (2011), then why didn't they demand that West African populations be afforded what bioethicists call "global security" rights?

I am convinced that before those of us who are interested in adopting critical legal rhetorical approaches can answer these types of questions we need to become familiar with the diachronic, as well synchronic, cultural or legal arguments of those who may have been worried about creating moral panic. For example, if we study the Ebola *dispositifs* that circulated in scientific spheres between 2013 and 2015 we may find that part of WHO's hesitancy to call this an "international" outbreak may have had something to do with their embarrassments—and their potential legal liability—that flowed from their ill-fated warnings about earlier flu epidemics. These were weighty matters that involved more than just conjectural mistakes—legal liability could flow from either the abdication of legal responsibility to warn *or* the circulation of illegitimacy Cassandra-like health warnings that later are characterized as moral panic, threat-inflation, or misguided. The agonizing choices that had to be made about human vulnerability involved human dilemmas, power disparities, and cultural assumptions that cannot be easily resolved by the updating of some health protocol or the passage of some universal legal edict.

It could be argued that none of this legal and cultural disputation took place in any moral vacuum, and that some of these debates about Ebola, infectious disease claims, epidemiological evidence, and argumentative warrants began with the reportage of the first case of "Patient Zero," who died in December of 2013 in southeastern Guinea.[41] While some today argue that we cannot be sure that the West African outbreak began when a two-year-old child in Guinea contracted EVD, others are convinced that this has been confirmed by DNA evidence as well as what is called "contract-tracing." This would then usher in debates about the lack of laboratories in Guinea, the need for the government to acknowledge the outbreak, and the possibility that experienced Ebola "hunters" from Europe needed to be called in to investigate matters.

Although sometimes journalists, writing in objectivist styles, create the impression that our historical legacy of all of this can be found in unvarnished, arhetorical chronicles of these affairs, the chapters in this book put on the display the contentious and ideological nature of the decisions that were made, dating back to the time of the discovery of "patient zero."

With this in mind, let me briefly explain the trajectory of the rest of the book, and how each chapter advances the arguments that I am making about the legal and cultural features of these Ebola landscapes and mediascapes.[42]

THE TRAJECTORY OF THIS BOOK AND
A BRIEF SUMMARY OF THE CHAPTERS

In chapter 2, I provide readers with an overview of the unique features of the organizational NGO *dispositifs* that are produced by leaders and doctors working for Médecins Sans Frontières (MSF). In that portion of the book I take up the question of how local populations in Guéckédou, Guinea reacted to some of their interventionism during the initial phase of the West African outbreak. Chapter 2 illustrates how MSF personnel were not just adopting the subject positions of doctors or public health care givers when they traveled to Guinea, Liberia, or Sierra Leone. They were also arguers who promoted the ideology of *témoignage*—or the witnessing of the tragedies of the other—at the same time that they were complaining about belated WHO intervention. This chapter also shows that while many communities outside of West Africa praised Doctors Without Borders there were also many Africans who resented the perceived elitism of this NGO, and they complained about the "illegality" of MSF interventionism.

MSF may have been a more radical organization but it nevertheless used variants of neo-liberal *dispositifs* as its members complained about West African denialism, problematic burial habits, and the physical threats that they received from those who believed that MSF brought Ebola to the region.

Chapter 3 provides a review of the storytelling and argumentative templates that were produced by West African contact tracers, other local health care workers, and their supporters. These were the volunteers who risked (and still risk) their lives in the name of trying to stop the spread of Ebola. This part of the book explains how they often complained about their ill treatment as they continued to work, even during times when they were not paid on time for their labor.

Chapter 3 also shows that at times these were some of the forgotten characters in the hagiographic tales that were told by those living the "North," that often celebrated foreign interventionism. This chapter is placed here so that we can see how the often-overlooked performances of the locals also raised some uncomfortable legal, moral, and economic questions about some of the labor practices of those on the "frontlines" of the Ebola outbreak.

Chapter 4 is a chapter that shifts gears so that we can study some of the legal *dispositifs* that were produced in America during the fall of 2014, when mainstream newspapers, radio outlets, and the blogosphere were talking about the role that politicians, lawyers, and the judicial system should play in the balancing of individual rights versus national public health interests. By presenting some of the contested rhetorics that swirled around the nurse Kaci Hickox, this particular part of the book illustrates how disputes that might appear to depend on resolving a single dispute, or the study of the "science" behind Ebola transmission, could impact the crafting of these particular Ebola *dispositifs*. There I highlight the ways that nurses, their legal representatives, governors, representatives of the CDC, and others could talk and write about the desirability and feasibility of travel restrictions, the "mandatory" quarantines, and preparedness and training for EVD at local hospitals and clinics.

Chapter 5 complicates matters by focusing on the role that economic *dispositifs* have played in Ebola debates. There I critique some of the key arguments that were made about how the "political economy" of World Bank or IMF policies impacted the ways that those in "the North" discussed the economics of the West African Ebola outbreak. This portion of the book explores the question of whether the use of austerity tactics by financial organizations helped or hurt the nations of Liberia, Guinea, and Sierra Leone, and whether they are legally culpable for their behavior. This is a chapter that allows readers to see some of the public and economic debates about the role that neo-liberalism played, or should play, when impoverished nations try to stop the spread of emerging infectious diseases.

Chapter 6 investigates the role that the mass media played during the legal and cultural disputation about the West African outbreak. Here, for example, I describe how various visual media, including books and films about Ebola helped with the crafting of Ebola expertise. At the same time, these text and visualities "anticipated" the latest outbreak. By this, I mean that they configured EVD, and the magnitude of Ebola epidemics, in ways that invited audiences to view Ebola outbreaks as if they were part of an "Ebola apocalypse." This part of the book also explores what happened when CNN tried to compare the securitization dangers of Ebola with those of ISIS.

Chapter 7 is a speculative chapter that uses a case study of the cordoning off of the Monrovian suburb of West Point, in Liberia, as a way of illustrating how fear of EVD can lead to rhetorical situations where police and military forces are used to try and coercive isolate entire "slums" in West African countries. In this particular case I point out how Liberians were doing all of this at the same time that they were complaining about how foreigners were restricting travel to their country.

Chapter 8 illustrates the continued rhetorical resonance of "military humanitarianism" rhetorics that put on display American leaderships, missions, and "exceptionalism." Here I explore how elites and publics reacted to the news from President Obama in late September of 2014 that he was asking for some $750 million to fight Ebola as he prepared more than 3,500 military doctors, engineers, and others to go overseas. This would later be dubbed Obama's "Ebola surge," and those who defended this intervention crafted militaristic *dispositifs* that clashed with more pacifistic ways of writing and talking about the management of infectious diseases.

Interestingly enough, the members of the military who traveled abroad had to live under a very different, stricter, quarantine regime than the civilians who were covered by the rules from the CDC and the Obama administration.

Chapter 9, the concluding chapter, illustrates the interconnectedness of these various *dispositifs*, and that portion of the book explains where we are today in the "battles" against the spread of Ebola. This chapter also takes up the question of how our current legal and cultural debates about Ebola may impact future discussions of how various nations and international communities handle MERS outbreaks and the spread of other infectious diseases.

By the time that readers reach the end of this book, I hope that they will have gained an appreciation of the complex legal and cultural arguments that circulate during times of perceived emerging disease emergencies. Sadly, I share the views of many doctors, researchers, and others who are convinced that we have not seen the last of Ebola outbreaks.

NOTES

1. Francesco Chiappelle et al., "Ebola: Translational Science Considerations," *Journal of Translational Medicine* 13, no. 11 (2015): 1–29, 11.

2. For an example of an argumentative study of some features of Ebola representations, see Kevin J. Ayotte, "A Vocabulary of Disease: Argumentation, Hot

Zones, and the Intertextuality of Bioterrorism," *Argumentation and Advocacy* 48 (Summer, 2011): 1–21. For more examples of Ayotte's work see Kevin J. Ayotte, Daniel Rex Bernard, and H. Dan O'Hair, "Knowing Terror: On the Epistemology and Rhetoric of Risk," in *Handbook of Risk and Crisis Communication*, edited by Robert L. Heath and H. Dan O'Hair (New York: Routledge, 2009), 607–628.

3. World Health Organization Staff, "Strengthening Health Security by Implementing the International Health Regulations, 2005," *World Health Organization*, last modified August 6, 2014, http://www.who.int/ihr/procedures/emerg_comm_members_20140806/en/. The International Health Regulations (IHR) were supposed to part of a comprehensive, multi-national effort that would be led by WHO, where each nation that was threatened by a major outbreak would use "event-based surveillance" to let the other nations know about the need for rapid risk assessment and event-based risk communications. What was called the Global Outbreak Alert and Response Network (GOARN) was supposed to ensure that the right technical expertise and skilled personnel were "on the ground" as quickly as possible where they were needed. In theory, WHO was supposed to help develop and provide tools, guidance and training for national public health communities who were supposed to follow IHR procedures.

4. Nick Childs, "WHO: Ebola 'An International Emergency.'" BBC News, last modified August 8, 2014, http://www.bbc.com/news/health-28700213.

5. See MSF Staff, "Ebola: Latest MSF Updates," *Doctors Without Borders* [November 1, 2015], http://www.doctorswithoutborders.org/our-work/medical-issues/ebola.

6. J. Benton Heath, "Global Emergency Power in the Age of Ebola," *Harvard International Law Journal* 57, July 6, 2015, http://papers.ssrn.com/sol3/papers.cfm?abstract_id=2587720.

7. I would like to thank one of my external reviewers for providing the short summary of the heuristic value of this investigation that appears in the previous two paragraphs.

8. See BBC News, "UK Ebola Aid Workers to Qualify for Medals Says Cameron," BBC News, last modified February 4, 2015, http://www.bbc.com/news/uk-politics-31133815.

9. By "critical cultural" studies I mean the ideological rhetorical investigation of the ways public cultures are involved in the formation of epistemic medical knowledge about Ebola. This type of an approach, that focuses on the power dimensions of scientific knowledge, invites investigators to explore how ordinary citizens, as well as scientific elites, are involved in the co-production of scientific knowledge. For an overview of some of the challenges that confront rhetoricians who study these cultural or public understandings of science, see Celeste M. Condit, John Lynch, and Emily Winderman, "Recent Rhetorical Studies in Public Understanding of Science: Multiple Purposes and Strengths," *Public Understanding of Science* 21, no. 4 (2012): 386–400. doi: 10.1177/0963662512437330. Some critical cultural investigations are satisfied with more descriptive studies of key structures and functions of the rhetorics that pass for scientific knowledge, while other research is more prescriptive in nature and might be influenced by post-structural, postmodern, or postcolonial perspectives that focus on the emancipatory desires of the disempowered. For example, empowerment of the weak may depend on

the recognition that there are always competing medical epistemologies. For some related studies that use Foucauldian approaches when they study Ebola or plague rhetorics but may not have authors that self-identify as "critical cultural" authors, see Liora Bigon, "Bubonic Plague, Colonial Ideologies, And Urban Planning Policies: Dakar, Lagos, and Kumasi," *Planning Perspectives* (August, 2015), doi:10.108 0/02665433.2015.1064779.

10. By "critical legal rhetorics" I mean those ideological investigations that look into the ways that the "rule of law" and judicial norms are co-constructed by hegemonic elites and empowered audiences. See Marouf Hasian Jr., "Critical Legal Rhetorics: The Theory and Practice of Law in a Postmodern World," *Southern Communication Journal* 60, no. 1 (1994): 44–56; Todd F. McDorman, "Challenging Constitutional Authority: African American Responses to *Scott v. Sandford*," *The Quarterly Journal of Speech* 83, no. 2 (1997): 192–209, doi: 10.1080/00335639709384180. Critical legal rhetorical approaches extend the work of members of the legal realist movements, critical legal studies movement, critical race theory movements, critical feminist movements, and other movements that have members who focus on the power dimensions of judicial relationships. For an example of a study on Ebola that draws on some the work of critical race theorists, see Carmela Murdocca, "When Ebola Came to Canada: Race and the Making of the Respectable Body," *Atlantis* 27, no. 2 (Spring/Summer 2003): 24–31.

11. Paul Farmer, *Infections and Inequalities: The Modern Plagues* (Berkeley: University of California Press, 2001).

12. Michel Foucault, The Confession of the Flesh," *in Power/Knowledge: Selected Interviews and Other Writings, 1972–1977,* edited by Colin Gordon (New York: Pantheon Books, 1980). 194–228, 194. I would like to thank one of the external reviewers of this manuscript for bringing this passage to my attention.

13. Gorgio Agamben, *"What Is an Apparatus?" and Other Essays* (London: Stanford University Press, 2009), 12–14.

14. Joseph J. Fins, "Ideology and Microbiology: Ebola, Science, and Deliberative Democracy," *The American Journal of Bioethics* 15, no. 4 (2015): 1–3. e DOI: 10.1080/15265161.2015.1023119.

15. Fins, "Ideology and Microbiology," 1.

16. Some of the important early legal and ethical discussions of the 2013–2015 West African Ebola Outbreak appear in Mark A. Rothstein, "From SARS to Ebola: Legal and Ethical Considerations for Modern Quarantine," *Indiana Health Law Review* 12, no. 1 (2015): 227–280.

17. The legal realists were social scientists and others who wrote during the 1920s and 1930s about how laws need to be written in ways that reflected actual public behavior instead of having the "rule of law" be based on "metaphysical" principles. For a recent example of how some in communication studies use "critical" approaches that extend some of the ideas that can be traced back to the legal realists see John Nguyet Erni, "A Legal Realist View of Citizen Actions in Hong Kong's Umbrella Movement," *Chinese Journal of Communication* 8, no. 4 (2015): 412–419.

18. The critical legal studies movement, that was popularized in law schools during the late 1970s and 1980s, sought to bring in some of the post-structural or postmodern ideas about epistemology and ideology into the realm of jurisprudence. For an overview of how some of these legal scholars tried to write critical

legal histories that extended the work of Michel Foucault and others see Christopher Tomlins, "The Presence and Absence of Legal Mind: A Commentary on Duncan Kennedy's "Three Globalizations of Law and Legal Thought, 1850–2000," *Law and Contemporary Problems* 78, no. 1 (2015): 1–2, http://papers.ssrn.com/sol3/papers.cfm?abstract_id=2557668.

19. For a fine example of a related critical security studies analysis that investigates the role the publics could play in critical security studies, see William Walters and Anne-Marie D'Aoust, "Bringing Publics into Critical Security Studies: Notes for a Research Strategy," *Millennium: Journal of International Studies* 44, no. 1 (2015): 45–68, doi: 10.1177/0305829815594439. "Biocriticism" is a related term that I will be using throughout this book as I explore the ideological and rhetorical features of Ebola narratives and other figurations circulated by empowered rhetors.

20. For an excellent example of a 2014 critical essay that extends the work of Michel Foucault in order to study the role that power plays in the crafting of our existential rhetorics of "insecurity," see Sung-Joon Park and René Umlauf, "Caring as Existential Insecurity: Quarantine, Care, and Human Insecurity in the Ebola Crisis," *Somatosphere*, November 24, 2014, http://somatosphere.net/2014/11/caring-as-existential-insecurity.html.

21. Sung-Joon Park and René Umlauf, "Caring as Existential Insecurity," paragraph 12.

22. In September of 2014 writers for the U.S. Centers for Disease Control and Prevention, in their *Morbidity and Mortality Weekly Report* (MMWR), were warning that cases in Liberia were doubling every 15,020 days, and those in Sierra Leone and Guinea were doubling every 30–40 days. They warned that without massive foreign interventionism or changes in West African community behavior the world might be looking at a total of 550,000 cases in Liberia and Sierra Leone. If one took into account the possibility that corrections were needed for possible underreporting of EVD cases, than it was possible that there might be 1.4 million victims in worst-case scenarios. In order to avoid these types of scenarios, the CDC was suggesting that approximately 70 percent of these cases needed to be treated in Ebola Treatment Units, or if those units were at capacity then homes and communities need to isolate the EVD victims and ensure that safe burial practices were followed. Martin Melzer et al., "Estimating the Future Number of Cases in the Ebola Epidemic—Liberia and Sierra Leone, 2014–2015," *Morbidity and Mortality Weekly Reports, Supplements* 63, no. 3 (September 26, 2914): 1–14.

23. See, for example, Lisa M. Brosseau and Rachel Jones, "Commentary: Health Workers Need Optimal Respiratory Protection for Ebola," *Center for Infectious Disease Research and Policy*, last modified September 17, 2014, http://www.cidrap.umn.edu/news-perspective/2014/09/commentary-health-workers-need-optimal-respiratory-protection-ebola. The University of Minnesota's Center for Infectious Disease Research and Policy (CIDRAP) made it clear when they published this article that this essay reflected the personal opinions of the authors, and did not represent the opinions of the University of Illinois at Chicago or any other organization. The authors were characterized as "national experts on respiratory protection and infectious disease transmission."

24. Image events are some of the resources for elite and public disputation that circulate during salient social controversies. For more theoretical discussion of the

ideological nature of these image events, see John W. Delicath and Kevin Michael DeLuca, "Image Events, the Public Sphere, and Argumentative Practice: The Case of Radical Environmental Groups," *Argumentation* 17 (2003): 315–333.

25. When legal positivists or legal formalists believe that there is a growing consensus of interpretations of the "rule of law" that can be found in similar interpretations of statutes or legal opinions, those convergent interpretations are said to make up the core of "settled" legal opinion. The more divergent, ambiguous, and contradictory features of legal interpretations are often called the "penumbra" that shadows that core. Those jurists and theorists who viewed themselves as legal scientists, like Oliver Wendell Holmes Jr., believed that the law was progressing when it moved from arbitrary and vague penumbras and toward more consensual cores. Holmes, like other scholars, was fond of using astronomical metaphors, and penumbras are literally "partial shadows." See Thomas C. Grey, "The Holmesian Judge in Theory and Practice," *William and Mary Law Review* 37 (1995): 19–45.

26. An ideograph is a key evocative term or phrase that puts on display the political consciousness or ideological allegiances of a rhetor or an audience. See Michael C. McGee, "The 'Ideograph': A Link between Rhetoric and Ideology," *The Quarterly Journal of Speech* 66, no. 1 (1980): 1–16, doi: 10.1080/00335638009383499. Examples of common ideographs include "liberty," "necessity," "freedom," or "equality." In Ebola contexts claiming that the spread of EVD constituted an "emergency" or a "security" threat would be examples of ideographic ways of trying to mobilize publics to take drastic action in the name of those ideographs.

27. See, of example, Hasian, *Critical Legal Rhetorics*," 44–56.

28. Priscilla Wald, "Panic and Precaution: Ebola and the Outbreak Narrative," *The Conversation.com*, last modified October 28, 2014, http://theconversation. com/panic-and-precaution-ebola-and-the-outbreak-narrative-32786.

29. At various points in *The History of Security of Sexuality, Volume 1: An Introduction*, Foucault alludes to *dispositifs* that are types of sedimented knowledges that can be contested. This might refer to an "apparatus," a type of "machinery," and/or an item that is deployed in contests over power. Michel Foucault, *The History of Sexuality, Volume I: An Introduction* (1976: London: Allen Lane, 1979). For a review of other ways of deploying the term "dispositive," see Jeffrey Bussolin, "What Is a Dispositif?" *Foucault Studies* 10 (2010): 85–107, as well as my other earlier commentaries on *dispositifs*.

30. For another example of a legal and public examination of rhetoric that I would characterize as an example of critical legal rhetoric, see Celeste M. Condit and John L. Lucaites, *Crafting Equality: America's Anglo-African Word* (Chicago: University of Chicago Press, 1993).

31. Lisa Keränen, "Review Essay: Addressing the Epidemic of Epidemics: Germs, Security, and a Call for Biocriticism," *The Quarterly Journal of Speech* 97, no. 2 (2011): 224–244, doi: 10.1080/00335630.2011.565785.

32. For related studies using Foucauldian methods in studies of biopolitics, see Stephen J. Collier and Andrew Lakoff, "Vital Systems Security: Reflective Biopolitics and the Government of Emergency," *Theory, Culture & Society* 32, no. 2 (2015): 19–51.

33. Michel Foucault, *"Society Must Be Defended": Lectures at the Collège De France, 1975–1976*, translated by David Macey (New York: Picador, 2003).

34. Michel Foucault, quoted in Stuart J. Murray, "Myth as Critique: Review of Michel Foucault's "Society Must Be Defended," *Qui Parle* 13, no. 2 (Spring/Summer, 2003): 203–221, 209.

35. For a critique of key Foucauldian thanatopolitical theories and practices see Stuart J. Murray, "Thanatopolitics: On the Use of Death for Mobilizing Political Life," *Polygraph* 18 (2006): 191–215.

36. See, for example, William P. Murphy, "Military Patrimonialism and Child Soldier Clientalism in the Liberia and Sierra Leonean Civil Wars," *African Studies Review* 46, no. 2 (2003): 61–87.

37. For an example of a review in one of the leading scientific magazines on the rapid response of MSF to the West African outbreak, see Erika Check Hayden, "MSF Takes Bigger Global-Health Role," *Nature* 522 (June 4, 2015): 18–19. One interesting question that needs to be asked—did the "reluctant" defense of military humanitarianism, and the MSF call for military support in the "war" against Ebola, help expand the base of MSF donors, and did this help with the growth of this particular organization?

38. Laura Wallis, "First U.S. Nurse to Contract Ebola Sues Texas Health Resources," *American Journal of Nursing* 115, no. 6 (June 2015): 16, doi: 10.1097/01. NAJ.0000466302.77895.c5.

39. For a nice overview of Esposito's work on these topics see Timothy Campbell, "'Bios,' Immunity, Life: The Thought of Roberto Esposito," *Diacritics* 36, no. 2 (Summer, 2006): 2–22.

40. Here I am using some of the nomenclature, and punctuation of time, that is used by Doctors Without Borders in their delineation of various stages of the 2013–2015 West African outbreak. MSF calls the period between March and July of 2014 the "initial phase" of the outbreak.

41. Denise Grady and Seri Fink, "Tracing Ebola's Breakout to an African 2-Year Old," *The New York Times*, last modified, August 9, 2014, http://www.nytimes.com/2014/08/10/world/africa/tracing-ebolas-breakout-to-an-african-2-year-old.html?_r=0. The first recorded indexical "Ground Zero" case for the 2013–2015 West African outbreak involved the death of a two-year-old child in Meliandou, Guinea in December of 2013. Within a matter of weeks, friends and relatives of the child become a part of a complex chain of transmission when they died or fell ill, but it would take almost three months before public health officials in Guinea and their regional and foreign advisers determined that they were dealing with "Zaire Ebola" and not cholera, Lassa fever, or some other infectious diseases.

42. "Mediascapes" were one of the five "scapes" that were popularized by Arjun Appadurai. A scape was a fluid or shifting essence that might come in the form of ideoscapes, mediascapes, ethnoscapes, technoscapes, or financescapes. Mediascapes where the ideologies that circulated in various media outlets and flows that put on display narratives and other images. See Arjun Appadurai, *Modernity at Large: Cultural Dimensions of Globalization* (Minneapolis, MN: University of Minnesota Press, 1996).

2

✛

NGO Organizational Tales, the Discovery of "Patient Zero," and MSF's Stories about the Origins of the 2013–2015 West African Ebola Outbreak

The pursuit of medical humanitarianism, especially after World War II, is an endeavor that has challenged many organizations, and Doctors Without Borders seems to be at the center of some of these key challenges. As Eyal Weizman has recently noted in his highly acclaimed *The Least of All Possible Evils* (2012), some of the logics of principled compromises of MSF have led it to promote "humanitarianism in its minimalist form . . . as the practice of "lesser evils" . . . [to sustain] life without seeking to govern or manage populations, [or to make] political claims on their behalf, [or to try] to resolve root causes of conflicts."[1] Having been accused of being used by Mengistu Haile Mariam's Ethiopian regime to draw out refugees that would be displaced during the 1980s' East African famines, the MSF sections during the following decades responded by declaring that MSF personnel were uninterested in revolutionary and counterrevolutionary entanglements. At the same time MSF would internationalize and become a medical organization that prided itself on keeping people alive long enough for them to be able to make up their own minds about governments and cultures. In theory, what Weizman might call the greater evils would come in the form of more coercive and intrusive forms of interventionism that smacked of the totalitarianism and imperialism that Hannah Arendt and others had been writing about during the post-Holocaust years.[2]

Yet what happens in situations where an organization like Médecins Sans Frontières finds itself in the center of a major epidemic in an impoverished region, where the absence of "official" global health care leadership creates a perceptual vacuum that needs to be filled? What if some major NGO—that constructs a "public image of neutrality," strategically deploys media, and practices specific forms of "humanitarian action"[3]—has to make some uneasy decisions that compromise some of that organization's founding principles? Is it possible that twenty-first-century public health discourses about austerity are forcing Doctors Without Borders to overcome "gaps" in privatization overseas, and that this in turn creates ruptures and fissures that allow for the empowerment of a few key NGOs in West Africa? How does a famous NGO empower itself so that it can provide needed "health security rights" for those trying to survive, and what happens in situations when it uses Cassandra-like warnings to try and avoid a major pandemic? Does MSF then set aside those vaunted principles of neutrality, minimalism, and the avoidance of militarism in the name of a more transcendent, and efficacious, medical humanitarianism?[4]

By now most readers who have kept up with what is presented to us in mainstream media outlets know something about the "origins" of the West African Ebola outbreak, and MSF's involvement is a key part of these origination tales. The basic plotline, and the rhetorical scaffolding for this particular narrative, looks much like a twenty-first-century version of the Ebola outbreak stories that were studied by Jeff Bass,[5] Rebecca Weldon,[6] Priscilla Wald, Melissa Leach,[7] and others who highlighted some of the ideological features of these "outbreak" tales. Although the particular features and geopolitical landscapes will always be slightly altered to fit the specific terrains of Liberia, Sierra Leone, and Guinea, the basic storyline endures, filled with protagonists, antagonists, discovered epidemics, and "lessons learned." Yet, as I noted in chapter 1, in this particular case, at some point during the first stage of the West African Ebola outbreak MSF would declare that they were overwhelmed and that military logistics were required to help control this massive EVD outbreak.

If readers synthesize some of the key fragments that are found in these popular, neoliberal versions of the Ebola outbreak *dispositifs*, they will find that it is relatively easy to put together what looks like an apolitical, coherent and objective medical "history" of what Médecins Sans Frontières (MSF) calls the "initial phase" of outbreak, that covered the period between March to July of 2014.[8] For example, we would typically begin to tell this tale by noting how public health officials in Guinea, working with personnel from Doctors Without Borders and a few other groups, were able to locate the beginning of this outbreak by tracing it back to the activities of a two-year-old in Guéckédou, Guinea, who supposedly came down with EVD in December of 2014.[9] As the story goes, it took a few weeks before health workers in that area determined that it was a strand of "Zaire Ebola" because the symptoms of the disease looked like cholera or Lassa fever.[10]

In this particular chapter, which critiques the roles that MSF sections played in the production and circulation of these popular medical narratives, I will be arguing that some of this telling hides the power and the cultural dimensions of some of these narrations. The conventional tales, that were often told from the points of view of a virologist, a clinician, or an epidemiologist, were turned into hagiographic archival accounts that valorized the role of foreign NGOs like MSF while treating local West African communities as obstructionists who hindered medical relief efforts. Moreover, some variants of these origination tales used explanatory rhetorical frames that argued that WHO, or the government of Guinea, initially *downplayed the dangers* in order to avoid causing panic. On April 25, 2014, for example, the regional WHO office in Brazzaville was reporting to the world that "overall, the epidemiological situation in Guinea has improved significantly over the last few weeks."[11] With the benefit of hindsight, that is almost always 20/20, the clear vision of MSF is juxtaposed with the myopia of WHO or West African governments.

As I will explain in more detail below, there were many global observers during these turbulent times who questioned this conventional wisdom, and they averred that MSF was actually just another elite organization from "the North" that thrived when they circulated hyper-inflating medical mythologies. While defenders of MSF might view this organization's collection of Ebola data and their timely reportage of officially reported cases as apolitical baseline information, many African intellectuals, who viewed Ebola as a pan-African problem, were equally convinced that the valorization of MSF interventionism was just another way of belittling local or regional public health initiatives.

The ideological nature of all of this biopolitics and thanatopolitics manifested itself as early as March 23, 2014, when Guinea made the first public announcement that European laboratories had confirmed that this was indeed Ebola virus disease.[12] "This was Zaire, the most deadly strain of Ebola, spread out in an unprepared region," noted Dr. Michel Van Herp, MSF senior viral haemorrhagic fever epidemiologist, and he explained how "even the dead were being transported from one village to another," and how all of this convinced him that there was "no doubt that it was unprecedented."[13] By that time, it was known that several people in Gueckedou, Guinea, including the two-year-old's mother, sister, and grandmother had contracted the same disease and had died.[14]

Within a matter of months, MSF—characterized by its supporters as the "first," and often only, line of defense against Ebola in West Africa—was configured as an efficacious organization that was treating almost a third of all of the cases of EVD on the continent.[15] This begged the question: Where were WHO personnel or World Bank employees when you needed them? Why didn't West African leaders declare this to be an emergency as soon as they realized that Ebola was spreading across a tri-state area?

Many arguers in these early debates agreed that epidemiologists could trace all of this back to "Patient Zero," but as soon as participants in this disputation tried to explain what happened next they invariably became entangled in political and cultural blame games. At this point divergent and polysemic stories were told about what happened next during the initial stage of the outbreak, and one's views regarding heroes and villains was often shaded by how one wanted to write or talk about global health responsibility, African social agency, the role of foreign medical interventionism, and the metrics that one used to determine when we were witnessing timely, as opposed to belated, medical interventions. Note, for example, how Lyle Fearnley wrote about the early presence of Médecins Sans Frontières and the supposed absence of WHO:

> The ongoing, devastating Ebola epidemic in West Africa has revealed, however, a troubling discrepancy between the relatively early detection of an emerging disease and the very late arrival of international public health response. By March 23, 2014 . . . the Ebola virus had been isolated in European laboratories. . . . Some might complain that those two weeks are too long, or blame the Guéckédou clinicians who were slow to identify and report the disease because they were not trained to anticipate Ebolavirus in their community. But these lapses in reporting and identification pale in comparison to the delays in international public health intervention as the epidemic grew in full public view. Incredibly, WHO did not declare the outbreak [to be a major problem] . . . [until] more than one month after Médecins San Frontières declared the epidemic in Liberia was "out of control."[16]

Smaller religious organizations, the International Committee of the Red Cross and Red Crescent, the U.N. Mission for Ebola Emergency Response, Cuban and Chinese doctors, and others would later become a part of all of this chaotic scenery, but earlier on it was often MSF that took center stage and served as the lightning rod for elite or vernacular controversy.

From the very outset, let me admit that I admire MSF and their efforts, but some of the paternalistic and chauvinist ways that they write and talk about the West African Ebola outbreak need to be critiqued. I will be arguing that we need to recognize the self-serving nature of some of this discursive strategizing, where future accounts of the origins of this latest outbreak will be used to empower MSF. If I am right, then it will be no coincidence that in the coming years MSF personnel will be consistently portrayed in varied media and public health outlets as some of the protagonists in medical humanities morality plays, while WHO leaders will play the role of the antagonists. Just one hint of what is to come can be found in Laurie Garrett's September/October 2015 assessment of WHO personnel decisionism:

> MSF officials were convinced that the decline in reported cases was a product not of a fading epidemic but of a reluctance by local villagers to engage with foreigners or national institutions. After the MSF Clinic in Macenta was attacked by a mob on April 4, MSF officials tried in vain to get the WHO to change its mind about withdrawing. When the 2014 WHA [World Health Assembly] convened in Geneva in late May, the Ebola epidemic garnered only a smattering of references in speeches. It was not on the agenda.[17]

Garrett, recognized as one of the leading medical journalists who was familiar with many Ebola histories, painted a picture of how nations that were in trouble wanted WHO to mobilize some of the world's top expertise to vaccinate Syrian refugees or stop cholera in post-earthquake Haiti. She then showed how those who desired this were let down by WHO inaction or incompetence, because communities like the World Health Assembly got sidetracked with their deliberations on "countless resolutions." Instead of leading those who wanted to mobilize immediately in the name of emergency military humanitarianism, the World Health Assembly got bogged down debating in their buildings about everything from international recognition of Palestine to the banning of tobacco company employees from public health meetings.[18] These types of *dispositifs* contrasted MSF foresight and experience with WHO cluelessness and detachment.

In theory, while WHO allowed national "politics" and regional squabbles to get in the way of the provision of much needed public health aid, MSF, with its activist agendas and expertise, jumped into the fray. This particular variant of the securitizing "do something" argumentative template made it appear as if MSF was the type of twenty-first-century organization that needed to lead those who believed in a medical responsibility to protect (R2P).

Granted, this comforting tale of having a "canary in the mines" may resonate with those who want to believe that there is at least one twenty-first-century NGO that can serve as the world's speedy caregiver during health crises, but as I noted above this ignores some of the power dimensions of the situation. Moreover, this deflects attention away from issues of African sovereignty, the accountability of governmental agencies, and the role that local citizens played in collecting EVD information.

In this chapter I will argue that MSF has indeed played a key role in the promotions of these neo-liberal narratives, and that we need to appreciate the fact that all of this mythologizing contributed to some needed publicity for those who wanted international support for the attempted containment of the West African Ebola outbreak of 2013–2015. Praising MSF did serve the function of creating catalytic, rhetorical events that altered international public health organizational relationships. The prospect of growth, and the hubris of those who worked for MSF, challenged that vaunted idea of medical humanitarian minimalism that Eyal Weizman and others have written about. There is little doubt that the stories that were told about MSF's early interventionism helped with the raising of some $1.24 billion last year, and this allowed it to deploy some 5,300 international and local workers to fight Ebola.[19] Yet we also need to be cognizant of the fact that the attack on WHO may have also created a crisis in organizational legitimation, that may or may not help with needed reformation.

The rising power of MSF need not be viewed as some material event that took place without the social agency of members of Doctors Without Borders. I am convinced that critical scholars can still laud the role that MSF placed during the various stages of the West African outbreak, while they raise a host of pointed questions about MSF rhetorical posturing and their exchanges with empowered African political leaders. We can respect them while we assess the *dispositifs* that they circulated that touched on matters of local burial habits, the eating of bushmeat,[20] the thanatopolitical hiding of bodies, or the dispensation of "modern" medicine.

This is an organization that has sections that pride themselves on self-criticism, and some of the leaders of MSF realize that many twenty-first-century observers seem to be at a loss about how to think about international health leadership and the inherent right to talk about global health security rights in impoverished nations. Joanne Liu, the president of Médecins San Frontières, has recently acknowledged that her organization now has a "voice that we have never had before,"[21] but what about the positions of those who *resent* this type of foreign medical humanitarianism? In other words, what do we do in situations where West Africans want to make their own decisions about how to deal with Ebola denialism, the refusal by some to seek medical care, or the Ebola fears and traumas that are associated with the spread of emerging infectious diseases?

With this in mind this chapter decodes the organizational discourses, and the persuasive images, that were produced by Médecins Sans Frontières, as well as this organization's critics during the early stages of this latest Ebola outbreak. My adoption of Foucauldian approaches allows readers and critics to see how the responses to an infectious disease outbreak can empower some while disempowering others. In this particular situation the MSF found itself entangled in debates about everything from the wearing of the proper protective gear to the best ways to avoiding the appearance of "neo-colonialism."

At the same time that I am critiquing many of MSF's strategic commentaries,[22] I will also be adopting synchronic approaches that evaluate the reactions of national and international audiences who responded to this particular NGO's unique rhetoric. MSF personnel would have an inordinate say in the rhetorical framings of that first stage of the latest Ebola outbreak, between March and June of 2014, and the very lack of Western media coverage only added to the luster of the reputation of the MSF doctors who did take vocal stances during these earlier periods.

Let me begin by discussing some of the muted criticisms that were sent in MSF's direction, and then I will take up the topic of how all of this impacted their (re)interpretation of MSF personnel's vaunted notion of "témoignage."

AFRICAN AND OTHER CRITIQUES
OF MSF GOALS AND TACTICS

Although many African intellectuals, academic communities, and public health authorities sometimes resent having to accept humanitarian aid tied with strings or help that comes in the form of patronizing moral sermonizing, they are not always sure what to make of MSF and their "rebellious" strand of humanitarianism.[23] This brand of humanitarianism is coproduced by MSF personnel who appear to claim that bright lines could be drawn between minimalist survivalist types of rescue efforts and more "political" approaches to global health, and MSF doctors marketed their organization as one that was interested in avoiding state intrigue and aid manipulation. In theory, those who espoused this particular type of humanitarian action did not close their eyes to injustice or potential war crimes, but on the other hand they asked to be allowed into "hot zones" because they were going to focus on saving lives and not on regime change. In some ways this echoed variants of medical argumentation that been around since the founding of Geneva's Red Cross.

African recipients of medical aid during epidemic outbreaks could understandably have ambivalent views when they listened to the promotion of a vision of what the French call "sans frontièrisme" (without borders), a geographic imaginary[24] where MSF would sometimes negotiate with nefarious rebels or state leaders in the name of pragmatism. After all, didn't it make sense that MSF personnel or leaders negotiate with Ebola denialists if they had to in order to keep alive as many humans as possible in "complex" disastrous situations?

From a critical cultural vantage point, it would be a mistake to view the organizational provision of foreign medical aid through apolitical, epidemiological lens that saw this a matter where MSF represented the spread of modern enlightenment principles while those who objected to this interventionism become symbolic ciphers for the darker forces of African incompetence of intransigence. As Rob DeChaine has explained, MSF often uses permutations of "humanitarian action" arguments as a form of advocacy, recruitment, and identity formation of humanitarian social movements, and all of this constitutive rhetoric can be linked to power relationships.[25] We therefore need to acknowledge the strategic nature of the discourse of *sans frontièrism* that can be twisted in strategic ways to rationalize and justify contentious forms of civilian medical interventionism.

Foucauldian critics have always been admonished to remember that they need to critique the flow of the power/knowledge/discourse, no matter who wields that power. If we apply these insights to the tale that is told about Patient Zero then we would notice how the narration of the plight of Guineans served a variety of functions, in that it helped Ebola victims as well as rescuers.[26] As Alberto Toscano recently noted, the "rhetoric of humanitarianism" has not "exhausted the attractions and ambiguities of the discourse of human rights,"[27] and this is certainly the case with MSF's interpretations of the provision of health care rights for West Africans.

As noted above, MSF workers have prided themselves on how they can pragmatically balance their principles of neutrality and impartiality with the need to remain relevant in humanitarian contexts, and the West African Ebola outbreak tested their abilities to juggle those various goals. Erika Hayden, writing for *Nature* magazine, has argued that MSF's mission may be expanding after the end of the West African Ebola outbreak,[28] and if this is the case then we need to see how their rhetorics, as well as their health care practices, may impact future public health interventionism.

MSF had been working in Guinea since 2001 on various public health projects, and many observers gave them credit for already being on the "frontlines" when the latest Ebola outbreak hit West Africa. However, it is also possible that MSF personnel *may have underestimated the socio-psychological impact that the sudden appearance of dozens of foreign workers*, wearing rubber boots, goggles, a face mask, and a Tyvek suit may have had on many rural and urban West African communities during the first stage.[29]

MSF was one of the organizations that complained about local misperceptions, but their personnel usually avoided commenting on how their own interventionism may have had the unintended consequence of contributing to the misreporting, and circulation of the miscalculations, that led to the premature "end" of the first stage of the outbreak in May of 2014. Sadly, this meant that it is very possible that some MSF personnel also had a hand in influencing the trajectory of the very WHO decisionism that they continually critiqued! After all, WHO personnel were not the only people who left West Africa thinking that they had contained this outbreak by the end of spring 2014.

I am not arguing here that we need to think of MSF personal as villains in twenty-first-century permutations of Ebola outbreak narratives or humanitarian interventionism tales. What I am arguing is that some of the MSF critiques of WHO, and the stories that were told about the "belated" interventionism of other foreign organizations, were self-serving and that this *realpolitik* strategizing is what rhetorically constructed select heroes and villains.

Moreover, we need to be aware that this magnification and eulogizing of MSF humanitarian action, that was often paired with critiques of WHO ineptitude in Ebola contexts, comes at a price. First of all, it begs the question, following critics, of who gave MSF personnel the right to cross sovereign Guinea borders and declare themselves the experts on Guinean health affairs? What about the efforts of the CDC personnel, the International Red Cross and Red Crescent, Western Africa doctors and nurses, and countless volunteers who were also on the scene?

Scientific hubris and ideological humanitarian interventionism that masquerades as neutrality cannot hide some of the moralism, the paternalism, and the Western-orientation of so many MSF discourses in Ebola contexts. Readers can understand the pride that many MSF personnel felt when they calculated the exact number of lives that they saved during the first months of the West African Ebola outbreak. We can understand some of the motivations of those who dwelled on how Doctors Without Borders warned others about the magnitude of this epidemic, but MSF also had critics who complained about this organization's elitism, its cultural insensitivity, and its unwavering defense of its own utopian creeds and protocols.[30]

While the vast majority of journalists, scientific writers, and others who wrote about Médecins Sans Frontières in Western media outlets often praised this organization, there would be others who would argue that they participated in fear mongering, that they used conservative Ebola therapies, and that they interfered with the daily operations of many African health campaigns. However, this is complicated by the reportage on how, by July of 2014 MSF had admitted some 891 of the 1,440 probable, suspected, and confirmed Ebola cases to their facilities.[31] We also need to keep in mind that several dozen members of this organization lost their lives during this period.

In order to provide one example of some of the political tensions that rose to the surface following MSF interventionism in West Africa, note the way that Guinea's president, Alpha Condé, responded to questions about the outbreak a year after the worst had passed. He supplied some representative fragments that needed to be unpacked when he told reporters in July of 2015 that Ebola "forced us to change completely."[32] At this point in the fight against Ebola, most journalists believed that the worst was behind us, and they applauded the fact that institutional and private donors around the world had pledged some $3.4 billion in aid to help with West African recovery. Not all of the aid would be forthcoming, but the aid that did flow into places like Guinea was needed and was appreciated.

President Condé was cautiously optimistic as he talked to reporters about the future, and yet one got the sense that he was circumspect in the ways that he responded to questions about how Médecins Sans Frontières had sounded the alarm about the nature and scope of the Ebola outbreak. Like other African leaders he hoped that the billions promised in aid would go to the *economies* of his nation instead of just providing an emergency fund, and his commentary on future economic policies transitioned into some reflections about what happened during the initial stages of the outbreak. As he reminisced about what had transpired, he talked about the adverse impact of the "isolation policies" of other nations that affected both the economies and the cultures of West Africa. "It's obvious that the international panic created severe damages to our economy," Condé explained, and he mentioned how it "not only made investors flee" but how these Ebola anxieties created situations where Guineans resented the efforts of those they felt had closed their borders and isolated their country.[33] One should isolate Ebola and not countries, he said, and then he talked about Guinea's declining economic situation.

Condé referenced how his country, along with Sierra Leone and Liberia, had suffered through travel bans, stopped flights, and widespread quarantine restrictions. He also mentioned how the very idea of Ebola was contrary to his nation's customs and habits, where a "warm people" who usually embrace were forced to change their funeral rights, their habits, and their "very natures and customs."[34] While he gingerly avoided directly responding to queries about WHO's belated help, he did express his thanks as he complemented the medical aid groups that came to his nation's aid.

Back in April of 2014 Condé had been accused of Ebola denialism for allegedly refusing to admit the scope of the Ebola problem in West Africa, but with the passage of time he could now respond to those who once claimed that Guinea and Sierra Leone had been reluctant to declare a state of emergency. "MSF has a tendency to exaggerate things," Condé explained, and although he was grateful for the help that they provided, he advanced the argument that it was the way that they tried to delivery messages about potential epidemics that bothered him. "They took the most risks to heal people everywhere," he conceded to reporters, but what Condé seemed to object to was the medical hubris, the relative status, and the evident power of MSF. "We just did not agree with them intervening," Condé averred, and he said that they were "not the official spokespeople."[35] Was Guinea's president implying that MSF personnel did not respect his presidency, the rights of his people, or African health care workers in general?

Was President Condé also implying that his country—without outside interference—had managed to walk that fine line between Ebola phobia and Ebola situational awareness, and that MSF was the wrong messenger during the initial stages of the outbreak? Was Guinea's president arguing that that MSF employees were acting hysterically and emotionally, and that Doctors Without Borders personnel were telling the world about an epidemic *before those claims were backed up with epidemiological evidence*? Or did his remarks provide us with subtle hints regarding Guinean embarrassment, that were signaling some disenchantment with the symbiotic relationship that existed between some NGOs and poor nations like Guinea that desperately needed MSF?

Western media outlets and MSF representatives responded to this by coming up with myriad reasons why President Condé did not immediately call for massive foreign medical interventionism in West Africa during the spring of 2014. A *New York Times* journalist was told by unnamed senior health officials that "health officials under him [Condé] massaged the numbers to avoid scaring off much-needed investors in his impoverished nation."[36] A senior MSF official complained that the Guinean officials' "first concern was not to scare outsiders" and so they wanted "to minimize" the Ebola cases.[37] This all made it appear as if WHO was not the only institutional authority that failed to be accountable during the outbreak.

The Western mainstream coverage of MSF Ebola efforts made it seem as though officials in the Guinean government, like some illiterate members of the population, were also engaging in a form of denialism that obstructed the efforts of MSF during the first stage of the outbreak. Adam Nossiter, writing in November of 2014, opined,

> Upset by the group's dire warnings, Mr. Condé publicly criticized Doctors Without Borders, despite its lonely efforts to blunt the disease on the front line. But as Mr. Condé played down the outbreak, Ebola was steadily entrenching itself in the Guinean forest villages where it surfaced nearly a year ago. Now, after more than a thousand deaths in Guinea, Mr. Condé has reversed course. Disturbed by the threat to his country's people and economy, he is grappling with Ebola nearly every waking moment. Having initially overlooked the crisis, he is now micromanaging it, some international officials say. "While shaving I think of Ebola, while eating I think of Ebola, while sleeping I think of Ebola," Mr. Condé, 76, said at the drab, concrete, Chinese-built presidential palace.[38]

Readers who read this account could reasonably conclude that Condé, like other West Africans, finally woke up from his dogmatic slumber and listened to the sage advice that was coming from MSF.

West African leaders were not the only Africans who objected to some of MFS's actions and those of other foreign interventionists. When MSF personnel visited some of the towns near Guéckédou, they encountered all sorts of resistance. By mid-June, 2014, for example, a rumor was spreading that the infection-control teams, that were wearing head-to-toe personal protection equipment, *were protecting themselves* as they spent their time "spraying the disease's causative agents."[39] Riots ensued in some places where MSF personnel were trying to work on isolation of suspected Ebola cases. In some cases all foreign medical doctors were lumped together and attacked as the purveyors of trouble. For example, there were reports that an army of some three thousand armed youths assembled in a mining town called Forécariah, leading a few WHO epidemiologists to flee for their lives.[40]

This clash illustrated the difficulties that came from assuming that everyone would automatically welcome the interventionist efforts of foreigners who started writing and talking about African scientific illiteracy, the eating of bushmeat, and problematic social practices. While many Africans appreciated the efforts of the MSF personnel, others objected to the ways that MSF leaders, doctors, and other public health workers talked and wrote about West African customs, burial traditions, and poverty.

Were MSF personnel being unfairly maligned? Was this the ungrateful reaction of those who were displacing blame and who were looking for scapegoats? Given the fact that many West African leaders were begging for aid, why would they object to the fact that MSF personnel built dozens of Ebola management centers, clinical trial sites, and training facilities? Would any of this criticism tarnish the reputation of MSF and would it hinder the growth of this organization?

The next section helps set the stage for the answering of those queries by investigating some of MSF's ideologies and practices.

UNDERSTANDING TÉMOIGNAGE AND MSF'S UNIQUE TAKE ON THE ROLE OF MEDICAL HUMANITARIAN INTERVENTIONISM

In many ways, the origination tales that are told about the discovery of Patient Zero reprise earlier Doctors Without Borders rescue tales. Those who want to laud MSF's interventionism and witnessing usually tell a tale of organizational origins that starts off by mentioning how some Parisian doctors, during the war between Nigeria and the ill-fated secessionist state of Biafra, worried about how famine might devastate that region. Concerned about the military might of the Nigerians, and worried about the plight of millions of suffering Biafrans who were caught between fighting forces, a group of about thirteen French doctors and journalists decided to form an emergency medical response organization that would work around the world, regardless of the politics of particular nation-states.[41] Regardless of whether a national was communist, socialist, capitalistic, and so forth, it was argued that the people should receive necessitous medical help when needed.

Over the years MSF oversaw the growth of a decentralized system of public health responders who, according to Peter Redfield, were trying to use their geographical imaginations as they thought about having a globalized version of France's emergency medical system.[42] During the 1980s they added six chapters, including some in Canada and Japan, and a decade later MSF personnel were conducting missions in many regions of the world, including Central America, the Middle East, Western Europe, and Southeast Asia. MSF eventually became the "largest independent medical relief organization in the world."[43]

Renée Fox has convincingly argued that in order to understand how MSF is trying to apply their more than forty years of experience in the current Ebola crisis, one must first understand their stance on the primacy of *temoignage,* or the act of bearing witness to injustice. For example, over the years MSF has clashed with large pharmaceutical companies over the price of the medications in "developing countries," and Fox contends that "people did not listen" during the initial phase of the outbreak when earlier on MSF called for a broader global response to what was happening in Guinea, Liberia, and Sierra Leone.[44]

In many MSF narratives the social actions of those who do not believe in *temoignage* become a point of emphasis. "We were reaching our breaking point, and we thought, surely there are countries that have civil protection forces, people who drill on chemical spills, who know evacuation and quarantine procedures, who've prepared for bioterror," remarked Christopher Stokes from Brussels when he was asked about the Ebola outbreak. Stokes went on to explain that he laughed at his optimist and concluded that they all woke up when they had to notice that only a few NGOs were in West Africa but "no one else came!"[45] Once again, in the same way that the French doctors had helped the Biafrans and circulated tales of Nigerian "genocide," the MSF personnel were bearing witness to the suffering of West Africans who had been abandoned by others in "the North."

In some cases MSF employees used visual argumentation to support their allegations as they circulated iconic images of MSF workers wearing yellow protective gear as the wrote about the treatment of suspected or confirmed EVD patients. One of the most popular images came from Paynesville Liberia, where an African child is held by a walking MSF worker. The image conveys the message that MSF personnel are willing to risk their lives and help anyone in need of care, regardless of their politic, their ethnicity, or their allegiance to particular border-states. Again, what is known as "minimalism" and survival becomes key, and the image of the small African child in the hands of the MSF worker puts on display the paternal but necessitous nature of MSF interventionism.

As hinted at above, some of the key fragments in these discourses and visual representations of *sans frontièrisme* appeared in the outbreak narratives that were told about the discovery of "Patient Zero" in Guinea.

MSF ARGUMENTATIVE PRACTICES, DISCOVERING "PATIENT ZERO," AND CHRONICLING OF DOCTORS WITHOUT BORDER'S CONTRIBUTIONS DURING THE 2013–2015 WEST AFRICAN OUTBREAK

More than a few researchers and journalists have noticed the unique style of arguing that comes from the ranks of those who join MSF. They often don't hesitate to articulate the position that the militarization of medical care is often problematic, and they supposedly loathe central bureaucratization. Renée Fox, a sociologist, contends that MSF leaders and personnel argue in pragmatic ways that prevent group-think, and they like to make sure that their executives have field experience.[46] Joanna Liu, their current leader, recently complained about having to meet with some international law experts because she was convinced that she was going to have to sit and listen to a "lot of people who haven't treated a patient." These legal types, she complained, considered themselves "world experts" on Ebola who were "going to give us lessons."[47]

MSF leaders and personnel often take the position that their own expertise, their voluntarism, and their efficacy speaks volumes about the beneficence of their vaunted principles. Other medical organizations talk while MSF acts. Two journalists, Brad Wieners and Makiko Kitamura, once described the organization as a place that "combines the *esprit de corps* of French Legionnaires (without weapons), the self-styled posturing of a graduate seminar, and the *bonhomie* of backpacking the developing world."[48]

MSF had a Swiss team of MSF personnel who were working on malaria control in the Guéckédou when they received a letter, on March 12, 2014, from Guinea's Ministry of Health. That correspondence explained that a mysterious illness had struck eight people, including a doctor who had died while caring for an EVD patient. The Swiss team alerted their superiors, and according to Hughes Robert-Nichoud, MSF headquarters then dispatched researchers to take blood samples, collect case histories, and investigate the symptoms.[49] Within a short period of time Robert-Nicoud had also looped in MSF Belgium, a place that had more Ebola veterans as well as a warehouse filled with "Ebola kits"—preprepared boxes of disinfectant, PPE suits, and medicines to help with the treatment of EVD symptoms.[50] All of this reportage underscored the unique preparation and response times of an organization that knew how to react when needed.

MSF chronicles of these Ebola events have recorded how some MSF personnel and Guinea public health workers initially suspected that they were dealing with Lassa fever, a disease that was endemic to the region. However, after about a week, the blood samples traveled to Conakry, Guinean, and then to the Pasteur Institute in Lyon, France. Near the end of March, 2014, MSF issued a statement that cited the eight cases in Conakry and called the outbreak "unprecedented."[51] This is often interpreted as the triggering event that should have catalyzed massive foreign medical aid.

MSF supporters used this chronicling of events to argue that one of first of many major mistakes that could be recorded took place in early January 2014, when the grandmother of "patient zero," traveled to a hospital in Guéckédou and sought care before she died. This was viewed as a rare, but lost opportunity to stop this transmission line in its tracks, because most people in that region might have sought out the help of traditional healers. Instead of detecting and stopping the disease, the Guéckédou hospital became another converging point that led to the transmission of new chains, as patients and health workers contracted the diseases and infected other communities.[52] Several months later, the outbreak had spread to the capital of Guinea, Conakry, and to neighboring countries.[53] This characterization of the Guinean hospital as another vector only reinforced the arguments of those who could argue about the necessitous nature of MSF Ebola centers.

In many of the rhetorical contextualizations of these affairs that are presented by MSF rhetors, this would be contextualized as a temporal period filled with "early misdiagnosis," where the "three most affected countries had already weak health systems that were unprepared and ill-equipped to deal with the crisis, fueling further spread of the disease."[54] To make matters worse, in April of 2014, when MSF personnel were adamant that the outbreak was already out of control, a WHO spokesperson insisted that was not the case, and during the next month a funeral of a traditional healer in Sierra Leone created the perfect storm for the spread of EVD to hundreds of people.[55]

The circulation of these types of self-serving, and partial accounts served several rhetorical functions. They highlighted the acumen of MSF doctors while belittling WHO efforts. They could also be used to underscore the magnitude of the challenges that were facing MSF, as well as the expertise, the will, and the knowledge that was needed by these West African countries. After listening to this for many months one could reasonably conclude that MSF personnel were "the" key players in West African Ebola outbreak narratives, especially in 2014.

To help make their *prima facie* case for more massive MSF intervention, this organization explained to readers on their web sites and in their publications that this latest outbreak, that had taken the lives of thousands, was nothing like the biggest previous Ebola outbreak that had totaled some 425 cases. MSF was configured as an organization that had helped control other Ebola outbreaks in nine countries over the span of the previous two decades, but they realized early on that this was different.

One clear argumentative strategy that was used to explain to readers both the magnitude of this latest outbreak, as well as the scale of the MSF response, involved the use of infographs and statistics that put on display the performative efforts of MSF employees. For example, one Doctors Without Borders publication mentioned how earlier outbreaks had warranted the use of only one Ebola Management Centre (EMC), but this time around MSF had had to manage some fifteen EMCs and transit centers. This involved the construction of buildings that could accommodate a 250-bed EMC, and readers were told about how MSF was quickly responding to reported EVD outbreaks in Mali, Senegal, Nigeria, and the Democratic Republic of the Congo.[56] All of this could be used for the collection of donations as well as recruitment.

Again, I am not arguing that all of these humanitarian communities painted totally inaccurate pictures of Ebola pathogenesis or material conditions during the first stage of the outbreak. Instead, what I am arguing is that all of these materials are presented in strategic fashion. These figurations convey epistemic information while valorizing the efforts of MSF personnel. Discovering Patient Zero, and helping diagnose these problems, only added to MSF's growing reputation.

Throughout both the first and second stages of this outbreak, from March until early October of 2014, MSF and a few other organizations were credited with staying on the frontlines of the Ebola battles. As noted above, not everyone agreed with some of their theories or their methods, but few openly disputed the fact that during the initial phase they played a major role in overseeing contact tracing, Ebola diagnostics, and treatment. MSF reportedly sent more than three hundred foreigners to this region during these stages, and they hired more than three thousand locals.[57] Later on (especially after the beginning of October), they would feel overwhelmed by the spread of Ebola contagion, but for many months this would be the organization that received a major share of the media spotlight.

The unnamed MSF authors of *An Unprecedented Year* (March 2015) marginalized the efforts of some of the other organizations involved in containing this outbreak at the same time that they trumpeted their own accomplishments. For example, in the introduction to this report, readers are told that when "large-scale international assistance was finally deployed towards the end of the year," this was a period that was already witnessing the beginning of a decline in "case numbers"[58]

MSF summary reports, research findings, and blog posts heralded the efforts of Doctors Without Borders personnel who had "repeatedly raised the alarm and called for additional support through public statements, media interviews, and stakeholder meetings."[59] The supposed inadequacy of the "the international effort" forced MSF to identify, and fill, "gaps" in "all aspects of response."[60] This was another example of the type of humanitarian action that DeChaine and others had written about.

To be sure, *An Unprecedented Year* is an impressive document, filled with startling statistics for readers who might not realize just how influential this organization was in West Africa between March and July of 2014. Unlike some of the other foreign interventionists who had trouble documenting the efficacy of their aid, MSF kept records of exactly how many people were admitted to their Ebola Management Centres. Representatives of this organization argued that they had admitted more than 8,500 people to their EMCs during the first year of the outbreak, and argued that they had trained more than 250 people from other organizations, including the U.S. Centers for Disease Control and Prevention, the World Health Organization, International Medical Corps, and Save the Children.[61]

For readers who might want to know exactly how these Africans and other EVD victims were treated, there were sections of *An Unprecedented Year* that outlined some of the key social and behavioral practices that were encouraged by MSF. For example, one reads of how EMCS were equipped to provide patients with both "supportive medical care and psychosocial support" for patients and families, and how the provision of "safe burials" allowed MSF to deal with "funeral traditions in which mourners wash or touch the bodies of the deceased."[62] After discussing MSF's involvement in disease surveillance and contact tracing, readers were told about how some five hundred health workers lives had been lost during this latest outbreak and how MSF had been forced to adopt "triage" methods to help maintain non-Ebola health care for those who needed antimalarial distributions.[63]

Given what I have written in chapter 1, readers can guess why MSF writers mentioned those "funeral traditions," and this begs the question of how to critique MFS responses to West African resistance.

MSF AND OTHER OUTBREAK TALES OF WEST AFRICAN
RESISTANCE, WITH A FOCUS ON BURIAL PRACTICES

One of the most controversial aspects of MSF interventionism during the West African Ebola outbreak had to do with the ways that MSF personnel worked alongside West African officials who tried to change local burial practices and other cultural "habits" in places like Sierra Leone, Liberia, or Guinea. Did overt critiques on these thanatopolitical activities violate those vaunted MSF principles of neutrality, or was this another dimension of the "lesser evil" humanitarian principles?

Foreign health care workers, including MSF personnel, tried to initially take into account the sensitivities of those who wanted to supervise elaborate burial rituals, but the spread of the outbreak created exigent situations where organizations like MSF had to oversee the cremation of many bodies. During one of the peaks of the outbreak, medical workers in places like Monrovia started to recognize a disconnect that once again underscored the point that local communities had their own priorities. While there was *epidemiological evidence* that pointed to the accelerated spread of Ebola, *there was cultural evidence* that the numbers of African bodies that were being collected sometimes dwindled. Were foreign interventionist efforts having unintended consequences, scaring away those who might have worked with local health care community workers?

For some reason, even those who worked on these disposal units in places like Monrovia sensed that some forms of foreign interventionism created backlash and burdens for the locals who were trying to contain the spread of EVD. Cokie van der Velde, a sanitation specialist working with MSF, explained to reporters that every day the corpses of those who died from EVD were collected from Ebola treatment centers and hospitals around the Liberian capital. The corpses were then stored in morgues, and then they were taken to a crematorium for burning in the evening. "Very, very few of those dying in the community are brought forward," der Velde explained, and by October of 2014 the number of bodies being collected was falling. She elaborated by noting that by late September the main crematorium in Monrovia had been running at full capacity, burning some eighty bodies at a time on a massive pyre, but that within a matter of weeks, the number of bodies that were being cremated had dropped to thirty or forty a day.[64] This type of calculus, a form of necropolitics, only underscored the point that not everyone was in a hurry to follow MSF cremation protocols.

MSF workers who tried to balance their appreciation of cultural relativism with their medical interventionist principles were convinced that something had to give, and they openly speculated about those who were resisting because of denialism or those who might be visiting local healers. However, as Almudena Marí Sáez explains, for many West Africans, the hasty disposal of potentially diseased bodies was not the personal or social priority that needed to be factored in here. How were the West Africans, who cared deeply about their own religious practices, supposed to benefit from medical survival if West African survivors were disconnected from their traditions, their ancestors, or their loved ones? MSF's Western orientations regarding cremation thus ran up against other ways of configuring bodily and spiritual gains and losses.

According to some Western African beliefs, burial of the dead represented a transitional stage for those believed in the spirit world of ancestors, and for them, "funeral is travel." A "good death" during this transitional stage meant that funerals were supposed to be emotive, personal, and tactic, and before Ebola ravaged the region, a dead person was wept upon, the corpse was "clutched, kissed, hugged and not let go."[65] Now, instead of a West African community coming together to mourn the loss of a loved one their way, "there were people in hazmat suits who spray the dead with chlorine before bundling them and their clothes in a body bag."[66] Again, from the point of view of some Africans, the presence of MSF personnel was a mixed blessing.

More than a few MSF writers had an intriguing way of dealing with contentious discussions of local Ebola denialism or the complaints about foreign intervention—*they used these complaints as even more evidence* that Doctors Without Borders was a needed presence in the region. For example, notice the commentary that circulated after MSF built a ten-bed transit center in Macenta during the initial phase of the outbreak. At that time local community hostility (April of 2014) forced this center to temporarily suspend its activities. Instead of viewing this as cultural or political evidence that some might consider this to be unwarranted interloping—a time to withdraw—MSF authors implied that this was just a small hindrance that demonstrated some temporary lack of African understanding.[67] Disagreement could be framed as ignorance.

Another rhetorical strategy that was used by many MFS personnel involved the recontextualization of some the *animus* that came their way. For example, they treated the distrust and hostility that they faced as a lingering influence that came in the aftermath of decades of "West African" civil wars. The corruption of state officials, and rebellious warfare, had purportedly created a social climate where populations were distrustful of their governments and anyone in power. Marc Poncin, a twenty-year MSF veteran of molecular biology, noted that by July of 2014 there were at least twenty Guinean villages that MSF couldn't safely enter in order to carry out needed contact tracing.[68]

Another strategy that was used by MSF authors to avoid grappling with the unintended consequences of their own actions had to do with

the ways that they discussed the premature ending of the first interventionism in late May of 2014. In the MSF chronicling of these events, after
the first cases were confirmed in Foya, near the border of Sierra Leone
and Guinea, an MSF team quickly set up isolation units in health care
centers as they trained health staff in Foya and Monrovia. We are then
told that reported cases "soon dwindled," without any explanation for
why everyone thought that the outbreak had been contained when there
were "no cases for more than 21 days (the maximum incubation period
of the virus)."[69]

Scholars, public health officials, and others who read other accounts
will soon find alternative stories that explain how this MSF recording of
dwindling cases had more to do with the fear and hiding of EVD victims
and suspects than with any actual empirical decrease in the numbers of
Africans contracting the disease. None of this was explained in texts like
An Unprecedented Year.

CONCLUSION

Rather than simply taking for granted the veracity of some of the binary
stories that I mentioned in chapter 1—that talked about the heroism of
MSF and the "belated" actions of WHO, the World Bank, the IMF, the
Americans, the Europeans, and so on—critical cultural and legal scholars
need to interrogate the theories and practices of all of those who were empowered to intervene during the 2013–2015 West African outbreak. If this
means that we have to critique MSF at the same time that we complain
about the practices of WHO or the World Bank, then so be it.

In order to accomplish this task, this chapter has invited readers to take
seriously the notion that MSF personnel were not just acting as apolitical
doctors or public health care givers when they traveled overseas. They
often adopted the subject position of humanitarian arguers who were ac-
tively promoting *témoignage* at the same time that the parent organizations
told the world that they were sending over more than 1,400 tons of equipment to countries affected by Ebola.[70] This active witnessing of suffering
could then be dealt with by MSF doctors and public health care workers
who knew all about the importance of contact tracing or cremation.

Yet this form of witnessing, which is supposed to help "the other,"
sometimes sounds jarring, especially when the alleged beneficiaries of
this medical aid may have different ways of configuring biopolitics and
thanatopolitics. In spite of all their talk about "neutrality" or "impartiality," MSF leaders and personnel need to be characterized as motivated
social agents who make selective decisions about how to configure EVD,
Ebola victims, African health care workers, and others as they witness

the suffering of others between 2013 and 2015. Their critiques of WHO or Guinean officials helped legitimate their own efforts, and this in turn created a situation where more global communities started to wonder, Should organizations like MSF be given even more responsibilities to make sure that everyone's global health security rights were protected? In other words, the supposed "gaps" or "vacuums" that existed when WHO fled the scene depended on accepting some of the rhetorics that were crafted by MSF rhetors who coproduced these mythic tales of MSF steadfastness and West African denialism.

Trying to provide ideological critiques of the theories, the strategies, and the practices of Médecins Sans Frontières is no easy matter, especially when critics identify with some of these principles, but this chapter shows that occasionally mainstream and alternative press outlets do provide critics with some clues that point to the tensions, the difficulties, and the agonizing choices that were made by MSF and other communities between March and May of 2014 in West Africa. However, many of these get papered over by noncritical readings of this events, and by November of 2014 countless journalists around the world were painting hagiographic pictures of MSF efforts. A few went so far as to praise this organization for showing the rest of the world "how to manage a plague."[71] This variant of what has been called the "savior" complex turns opinions into facts.

With the benefit of hindsight, critical cultural and critical legal scholars can see that the MSF narration of these events was just one of the many ways that we can contextualize the "initial" phase of the outbreak. Moreover, MFS's talk of "belated" global interventionism was one of many threads that were a part of these complex Ebola *dispositifs*. For example, if we wanted to take into account other plausible framings of these affairs, we could dwell on the ways that local health officials and Doctors Without Borders personnel missed a major chance to diagnose Ebola after "seeing bacteria in blood samples" and concluding that "cholera might be [the] culprit."[72] We could concentrate the cultural and social mistakes that were made by those who wore hazmat suits to protect themselves, while terrifying some of the West African "others."

There is little doubt that MSF was a major player in the "war" that was fought against Ebola during 2014 and 2015, but I have argued in this chapter that critics also need to reflect on the complex legacies that have been left by those who worked for Doctors Without Borders during these difficult times. Joanne Liu, in spite of the donated money that is coming MSF's way from private and institutional donors, continues to insist that MSF cannot become "the world's doctor," but this is belied by the fact that the latest Ebola outbreak "catapulted" this organization to "a new prominence in the international health community."[73] In other words, during the next Ebola crises others outside of MSF may expect their personnel to be the public health leaders who need to be in charge of foreign interventionism. They may be trapped by some of their own rhetoric.

This prominence has also resulted in some new interrogations of *témoignage*, as well as the protocols and the attitudes of the MSF. For example, during a May 20, 2015, meeting that was organized by MSF, health care workers from other countries voiced their opinions about some of the elitism and the difficulties that were posed by the presence of MSF workers who defiantly stood by their own protocols, their own results of their own laboratory research, and their own treatments for Ebola. In an open exchange with Joanne Liu, Miatta Gbanya, the coordinator of the Liberian Ebola response, said that she hoped the outbreak would allow MSF personnel to "examine the way" that they worked with other colleagues and governments.[74] Paternalism was in the air, and Africans were aware of some of the costs that came with dependence on foreign medical aid.

NOTES

1. For more on MSF decisionism and these "lesser evils," see Eyal Weizman's chapter on Rony Brauman of MSF during the 1980s' African famines. Eyal Weizman, *The Least of All Possible Evils* (London: Verso, 2011).

2. Hannah Arendt, *The Origins of Totalitarianism* (1951: New York: Harcourt, Inc., 1973).

3. D. Robert DeChaine, "Humanitarian Space and the Social Imaginary: Médecins Sans Frontières/Doctors Without Borders and the Rhetoric of Global Community," *Journal of Communication Inquiry* 26, no. 4 (October, 2012): 354–369, 357–358.

4. For a fine discussion of some of the tensions that face MSF doctors in contemporary humanitarian situations when they deal with everything from "sentimentality" to realpolitik negotiations, see Alberto Toscano, "The Tactics and Ethics of Humanitarianism," *Humanity* (Spring, 2014): 123–147.

5. Jeff D. Bass, "Hearts of Darkness and Hot Zones: The Ideogeme of Imperial Contagion in Recent Accounts of Viral Outbreaks," *The Quarterly Journal of Speech* 84 (1998): 430–447, doi: 10.1080/00335639809384231.

6. Rebecca A. Weldon, "The Rhetorical Construction of the Predatorial Virus: A Burkian Analysis of Nonfiction Accounts of the Ebola Virus," *Qualitative Health Research* 11, no. 1 (2001): 5–25, doi: 10.1177/104973201129118902. See also Hélène Joffe and Georgina Haarhoff, "Representations of Far-Flung Illnesses: The Case of Ebola in Britain," *Social Science and Medicine* 54 (2002): 961, doi: 10.1016/S0277-9536(01)00068-5.

7. Melissa, Leach, "Time to Put Ebola in Context," *Bulletin of the World Health Organization*, 88, no. 7 (July 1, 2010): 481–560. doi: 10.2471/BLT.10.030710.

8. For MSF's own organizational narrations of the "initial phrase" periods, see Médecins Sans Frontières staff, *An Unprecedented Year: Médecins Sans Frontières' Response to the Largest Ever Outbreak*, March, 2015, 7–8, http://www.msf.org/sites/msf.org/files/ebola_accountability_report_final_july_low_res.pdf.

9. Sylvain Baize et al., "Emergence of Zaire Ebola Virus Disease in Guinea," *New England Journal of Medicine* 371, no. 15 (2014):1418–1425, http://dx.doi.org/10.1056/NEJMoa1404505.

10. Although many more people contract Lassa fever, it is not usually fatal, in part because of the existence of a drug called Ribavirin, an effective antiviral.

11. Laurie Garrett, "Ebola's Lesson: How the WHO Mishandled the Crisis," *Foreign Affairs*, September/October, 2015, paragraph 41, https://www.foreignaffairs.com/articles/west-africa/2015-08-18/ebola-s-lessons.

12. For a typical example of the telling of this tale that appears in many medical or public health texts, see Anna Petherick, "Ebola in West Africa: Learning the Lessons," The *Lancet* 385, no. 9968 (February 14, 2014): 591–592.

13. Michel Van Herp, quoted in Médecins Sans Frontières staff, "Pushed to the Limit and Beyond: A Year into the Largest Ever Outbreak," *Médecins Sans Frontières* March, 2015, https://www.doctorswithoutborders.org/sites/usa/files/msf143061.pdf.

14. E. E. Etuk, "Ebola: A West African Perspective," *Journal of the Royal College of Physicians, Edinburgh* 45 (2015): 19–22, 19.

15. Makiko Kitamura and Naomi Kresge, "Ebola Front-Line Doctors at Breaking Point," *Bloomberg*, last modified October 19, 2014, paragraph 4, http://www.bloomberg.com/news/articles/2014-10-19/ebola-front-line-doctors-at-breaking-point.

16. Lyle Fearnley, "The Disease That Emerged," *LIMN*, last modified January, 2015, paragraphs 4–5, http://limn.it/the-disease-that-emerged/.

17. Garrett, "How the WHO Mishandled the Crisis," paragraph 43.

18. Ibid., paragraph 37.

19. Erika Check Hayden, "Ebola Outbreak Thrusts MSF Into New Roles," *Nature* 572 (7554 (June 3, 2015): 18–19.

20. See, for example, Jason Beaubien, "Why Is Guinea's Ebola Outbreak So Unusual?" NPR.com, last modified January 14, 2015, http://www.npr.org/sections/health-shots/2014/04/01/297884573/why-is-guineas-ebola-outbreak-so-unusual; Lisa O'Carroll, "Ebola Crisis Brutally Exposed Failures of the Aid System, Says MSF," *The Guardian*, last modified March 23, 2015, http://www.theguardian.com/global-development/2015/mar/23/ebola-crisis-response-aid-who-msf-report-sierra-leone-guinea.

21. Joanne Liu, quoted in Hayden, "MSF Takes Bigger Global-Health Role," 18.

22. One of the most important of these commentaries came out in June of 2014, when MSF argued that the outbreak in West Africa required massive deployment of resources. It was near this point in time when they began arguing that MSF had reached the "limits" of what its own teams could do. Médecins Sans Frontières staff, "Ebola in West Africa: Epidemic Requires Massive Deployment of Resources," MSF.org, last modified June 21, 2014, http://www.msf.org/article/ebola-west-africa-epidemic-requires-massive-deployment-resources.

23. Françoise Bouchet-Saulnier, "The Theory and Practice of "Rebellious Humanitarianism," Humanitarian Practice Network, June 2003, http://odihpn.org/magazine/the-theory-and-practice-of-%C2%91rebellious-humanitarianism%C2%92. For a critique of some of this, see Michael Barnett and Thomas G. Weiss, *Humanitarianism Contested: Where Angels Fear to Tread* (New York: Routledge: 2011).

24. DeChaine, "Humanitarian Space," 355.

25. Ibid., 354–356.

26. I also want to argue that combatting EVD in West Africa brought to the surface some of the inevitable contradictions that have often shadowed MFS's underscoring of the witnessing function of this organization.

27. Toscano, "The Tactics and Ethics of Humanitarianism," 123.

28. Hayden, "MSF Takes Bigger Global-Health Role," 18–19.

29. MSF would later report that they had distributed hundreds of thousands of protective suits to public health care workers and others in Liberia, Guinea, and Sierra Leone. For an intriguing discussion of how various communities were even willing to debate about which community's protective gear was the best in the fight against Ebola, see Jason Beaubein, "Gear Wars: Whose Ebola Protective Suit Is Better?" NPR.com, last modified October, 25, 2014, http://www.npr.org/sections/goatsandsoda/2014/10/25/358898029/gear-wars-whose-ebola-protective-suit-is-better.

30. For an excellent overview of some of these criticisms, see Erik Check Hayden, "MSF Takes Bigger Global-Health Role," *Nature* 522 (June 4, 2015): 18–19.

31. Médecins Sans Frontières staff, *An Unprecedented Year*, 7.

32. Alpha Condé, quoted in Raya Jalabi, "Guinea's President on Global Aid Push: 'Ebola Forced Us to Change Completely,'" *The Guardian*, last modified July 12, 2015, http://www.theguardian.com/world/2015/jul/12/guinea-president-alpha-conde-ebola-aid.

33. Condé, quoted in Raya Jalabi, "Guinea's President on Global Aid," paragraph 8.

34. Ibid., paragraph 23.

35. Ibid., paragraphs 27–29.

36. Adam Nossiter, "Ebola Now Preoccupies Once-Skeptical Leader in Guinea," *The New York Times*, last modified November 30, 2014, paragraph 7, http://www.nytimes.com/2014/12/01/world/africa/ebola-now-preoccupies-once-skeptical-leader-in-guinea.html.

37. Nossiter, "Ebola Now Preoccupies," paragraph 8.

38. Ibid., paragraphs 9–11.

39. Ann Petherick, "Ebola in West Africa: Learning the Lessons," *The Lancet* 385, no 9968 (February 14, 2015): 591–592.

40. Ibid., 591.

41. Kitamura and Kresge, "Ebola Front-Line Doctors," paragraph 6.

42. Peter Redfield, *Life in Crisis: The Ethical Journal of Doctors Without Borders* (Berkeley: University of California Press, 2013).

43. DeChaine, "Humanitarian Space," 356.

44. Renee Fox, quoted in Kitamura and Kresge, "Ebola Front-Line Doctors," paragraphs 8–9.

45. Christopher Stokes, quoted in Bradford Wieners and Makiko Kitamura, "Ebola: Doctors Without Borders Shows How to Manage a Plague," *Bloomberg*, last modified November 13, 2014, http://www.bloomberg.com/bw/articles/2014-11-13/ebola-doctors-without-borders-shows-how-to-manage-a-plague, paragraph 5.

46. Wieners and Kitamura, "Ebola: Doctors Without Borders Shows How to Manage a Plague," paragraph 18.

47. Hayden, "MSF Takes Bigger Global-Health Role," 19.

48. Kitamura and Kresge, "Ebola Front-Line Doctors," paragraphs 21.

49. Ibid., paragraphs 12.

50. Wieners and Kitamura, "Ebola: Doctors Without Borders Shows How to Manage a Plague," paragraph 12.

51. Médecins Sans Frontières staff, *An Unprecedented Year*, 3; Kitamura and Kresge, "Ebola Front-Line Doctors," paragraphs 14–15.

52. Marylynne Marchione, "Mission Unaccomplished: Containing Ebola in Africa," Yahoo.com, last modified October 19, 2014, paragraph 13, http://news.yahoo.com/mission-unaccomplished-containing-ebola-africa-140654240.html.

53. Elhadj Ilbrahima Bah, "Clinical Presentation of Patients with Ebola Virus Disease in Conakry, Guinea," *The New England Journal of Medicine* 372 (2015): 40–47, 40. As Bah and the other coauthors of this essay explained, once EVD got to the large urban settings, this presented "special challenges to emergency health care facilities, and nosocomial transmission among health care staff members and patients" that led to amplification of the problem and new lines of transmission (p. 45).

54. Médecins Sans Frontières staff, *An Unprecedented Year*, 3.

55. Marchione, "Mission Unaccomplished," paragraph 14.

56. Médecins Sans Frontières staff, *An Unprecedented Year*, 3.

57. Kitamura and Kresge, "Ebola Front-Line Doctors," paragraph 17.

58. Médecins Sans Frontières staff, *An Unprecedented Year*, 3.

59. Ibid., 3.

60. Ibid., 3.

61. Ibid., 4.

62. Ibid., 5.

63. Ibid., 6.

64. Cokie van der Velde, quoted in *Global Post* Staff, "Some People Would Rather Die," paragraphs 4–8.

65. *Global Post* Staff, Some People Would Rather Die of Ebola Than Stop Hugging Sick Loved Ones," *Global Post* [Nairobi, Kenya], last modified October 10, 2014, paragraphs 10–11, http://www.globalpost.com/dispatch/news/health/141010/familes-cant-mourn-ebola-victims-liberia. See Almudena Marí Sáez, Ann Kelly, and Hannah Brown, "Notes from Case Zero: Anthropology in the Time of Ebola," Somatosphere, last modified September 16, 2014, http://somatosphere.net/2014/09/notes-from-case-zero-anthropology-in-the-time-of-ebola.html.

66. *Global Post* Staff, "Some People Would Rather Die," paragraph 21.

67. Médecins Sans Frontières staff, *An Unprecedented Year*, 7

68. Marc Poncin, quoted in Wieners and Kitamura, "Ebola Doctors Without Borders Show How to Manage a Plague," paragraph 9.

69. Médecins Sans Frontières staff, *An Unprecedented Year*, 8

70. Ibid., 4.

71. Wieners and Kitamura, "Ebola: Doctors Without Borders Shows How to Manage a Plague."

72. Marchione, "Mission Unaccomplished," paragraph 13.

73. Hayden, "MSF Takes Bigger Global-Health Role," 18.

74. Miatta Gbanya, quoted in Hayden, "MSF Takes Bigger Global-Health Role," 18.

3

✝

The Legal and Ethical Duties That Are Owed to "Contact Tracers" and Other West African Volunteers

During the late summer months of 2014 many of the streets of Liberia's capital, Monrovia, were deserted. By this time dozens of leading West African doctors and nurses had given their lives in the fight against the spread of Ebola, and more than a few tears were shed as helpless Liberians realized that they were on their own. Miatta Zenabu Gbanya, a Liberian who had spent a decade doing relief work in Darfur, South Sudan, and the Democratic Republic of the Congo, had come home during mid-2013 to help her nation cope with this latest crisis. She was assigned by President Ellen Johnson Sirleaf the task of heading up what was called the "Health Sector Poor Fund," a health-care initiative that tried to help Ebola fighters by bringing together the limited resources that were coming in from a dozen donors. When Gbanya arrived on the scene she found that this Health Sector Pool Fund only had about $65 million in the bank, in part because the U.S. Congress does not permit the pooling of American financial resources.[1] Gbanya was one of the Liberian administrators who had to explain why many public health volunteers could not all be paid, or couldn't be paid on time, during the worst of times. "We were dealing with a tough work force," she later recalled, "that was dissatisfied, from top to bottom,"[2] and yet Gbanya went about trying to fight governmental corruption, begged donors for more aid, and she did her best to placate those who were constantly threatening to strike or to walk away from their jobs.

This chapter tells the story of many of the nameless or forgotten Liberians and other West Africans who made incredible sacrifices in order to stop the spread of EVD. In chapter 2, I outlined some of the contributions of foreign NGOs like Médecins Sans Frontières (MSF) who helped in the fight against Ebola, but oftentimes the glare of the media spotlights that underscored the importance of medical humanitarian intervention cast a shadow on the deeds of those who had to treat emerging infectious diseases as both endemic and epidemic problems. Although it may be months, or even years, before medical researchers and others can empirically evidence the impact of all of their local volunteering and community work, a critical cultural critique of their efforts reminds us that we should not forget either the symbolic or the material consequences of their labor. Although it must have seemed at times during the latest Ebola outbreak that they were engaging in acts of futility, they persevered and they were able to track, and to isolate, enough patients in urban and rural communities to contain the 2013–2015 outbreak.

As I noted in chapter 1, one of the major arguments that I advance in this book is that foreign interventionists like to take primary credit for the work that was accomplished by many social agents, empowered and disempowered, including those who worked at the grass-roots levels. I realize that at the present time—when many want to uncritically celebrate the heroism of foreign expatriates and other Western interventionism— this spotlighting of the efficacy of West African volunteerism and public health efforts may constitute a minority view. However, I am not the only observer who senses that some social agents' rhetorics don't always mesh with concrete material realities. "Charts of the rates of infection and fatalities," noted Laurie Garrett during the fall of 2015, "show that Liberia's plague was on its downward course *before* the world mobilized to help" (my emphasis).[3] Garrett went on to elaborate by noting that Liberia was somehow about to "turn the tide of its epidemic largely without" the help of the U.N. Mission for Ebola Emergency Response (UNMEER), the U.S. military, or the promises of hundreds of millions of dollars from the World Bank or other forms of multinational aid.

These, however, are not the dominant tales that are usually told about general Ebola efforts or the "battles" that were waged during this particular Ebola outbreak. Eulogistic purveyors of Western-oriented *dispositifs* focused on the beneficence of belated foreign intervention in West Africa, despite the fact that as late as February of 2015, after the worst of the Ebola crisis had passed, less than half of the promised supplies, personnel, or finances actually arrived on the ground in time to help the spread of EVD during these key moments in time.

Moreover, it could be argued that a critical review of the situation shows that Garrett was merely summarizing the views of other scientific journalists when she circulated a permutation of investigative journalists' Ebola rhetorics when she argued that "if the aid had arrived earlier, the epidemic would undoubtedly have been contained faster and with fewer fatalities."[4] The West Africans did their best with limited resources, and they were some of the major figures who helped stop the rampant spread of EVD, but the final mortality tallies speak volumes. They remind us of what life was like when impoverished African nations lacked everything from vaccines to isolation wards in their postcolonial hospitals or clinics.

To some readers this may sound like Monday-morning quarterbacking and retrospective critique, but remember who ended up trying to take credit for "ending" the outbreak during the fall of 2014 and throughout 2015. Notice how many media commentaries on this containment celebrity the "rescue" efforts of foreigners while local Africans make cameo appearances in these hagiographic accounts of the West African outbreak.

What do scholars, cosmopolitan citizens of the world, decision makers and others owe those who often stayed on the job throughout 2014, even after newspapers wrote about their strikes? For example, do we simply congratulate Liberian elites for having deployed the weapons of modern medicine as they tried to educate a largely "illiterate" population? Do we just thank them for ensuring that the Ebola virus did not "travel from *there* and infect us *here*" (emphasis in the original)?[5]

Administrators and nurses like Miatta Zenabu Gbanya were not just having to cope with payroll issues and resource scarcity-they were also having to deal with perceptual emergency contexts that raised a host of human rights and jurisprudential issues. Oftentimes during "emerging" infectious disease outbreaks legal scholars and bioethicists regularly debate about the importance of maintaining civil liberties of human rights when others want to impose harsh quarantines, cordons, and travel restrictions, but there are many other legal and ethical issues that were raised by this particular outbreak. James Hodge Jr., Gregory Measer, and Asha Agrawal recently wrote,

> Despite the availability of appropriate infection control protocols and equipment, treating Ebola patients creates a higher risk of exposure for healthcare workers ("HCWs") and raises personal safety concerns that implicate ethical and legal duties to treat. Providing workers with adequate training, personal protective equipment ("PPE"), and supervision mitigates some of these concerns. Public health laws, disability protections, employment contracts, and medical licensure standards can mandate treatment of Ebola patients through legal recourse or sanctions. Though voluntarism among HCWs is highly preferable to imposing legal mandates, workers may be pressed into action if cases of Ebola mount.[6]

Hodge, Measer, and Agrawal were writing for Anglo-American audiences who read materials produced by the American Bar Association who were interested in health law, but they were nevertheless pointing out some of the reasons why some of the "legal preparedness issues related to emerging infectious diseases like Ebola are dynamic."[7]

While detailed legal discussions of the rights of West African contact workers, nurses and others are rarely discussed in Western jurisprudential outlets, I want to argue in this chapter that Liberia, Sierra Leone, and Guinea, as well as foreign governments, need to respect the express and implied contracts that they have made with African volunteers and health care workers. These parties have legal and ethical duties that should guide their behavior during future Ebola outbreaks. At the same time, a critical cultural or a critical legal framing of these issues remind us that we need to recognize the importance of the rhetorics of differentiation or of similarity that circulated in some of these rhetorical cultures during these Ebola crises. For example, critical observers need to notice that when Western doctors and nurses who contracted EVD were medevacked out, their African counterparts often had to stay behind. At the same time, it is not only bothersome, but dangerous, when Ebola volunteers—contact tracers, ambulance drivers, and others—are not provided with some of the same PPE that is worn by foreign medical interventionists. Many Western presses seem to have assiduously avoided discussing this disparate treatment as they sought to recognize the heroism of those who were wearing proper gear.

As I note in other chapters, when researchers, doctors, administrators, or others mention the specific names of individuals in Ebola contexts and treat them as protagonists or antagonists in their contagion tales they often highlight the activities of high-profile public intellectuals or Western survivors who lived to tell about their near-death experiences. For example, Kent Brantly, a U.S. medical missionary who contracted EVD in July of 2014 (while he was working as a doctor in Liberia), watched as countless stories were written about his survival. He became a minor celebrity who was asked to appear before a joint U.S. Congressional hearing so that he could talk about conditions on the ground in West Africa.[8] Brantly was encouraged to provide experiential testimony about the suffering of the voiceless, who theoretically needed foreign interventionism, and he dutifully regaled his listeners in Washington, D.C., with commentaries that would have been familiar to those who had read about the 1976 exploits of Peter Piot or Richard Preston's *Hot Zone*:

> [I] witnessed the horror that this disease visits upon its victims—the intense pain and humiliation of those who suffer from it, the irrational fear and superstition that pervades communities, and the violence and unrest that now threaten entire nations. . . . I came to understand firsthand what my own patients had suffered. I was isolated from family and unsure if I would ever see them again. Even though I knew most of my caretakers, I could see

nothing but their eyes through my protective goggles. . . . I experienced the humiliation of losing control of my bodily functions and faced the horror of vomiting blood—a sign of the internal bleeding that could eventually lead to my death.[9]

Brantly's frank admissions about his bodily struggles only added to the authenticity and the emotive nature of his peroration, because now geographic time and distance was removed as Congressional leaders and others could understand some of the sense of urgency that was a part of his witnessing.

Brantly, like many Ebola survivors, used this image event as an opportunity to plead for hasty foreign intervention in West Africa. He explained to his listeners that treating Ebola was different from caring for other patients, because it involved grueling work. He went into great detail explaining that the personal protective equipment that doctors wore overseas became "excruciatingly hot," with temperatures inside the suits sometimes reaching up to 115 degrees.[10] All of this commentary was meant to underscore the point that the PPE could only be worn for about an hour-and-a-half at a time, which meant that only so many victims could be treated in any given period. Was Brantly hinting that more equipment needed to be sent overseas if his listeners wanted to see the containment of EVD?

Many parts of Brantly's testimony put on display the precarious nature of the spread of Ebola once this viral epidemic reached the capital of Liberia. He explained that his hospital, the ELWA Hospital in Monrovia, was the capital's only Ebola treatment center when the disease broke out. "The disease was spiraling out of control," Brantly explained, "and it was clear we were not equipped to fight it effectively on our own. We began to call for more international assistance, but our pleas seemed to fall on deaf ears."[11] One of my arguments, of course, is that he could not have known that by this time the West Africans had successfully isolated and treated those who needed help.

Brantly's visit to Washington, D.C., that allowed him to testify about the ravages of Ebola, symbolically and materially linked together conditions in Monrovia, Liberia—a town named after former President James Monroe—with a twenty-first-century collection of American congressional leaders who were now being asked to listen to tales that were allegedly being ignored by others. The implicit message that was being conveyed by this self-sacrificing medical missionary was clear—an exceptional nation needed to rise up and share Brantly's missionary zeal, take up the responsibilities associated with world leadership in public health, and help those who were losing the battle against EVD in places like Liberia. To be sure, a variant of Rudyard Kipling's old "White Man's Burden,"[12] but was this neoliberal medical humanitarian tale conveying something that was actually needed?

Brantly's type of medicalized Ebola *dispositif* thus served a host of rhetorical functions for both immediate and implied audiences in America and elsewhere. First of all, it served witnessing functions when it allowed his congressional listeners to visualize the pain and agony of those Africans who had been suffering from EVD throughout the summer of 2014—before the world took this threat seriously. It served a second, pedagogical function that allowed Brantly to talk about "irrational fears and superstition" that were pervading West African communities. This, in turn, implied that he, and other medical missionaries, were the ones who could bring the light of modern medicine to the darkness of those who suffered from scientific and public health illiteracy. This type of narrative also served a third function when it became a vehicle for the establishment of religious and nationalistic identification and connectivity. Brantly, after all, got to explain the rationale beyond his personal missionary decisions and how he felt that he was doing God's work, in spite of his "isolation" from country and family.

Much of this sounds like an echo of the personal, technical, and public commentary of colonial doctors like David Livingstone, and the hagiographic discourse that swirled around him for decades in British imperial circles during the nineteenth century or early twentieth century as generations of "Anglo-Saxons" dreamed of the day they would be old enough to follow in the footsteps of the next Burton, Livingstone, or Albert Schweitzer.[13]

Now, of course, altered power relations and political geographies had changed the specific names of the particular nations that were expected to carry on civilizing missions and rescue the downtrodden, but the dominant argumentative claims, warrants, and evidentiary expectations remained the same. Could Brantly, and many other social agents worried about the spread of Ebola, produce the types of convincing arguments that respond to what John Stuart Mill once called the presumptions behind "non-interventionism"?[14]

Granted, studying the words and deeds of empowered rhetors like President Ellen Johnson Sirleaf or witnesses like Kent Brantly serve their purposes, but in the rest of this chapter I want to put on display the textual arguments and the visualities about the latest Ebola outbreak that were produced by those who did not have the chance to appear before congressional audiences or other elite forums. As Professor Dana Cloud once argued in her essay on the "null persona," there are often times when workers' efforts involve some "silence" that is "audible only in relief from the sound" of voices of the empowered, and she highlighted the importance of studying the efforts of laborers who face "long hours, work hazards" and other dangers in order to survive.[15]

My analysis of the legal and cultural dimensions of workers' efforts in Ebola contexts is meant to supplement, and to extend, the work of Dana

Cloud, Philip Wander,[16] Raymie McKerrow,[17] and others who have written on the importance of critical rhetoric in salient public controversies. Here I want to follow up on Michel Foucault's notion that scholars need to be producing critical genealogies that attend to the fragmentary relics that appear in our various elite and vernacular archives that hint at the "gray," "patient," and "meticulous rituals of power."[18]

If it is indeed the case that our contemporary archives are filled with shards left over from winning and losing medical campaigns, fragments from all sorts of public health controversies, then we need to pay attention to the voices of workers and others who actually have to implement the strategies and tactics that are proposed by their superiors in places like Liberia. This way, readers can see the human contradictions, the sacrifices, and the other dimensions of some of this grayness that is produced by lay persons as well as elites during Ebola crises.

Later on in this chapter I will be citing multiple mainstream and alternative press sources who wrote about strikes of nurses in West Africa and the United States, but what they often failed to mention is that many angered and frustrated workers stayed on the job, and that "paid health-care workers" in Liberia "shared their salaries with the unpaid, on the assumption that someday their clinical comrades would finally earn enough to reimburse them."[19] They were sometimes harassed or attacked by communities who thought that the workers were the ones bringing Ebola, and yet they continued to fight for what Miatta Gbanya called "mother Liberia." The contact tracers who initially faced resistance eventually won over many rural residents, who, instead of touching and hugging the dead, learned that they needed to bring their dead to West African authorities.[20]

These contact tracers, and thousands of other African volunteers and health care workers, risked their own lives as they traveled to villages and the "slums" of West Africa between 2013 and 2015, and along the way they helped co-create a number of legal and ethical issues.[21] These were some of those who did the "painstaking detective work"[22] that was needed to treat potential Ebola victims, and it behooves us to listen to some of their stories about their trials and tribulations at the same time that we hear the admonitions of empowered social agents like Kent Brantly.

Granted, as I note below, many of the stories that these contact tracers and West African health care workers will tell do not always look like the coherent, logical, and pristine reports on EVD that are cobbled together in the linear assemblages that appear in the pages of scientific outlets like *Nature*, *Science*, *The Lancet*, or *The New England Journal of Medicine*. Their stories of Ebola denialism, obstruction, lack of government pay, and so on, may have affective dimensions that highlight the contradictions of the human condition. They put on display the partiality of vision, and the

select nature of the public health care workers' recollections of their experiences. These African health care workers were often the ones who told
others about how rural communities, over time, "without any push from
government," took "matters into their own hands, setting up temporary
isolation places," usually houses or sheds, that allowed the communities
to order that visitors and "returnees from the cities be quarantined."[23]
Conventional Western tales, that wanted to vilify locals while valorizing
foreign efforts, rarely admitted any of this.

These alternative Ebola *dispositifs* have protagonists who are West Africans, and their rhetorics are not easily folded into some of the Western-
oriented narrations that contain black-and-white binary ways of viewing
Western heroism during outbreaks. Yes, the contact tracers, and the local
nurses and others who occasionally went on strike played small parts
in Eurocentric rescue tales, but their own renditions of what happened
during this same period also circulated in the blogosphere and served as
alternative ways of thinking about Ebola counternarratives, counterhistories, or countermemories.

Contact tracers, when they appeared in most mainstream accounts
from "the North," were usually characterized as some of the background
figures who aided in the pursuit of Patient Zero, or they appeared as
nameless individuals who helped with the isolation of recalcitrant EVD
patients before the Obama "surge." The real focus of attention of mainstream Western newspapers was on the actions of the belated rescuers,
and not on the everyday world of those who washed their hands with
chlorine or talked to victims' families.

Occasionally the contact tracers were thanked by foreign doctors
or Western science journalists for the contributions that they made in
helping with social or behavioral changes, but these were often framed
in ways that valorized the mystical power that came with twenty-first-
century medical modernity or enlightenment. "Lost in much of the panic-
churning coverage of the Ebola epidemic," argued Michael Bonner in
November of 2014, "is a palpable sense of treating the sick" that was "the
at once basic and sometimes perilous care being administered by teams of
local and international medical workers."[24] For others, respecting needed
interventionism, even if belated, was deemed to be one of the precondi-
tions for garnering this rare praise, and accepting Western orientations
was viewed as a precondition for halting the spread of EVD.

While foreign accounts rarely went into great detail explaining the day-
to-day struggles of the contact tracers, they were at least given credit for
bravely facing hostile populations in Liberia, Sierra Leone, and Guinea.
As Ranu Dhillon and Daniel Kelly wrote in their study of community
trust in Guinea in July of 2015, "community distrust enables Ebola to
persist in areas where people continue to hide the sick, conduct funerals

in secret and elude contact tracing."[25] Those who were uncooperative in Guinea, argued Dhillon and Kelly, were not doing so because they were "backward or uneducated," but because their harboring of distrust of Ebola response efforts had everything to do with "their experience during recent decades of misrule and political tumult."[26] Commentary about the contact tracers could be written in forms that focused on intentionalism, but the Dhillon and Kelly analysis hinted that others could also adopt more functional or structural ways of conceptualizing this outbreak.

What activities did contract tracers engage in that prevented this from being an outbreak that might have taken hundreds of thousands of lives? How did they themselves view their activities, and why would nurses and other care workers talk of going on strike while patients were dying all around them? How did media outlets, in West Africa and in the Anglo-American communities, characterize their efforts, especially near the end of 2014 when WHO, the UN, and other organizations argued that we were nearing the "end" of this latest outbreak?

In order to answer those types of questions we need to be able to go back in time and survey a period when only a few public health care workers were looking for the "index" case in Guinea in December of 2013. Only then can we trace the evolutionary nature of some of the arguments and Ebola *dispositifs* that were produced by these African laborers. We need to listen to them and watch how they were characterized by their friends and neighbors, so that we get some needed insight into the day-to-day struggles of those whose efforts are glossed over in most Western neoliberal tales that intended to highlight the beneficence of the empowered.

As David N. Livingstone explains, one of the advantages of using a critical genealogical approach when scholars study tropical diseases stems from the way that this allows us to "peel back" overlapping "layers" of sedimented public health knowledge so that we can see the contested nature of the rhetoric that became more persistent "over time."[27] This is especially important in the study of what critical rhetoricians call "vernacular" studies of everyday worlds.[28]

This type of a cultural, post-structural approach allows the critic to see some of the historical and contemporary debates in ways that accentuate the contingent, the partial, and the fragmentary so that we can "elucidate" multiple significations that circulate during salient public health controversies. Professor Livingstone has elaborated by noting that this type of perspectival critique employs a "tropical hermeneutics" that allows for the "textual interrogation" of theories and practices that can be found in all sorts of reports, including those implicated in the "moral stigmatizing of people who inhabited certain regions or zones."[29]

Regardless of our choice of outbreak *dispositifs*, there is little question that all of these Ebola tales have to take into account the unique ideological and cultural features of this particular outbreak. The African health care workers sometimes had to deal with many members of local communities in West Africa who once thought that Ebola was some governmental hoax, invented by administrators to bring in foreign aid that only helped those living in places like Monrovia. Ranu Dhillon and Daniel Kelly's commentary on "shock" perhaps gets at some of the material realities that helped change some opinions:

> In Liberia, Sierra Leone and areas of Guinea affected earlier in the epidemic, "apocalyptic" transmission—dead bodies in the street, entire villages nearly wiped out—jolted communities into believing in the reality of Ebola and cooperating with response efforts. The shocks generated abrupt change, but how can buy-in be garnered without communities first enduring such intense suffering?[30]

Dhillon and Kelly hoped that their own work, and the recognition that public health workers needed to gain the trust of populations during Ebola outbreaks, would help make us aware of the contributions that led to these psychic and social changes.

Critical cultural scholars or critical legal rhetoricians may not be able to pinpoint the exact temporal moment when reluctant families in Guinea, Liberia, and Sierra Leone grudgingly admitted that it was in their own best interest to work with contact tracers and Ebola response teams. These critics can admit that we may never be able to definitely point to some specific hour or day when Ebola denialists changed their minds or when skeptical communities decided that their governments were not the only ones that might profit from Ebola eradication. However, what a "bottom-up," critique of elite and vernacular rhetorics allows us to do is keep track of changes in discursive and visual signification at the "micro" level, that in turn provide us with some clues regarding altered *dispositifs*.

I'll begin my critique with an analysis of some of the diachronic features of this rhetorical landscape that were produced during the first stage of the outbreak, and I will be concentrating on the micro-level social agency of contact tracers

THE ROLE OF CONTACT TRACERS AND
OTHER LOCALS DURING THE FIRST STAGE OF
THE EBOLA OUTBREAK, MARCH 2014 TO JULY 2014

The term "contact tracer" probably entered many Anglo-American vocabularies after mainstream newspapers reported that in March of 2014 the Guinean Minister of Health had called Médecins Sans Frontières and let them know that an outbreak of Ebola virus disease was believed to have started in a village of the Guéckédou Prefecture in the south of Guinea. In order to help Western audiences visualize what was happening they were told that in Guéckédou there was an Ebola treatment center where contact tracers worked with scores of local West African personnel and MSF at the "front lines fighting the epidemic."[31]

In these early accounts science reporters and others explained that contact tracers were trained to make sure that villagers and other Africans knew about the importance of "isolating" those who had EVD or were suspected of having the virus. Readers were informed that the contact tracers were some of those who had to visit the afflicted and they were supposed to check-in with individuals who are quarantined for twenty-one days in their West African homes. Kadiatu Lansa and other contact tracers, noted Amrai Coen and Malte Henk, "have become detectives of sorts in the midst of this chaos," and when anyone in rural or urbans areas fell prey to, or died of, EVD, it was "their job is to monitor anyone who came in contact with that person."[32] The contact tracers, by their incessant questioning of villagers who might complain about fear, headaches, diarrhea, or vomiting, thus became the parties who helped render visible the efforts of those who labored away in intensive, diffuse, massive surveillance and detection systems.

In some cases foreign commentators who wrote about the contact tracers treated them as important subordinates who understood the importance of managing Ebola risks. For example, Carissa Guild, a doctor working with MSF in Guinea, wrote about how the "hands-on" efforts of those who worked at community levels helped EVD patients, even as "casualties" fell all around them. "The vibe in the treatment center" in Guinea was very different from the "American-style ER," explained Guild, because in rural Guinea the latest in gadgetry was not going to save patients. The smaller EVD treatment centers relied on the provision of individuated human comfort, human dignity, and the personal easing of pain.[33]

Carissa Guild, who was a part of what MSF calls the "first stage" of containment efforts, was able to explain how foreign interveners who thought that they had everything under control in April of 2014 quickly changed their minds when the Guéckédou Ebola treatment center started hearing from Sierra Leonean refugees who told their own stories of EVD outbreaks *across the border*. During a previous 2012 outbreak in another part of Africa, Guild had dealt with about a dozen and half patients, but now she had to watch as hundreds of beds in Guéckédou started filling up.[34]

In Guild's account it would be the local public health care workers who took center stage. She explained that on a typical day in Guéckédou teams of contact tracers would be sent out every morning to collect needed information, and they and others would then send along this information to the Department of Health in Guinea and to the ambulatory services. In theory, Guinean health officials would process this information and send out ambulances to either pick up suspected Ebola victims or try and convince the people in "hot spots" to come into the treatment centers.

These types of frontline accounts contained descriptive information that enabled sympathetic writers to comment on the pedagogical duties of the tracers. During one lengthy interview, Carissa Guild told an intrigued reporter about the everyday world of the tracers:

> Contact tracers create a list of people who had physical contact with an Ebola patient while that person presented with symptoms. They go to the villages every day for 21 days to personally check on all of these contacts, making sure they feel well, with the purpose of identifying and isolating cases in the community as fast as possible after the onset of symptoms, and thus as soon as they become contagious. Then there is also the team of "health promoters" who would also be dispatched. They teach local communities by explaining what Ebola is and how to avoid transmission.[35]

So far, Carissa Guild's Ebola outbreak tale looks fairly mundane, the type of commentary that might appear in a recital of what happened in Dallas or Lagos. However, as soon as Michael Bronner, her interviewer, started to ask about the gear that is typically worn by these African volunteers we begin to see some of disparate treatment, differential economics, and ethnic features of the Ebola outbreak that may be papered over in some other biological or epidemiological accounts of the epidemic. Dr. Guild tells Bronner that neither the contact tracers nor the "health promoters" were wearing protective gear, and that the ambulance drivers who were using pickup trucks also worked without PPE. This was part of the reason why so many contracted EVD during this initial stage of the outbreak.

Once the ambulance drivers or the health promoters felt that they had found an Ebola patient who tested positive for EVD, then that same team would get dressed in personal protective gear and decontaminate the house. Dr. Guild goes on to explain how West African contexts created challenges that might not be faced by workers in other geopolitical regions:

> We had a bit of flak in Guinea because we were using pickup trucks. They thought this was like transporting animals, but we actually chose those specifically because they're really easy to decontaminate when we drop the patients off. You can just take off the mattress, you spray the whole pickup bed—there are no nooks and crannies—and then you put a fresh mattress in.[36]

Some West Africans, like many other global denizens, commented on how some of these practices might look dehumanizing, and yet this talk of pick-up trucks brought to the surface all types of latent tensions regarding how one factored in the frontlines needs of those battling contagion. This welter of worries about diverse forms of stigmatization had to be juxtaposed with medical necessities and the medicalized practicalities of daily life fighting Ebola.

These types of "frontline" commentaries supplemented the information about the contact tracers that appeared in more scientific and mainstream Western outlets. For example, as Daniel Cooney, Vincent Wong, and Yaneer Bar-Yam explained in May of 2015, "contact tracing is the accepted method for public control of infectious diseases."[37] Given the fact that early detection of Ebola-like symptoms helped limit the number of new infection cases, the contact tracers were said to use a structure that began with the identification of an "index" case, and then that person was linked with all of the people that the patient may have interacted with.

While many journalists in mainstream Western presses harped on the supposed ignorance of West African populations and their denialism, interviewees like Carissa Guild commented on how local community observation of the spread of EVD taught some life lessons to observant communities in Guinea, Liberia, and Sierra Leone. Dr. Guild was aware that in Wome, not far from Guéckédou, some eight health workers had been killed by angry villagers, but she goes on to explain that "Ebola does its own health promotion and education." Ebola would first hit a town, then the people watch who gets sick, observe who is taking care of that person, and they could watch how that caring person gets sick. After "two weeks or three weeks," averred Guild, the "population starts to see and understand how it works."[38] This put on display the reasonableness and savvy, and not the ignorance, of local African communities who adapted to their changing environment.

This type of "on the spot" vernacular explanation looked nothing like the vilifying and primitivist accounts that sometimes circulated in Western media outlets. While Guild would go on to explain that MSF and local volunteers had to deal with viral "dead bodies" that were moving across towns and borders, she thought that local communities still needed more treatment centers, that the world needed to know more about the health care workers who were dying, and that lessons still needed to be learned about the continued need for more vaccines and more personal protection equipment. As far as she was concerned the West African families who appeared to be suffering from emotional trauma were the ones who had to watch as foreign people came to their aid "dressed up like space men." These medical interventionists were covered in chlorine and were dripping wet, while these same social agents constantly harped on what families of EVD victims could not touch. All of this was physically and emotionally draining.[39]

Dr. Guild and others have commented on how, in May of 2014, the West African Ebola outbreak was supposed to burn itself out and end like dozens of other outbreaks on the African continent, but within weeks, as Ebola spread to places like Monrovia, worried observers found that they were in what Amrai Coen and Malte Henk called a "nihilistic biological relay race."[40]

As noted above, I am arguing that West African countries have legal and ethical responsibilities and duties that should not be set aside during times of emergency, and the risks that many of the volunteers took the first phase of the outbreak simply underscored their sacrifices.

At one time it looked as though Liberians were faced with an impossible situation as they tried to track down thousands of different people who had been in contact with patients. Kai Kupferschmidt, a journalist for *Science* magazine, who was working on a story about contact tracers, followed along as an Ebola-tracing team tried to find a woman who had gone to a hospital seeking medical care. When the doctors called an ambulance to take her to one of the treatment units so that she could be tested for EVD, she reportedly fled into the jungle. Locals suggested that she had headed toward a village in Guinea called Fenemetaa. Kupferschmidt's particular team—made up of an epidemiologist from Uganda, a county surveillance official, and two people from Doctors Without Borders packed some water and set off to find her.[41]

Stories about rural tracking are complicated enough, but imagine what happens when travelers cross borders and move into populated areas. Cooney, Wong, and Bar-Yam pointed out that some of this tracing is "made nearly impossible in urban environments with more than a few cases,"[42] but they may be underestimating the material and symbolic power of these tracers. The tracers efforts may have had what some call a "multiplier effect" when they help educate local communities, families, and neighbors at the same time that they are tracking down potential EVD victims.

Until West African governments, NGOs, or foreign powers are willing to pay for more elaborate community-based monitor centers, it is the labor-intensive efforts of the contact tracers that play essential roles in helping stop the spread of Ebola virus disease.

When we read about the valor of individuals like Kent Brantly, it is easy to forget that tens of thousands of contact tracers, local religious groups, NGO volunteers, village leaders, and others in Liberia, Guinea, and Sierra Leone who tried to persuade taxi drivers, families, neighbors, and others that it was in their best interest to report suspected cases, engage in isolationist practices, and at least tolerate some form of government help. While a vocal minority of skeptics and deniers conjured up conspiracy tales about the non-existence of the virus or the governments' strategic use of Ebola to collect more foreign aid, *most West Africans*—especially after June of 2014—started to realize that they had to try and stop an existential threat.

Those who were contacted by the tracers may not have known that the Ebola virus was what some in the West called a "Biosafety Level (BSL) 4 pathogen,"[43] but they got out their buckets of chlorine, listened to lectures on Ebola pathogenesis, and tried to modify some of their cultural practices to help end the ravages of these diseases. All of these efforts belied the claims of many Western journalists, foreign public health specialists, and others who argued that massive "military humanitarianism" provided the best, or only hope for those wishing to prevent this from turning into a viral apocalyptic disaster.

FOREIGN INTERVENTIONISM AND THE BEGINNING OF THE "END" OF THE 2013–2015 WEST AFRICAN OUTBREAK, AUGUST 2014–FEBRUARY 2015

By August of 2014, the nations of Guinea, Liberia, and Sierra Leone faced what WHO would call a "Public Health Emergency of International Concern" (PHEIC). This signaled that some extraordinary event had taken place that constituted a public health risk that could not be contained by a single nation-state, to the point where it needed some type of coordinated international response.[44]

Many WHO officials and national leaders are reluctant to call for this type of help because it is often interpreted as a type of state failure. For example, doctor Hans Rosling, a WHO statistician, once argued in July of 2014 that Ebola was a "small problem" and that West Africans should not scare away national health talent from the greater threats of malaria, pregnancy complications, bacterial infections, or diarrheal disease. A contrite Rosling would later say, "If you want to blame someone for this epidemic, blame me. . . . It was my mistake," and he later volunteered to work in Liberia counting the sick and the dead.[45] As noted in chapter 2, leaders in Guinea bickered with MSF doctors about the scale of the outbreak, but they also debated about the numbers of trained doctors, nurses, and others that might be needed to control the outbreak.

With the benefit of hindsight, it could be argued that from an empirical standpoint the contact tracers and the African health care workers had contained most of the outbreak before foreign interventions, but imagine the difficulties that would be raised if potential donors heard that type of talk. There are perhaps substantive, consciousness-raising, and commodified reasons why Western news outlets circulated *dispositifs* that made it appear as though only aid that might come for China, Cuba, the United States, the United Kingdom or elsewhere could prevent this from turning into a pandemic that threatened the lives of millions.

By September of 2014 countless newspapers, radio programs, televisions stations, and blogosphere sites contained stories of Western African attacks on public health care workers and MSF personnel. Journalists and pundits complained that illiterate and obstinate communities in Guinea, Liberia, and Sierra Leone were continuing to eat bushmeat and were still attending funerals where they touched those who died of Ebola.[46] More than a few were convinced that elite nepotism, corruption, African denialism, conspiracy rhetorics, and mistrust of government were pervasive and intractable problems that could not be handled by the West Africans. No wonder that statisticians of the U.S. Centers for Diseases Control and Prevention and WHO started to come up with scenarios and extrapolations that tried to factor in the possibility that *there would be little change in the behavior* of many West Africans, and based on these worse-case scenarios they predicted that the number of EVD cases might rise up to 1.4 million by the middle of January 2015.[47]

The cultural and ideological features of this particular rhetorical usage of statistics are fascinating. As Alexander Kekulé explains, the CDC arrived at this figure by estimating that there would be more than 550,000 reported cases in Liberia and Sierra Leone alone, and then they factored in the possibility that all of this was *underreporting* Ebola incidents by a factor of 2.5. Ebola victims and their families, in other words, might be hiding their disease, or refusing to visit Ebola Treatment Centers (ETCs). "On the basis of these pessimistic forecasts," argued Kekulé, many countries "devised long-term aid programs, with the result that most of the treatment centers were only completed when the epidemic had already abated."[48]

Why, during this period, didn't organizations like MSF, WHO, the World Bank, and so on, use their neoliberal ideologies to back a system of much higher payments to contact tracers, nurses, doctors, and other volunteers who would then have greater incentives to track down those who needed to be isolated? Why was so much attention being lavished on Obama's billions and his "surge," that was geared toward the provision of logistics or the building of treatment centers? Why not put in place legal and ethical codes that protected the African workers who risked their lives on those "front lines"?

Part of this reluctance to focus on the needs of contact tracers may have something to do with the Western-oriented focus on the perceived need for "mobile" foreign interventionism. Since the identification of "Patient Zero" in December of 2013, the rapid deployments of international mobile laboratories through WHO networks—like the Global Outbreak Alert and response Network (GOARN) and Emerging and Dangerous Pathogens Laboratory Network (EDPLN)—were viewed by those in the "North" as the key activities that played an important role in trying to stop the 2013–2015 West African outbreak. Some of the organizations that provided these types of laboratories included China Centers for Disease Control Lab, European Union Mobile Laboratory Consortium (EM Lab), Institute Pasteur Dakar, Institute Pasteur Lyon, Institute Pasteur Paris, Institut National de Recherche Bio-Médicale Mobile lab in Democratic Republic of Congo, National Institute for Communicable Diseases in South Africa, Public Health England Mobile lab, Public Health Canada Mobile Lab, Russian Rospotrebnadzor Mobile Lab, United States Centers for Disease Control (CDC), U.S First Area Medical Laboratory, U.S. National Institutes of Health, and the U.S. Naval Medical Research Center Mobile Lab.[49] These mobile labs were supposed to help confirm disease in patients with suggestive symptoms so that this can trigger isolation, contact tracing, and the documentation of accurate records for those who either did, or did not, have EVD. Someone, of course, had to pay for all of this medical knowledge, laboratory equipment, and infrastructure.

Stigmatization, fear of these volunteers, and the lack of status may also have influenced the marginalization of these African health workers. For example, by October of 2014, many Liberian nurses who had been risking their lives had had enough. During this period the average Liberian health care worker's base salary was somewhere between $200 to $500 per month, and members of Liberia's National Health Workers Association threatened to strike unless a demand for an increase in hazard pay was met.[50]

By this time some two hundred health workers in Liberia had contracted EVD, and ninety-five had died, and although nurses and medical workers understood the importance of their work, they faced an administration, led by assistant health minister Tolbert Nyenswah, that treated this as an ultimatum that placed a "huge financial burden on the state."[51] "Ordinary citizens" in Liberia, reported *Al Jazeera*, "expressed alarm" at the prospect of the strike, that might "cripple the campaign against Ebola just as the international community ramped up assistance."[52] What these commentaries often failed to mention were the numbers who stayed on the job, those who worked without pay, and those who suffered while on the job.

Cultural differences, contested economic statuses, and competing political needs were at play here as nurses and other workers fought for their contractual rights. This, however, could be configured by fiscally strapped governments as individuated selfishness during periods that required collective sacrifice, national courage, and delayed gratification. The nurses and other workers involved in these potential strikes responded to these worries by noting that since EVD was spread via the bodily fluids of infected Ebola victims, public health care workers who treated Ebola patients were especially vulnerable, and therefor needed to be paid for taking these higher risks.

Before the health minister provided assurances that hazard pay would be handed out, these health care workers walked out of several hospitals and clinics that had to be temporarily closed. In places like Monrovia's Island clinic, "go slow" policies were linked to governmental refusals to pay the extra hazard pay, and this in turn was credited with having led to the deaths of dozens of Ebola patients.[53] Months later, in places like the clinic in Bandajuma (that was the only Ebola treatment center in the Southern part of Sierra Leone), staff felt they had to go on strike when the government failed to pay an agreed-upon weekly $100 "hazard payment."[54]

By not fulfilling their contractual duties West African officials were not only impacting the lives of the volunteers but the lives of Ebola victims. In late November of 2014, the contact tracers who were supervised by the Ministry of Health had some new challenges when they tried to encourage suspected EVD victims in Monrovia to stay in their homes in order to help with the isolation of the disease. One of the many problems that the tracers faced is that no one had put together any system to provide those who were being quarantined with any food. In some cases the contact tracers did not even have the thermometers that they needed to check these individuals for fever.[55]

Paid and unpaid contact tracers raced through towns and villages, but they were having to compete with a virus that was spread by equally mobile travelers. In some cases during this period, modern means of transportation worked to hinder relief efforts. For example, Adam Bjork, an epidemiologist working with the CDC in Atlanta, spent two weeks in September and early October in the Southwest corner of Liberia trying to help contain the outbreak. He explained that he worked in an area that was a three-day drive from Monrovia during the rainy season, and that he and the other CDC employees who worked with him were supposed to be the "eyes and ears on the ground" that gave their bosses in Monrovia some sense of the situation in their area.[56] Bjork told the story about a sick family, that was traveling around from place to place in a taxi, trying desperately to get some care. While these well-intentioned efforts involved a search for medical care, this family was inadvertently spreading the disease as they traveled along in that taxi.

Bjork used the story of the toxic taxi as a way of conveying both the nature of Ebola pathogenesis as well as the hurdles that were inadvertently placed in the paths of the CDC and others who worked on this outbreak. The taxi narrative began when the pharmacist from Grand Kru and his son fell ill. They took a taxi with three other family members, who set out to seek care in Monrovia. First they tried to drive through River Gee County toward Zwedru, the capital of Grand Gedeh County, but they were turned away at the border by some of those who had been ordered to set up cordons. The taxi driver and family members spent a night in River Gee, and eventually the dad and son died in the taxi. All three of the remaining family members became Ebola cases, along with the driver. Two made it to Monrovia, where they died.[57]

Part of Bjork's job involved making sure that contact tracers in the region knew what to do, but he argued that they were already doing most of what he would have wanted, but that they were short on motorbikes and other vehicles. "They know what to do, but they don't have the resources," explained Bjork, and he went on to note that they sometimes had difficulties communicating with nearby communities that did not always accept them.[58]

Bjork's micro-narrative rendered visible would have happened countless times in the coming months. At first the contact tracers in Gee River County were met with some hostility and one town even threatened to burn some of the ambulances of the health care workers. Yet when the team of contact tracers held a community meeting that included town leaders, the mood suddenly shifted as those who gathered together allowed the local residents to have their say, and in the process they were able to get the information about Ebola that they needed.[59]

The incremental nature of these attitudinal or behavior changes may have gone unnoticed in most Western circles, but there were a few foreign journalists who realized that "those on the spot" were being mistreated. By November of 2014 Laurie Garrett was reporting that some 2,700 Liberians had died of EVD, but that hundreds of angry contact tracers were surrounding Liberia's Ministry of Health because they hadn't been paid since early September. Some of the "ministry employees," reported Garrett, "who track down anyone who may have come into contact with an Ebola victim," have "never received a dime."[60]

For several hours Garrett watched as angry workers shouted at those who ended up processing the payments of only a few dozen workers. Many held up cellphones so that they could show pictures that supported their assertions that they had forded raging rivers in dugout canoes, hiked through knee-deep mud, and hunted for long hours in the hot sun through neighborhoods that had no known addresses.[61]

One contact tracer, Tamba Korkor, told the story of how he, and his family, had been put at risk because of his work efforts. Shortly after he started working as a contact tracer, Korkor and one of his colleagues discovered an Ebola suspect in Monrovia. They sent for the supervisor to call for an ambulance, and after receiving this ambulatory care the victim died. The family and friends of the victim confronted Korkor and accused him of selling the man's body for money, and Korkor averred that he had not gone home for some two months after the aggrieved family members attacked his own family.[62]

When Garrett heard these stories, she reported that Liberia was "stiffing its contact tracers," at the very time that the Ebola epidemic was continuing to spread. She admired the fact that the tracers risked their lives, didn't wear the right protective gear, and continued to work under harsh conditions, and she characterized them as patriots who were trying to protect Liberian lives. "We have been working very hard against this virus and we're not getting no pay," Andrew Lewis Jr., told Garrett, and he asked that President Obama use some of his diplomatic power to "tell the people here to give us our money."[63]

To give readers some sense of the compensation that these tracers were owed, note that after several months of work the average amount owed these workers was around $240. Some were so poor at this point that they did not have the money to pay for their transportation back home after they joined the picketing.

By November and December of 2014 the number of reported EVD cases had declined sharply, and this in turn helped with the contact tracing. The reproduction rate of EVD was 1.51 for Guinea, 2.53 for Sierra Leone, and 1.59 for Liberia,[64] and it required an immense amount of "manpower" to try to track down potential victims, and countless Africans put their lives on the line as they worked to halt the spread of disease.

However, it would be the foreign interventionists that grabbled the media headlines. "At the height of the epidemic," reported Pentagon Press Secretary Rear Admiral John Kirby, "there were 2,800 DoD [Department of Defense] personnel deployed to West Africa," and by February of 2015 he could tell CNN viewers and readers that "given the success of the U.S. responses to the crisis," the majority of the Department of Defense personnel could return home.[65]

While there is little question that this DOD help, though belated, was appreciated by some leading members of West African governments, these types of statements magnified the social agency of the military interventionists while they obfuscating the role that relatively poor contact tracers, nurses, and other Africans played in controlling the spread of EVD.

CONCLUSION

Throughout 2014 and most of 2015, contact tracers in Guinea, Liberia, and Sierra Leone tried to find every patient, and tried to identify everyone who may have interacted with someone who had Ebola virus disease. The operative idea here was that if you identified these select individuals, and if you then monitored their behavior during Ebola's twenty-one-day period, then you could isolate them before he or she infected others.[66] This all required the cooperation of villagers and others in West Africa who would stop hiding their relatives in homes.

The early protocols for contact tracers were formulated after the 1976 discovery of the "Zaire" Ebola virus, and the lack of a vaccine created the material conditions for heavy reliance on this contact tracing approach. Like many infectious disease protocols, contact tracing has its own strengths and weaknesses, and the efficacy of this approach depends on having populations that are willing to work with public care workers.

Contact tracing apparently works best when volunteers feel that they are treated fairly, when members of the community don't feel stigmatized or marginalized, and when Ebola suspects understand why they are being tracked down and why they need to be traced. The contact tracers, in other words, need to be culturally sensitive to the particular needs of indigenous populations, and they cannot simply assume that West African communities are going to immediately change all of their habits and their cultures and automatically embrace Western notions of medicine or biosecurity treatments of EVD.

Before the summer of 2014, many health care workers and contact tracers ran into trouble because the early prevention messages that were being circulated emphasized the high mortality rates associated with the disease. Instead of encouraging people to seek help from Doctors Without Borders or West African health officials, these discouraging messages made it appear as if seeking care was some hopeless endeavor, and many of those who were afraid of the contact tracers fled into the jungle and sought the help of "traditional healers." Marí Sáez, an anthropologist who has worked in Guinea and Sierra Leone, explained that these messages were counterproductive in that they gave the impression that EVD was incurable. She explained that the local indigenous populations reasoned that it would do little good to seek aid from those disseminating these types of messages.[67] The problem, she argued, was in the nature of the messaging, and not the supposed irrationality of West African populations.

In this chapter I have underscored the dangers and the difficulties associated with contact tracing, and I have highlighted the need for West African governments to carry out their legal and ethical duties as they contract with contact tracers and other volunteers. They are the ones who were there before, and after, the appearance of the foreign interventionists, and they helped track down and isolate EVD patients. Moreover, they also helped with the reduction of stigmatization, the calming of fears, and the behavior modification of entire communities and populations. At the same time, they worked to persuade suspicious groups in Liberia, Sierra Leone, and Guinea that Ebola represented a real threat and that it was in families' own interest to cooperate with those who asked that they use chlorine and change a few of their habits.

Granted, the people of West Africa needed mobile Ebola treatment centers, beds, gloves, the right personal protective equipment (PPE), and many welcomed the funding that came from places like America, Europe, China, and elsewhere. However, we all need to admit that many of those who arrived on the scene during the fall of 2014 *rarely came in contact with many actual Ebola victims or their families*. Diagnostic work is important, but we owe a great deal to those who follow up on the laboratory reports, those who put their lives on the line as they try to help other health care workers.[68] Arlene Chua and her colleagues, writing for *Neglected Infectious Diseases*, have recently reported that more than eight hundred health care workers have been infected with EVD, and that early analysis of the data shows that a substantial portion of these infections occurred "outside the context of Ebola treatment and care centers."[69]

With the passage of time one hopes that vernacular Ebola *dispositifs* will impact the ways that decision makers think about the rights and duties of those who work with these contact tracers. Centers for Disease Control director Tom Frieden attributed much of the success of the Liberians when they announced that they were "Ebola free" in May of 2015 to those local teams that followed the principle of RITE (Rapid Isolation and Treatment of Ebola),[70] but Daniel Cooney, Vincent Wong, and Yaneer Bar-Yam are more skeptical and they argue that the "direct cause of the reduction is not well-documented."[71]

All of the ambiguity, mysticism, and politics that swirls around the Ebola prevention, treatment, and eradication programs has created a rhetorical situation where many different communities want to take credit for helping "end" the last outbreak. It is understandable that mainstream presses in the West, who wanted to be patriotic and who wanted to applaud the efforts of the medical or military humanitarians would focus on the social agency of the foreigners who intervened to stop the spread of Ebola. Yet the symbolic magnification of those who belatedly intervened during the fall of 2014 unintentionally often slights the works of thousands of nameless contact tracers and others who did a great deal of the everyday work that had to be done to contain the latest Ebola outbreak. One of the many ways that contact tracers help is by the avoidance of treating West African traditions as if they were "exotic behavior."[72]

For many foreign observers, the epidemic abated when Liberia was declared to be (erroneously) "Ebola-free" in May of 2015. By that time WHO had registered some 27,500 EVD cases, and more than 11,220 deaths, but this was nowhere near the figure that appeared in the apocalyptic rhetorics of the CDC and WHO. So, if this is the case, then *what happened between September of 2014 and May of 2015?* Did the EVD epidemic burn itself out on its own? Did the massive "surge" of some 2,700 military personnel from the United States lead to the treatment of all of the suspected Ebola cases in Liberia? Did foreign NGOs suddenly appear on the scene with hundreds of doctors who tracked down thousands of patients? Did the use of coercive quarantines and *cordons sanitaires* at the borders of West African nations make the difference?

If I am right then many of these self-serving Ebola *dispositifs* from "the North" slight the contributions of the contact tracers, nurses, and others who worked in neighborhoods, on the road, and in Ebola treatment centers. From a critical cultural or critical legal vantage point, perhaps we need to support the adoption of West African variants of what U.S. nurses call the "National Nurse Act of 2013."[73] This bill, if it was passed in the United States would make sure that a new position, called the "National Nurse," would be set up so that empowered nurses could work with, and complement the work of, the "surgeon general in public health campaigns, including Ebola transmission, the need for flu shots, or worries about enterovirus."[74] In the same way that American health workers are trying to take advantage of the massive media coverage of the Ebola infections of Nina Pham and Amber Vinson in Dallas, West African health care workers and contact tracers would seek national legislation that provided them with some say in future infectious disease preparedness.

Regardless of the efficacy of these types of legislature initiatives, it would be a mistake to forget about the contributions that were made by Kadiatu Lansana and many other contact tracers. If the 2013–2015 West African outbreak "ended," they played an underappreciated role in making that happen.

NOTES

1. Laurie Garrett, "Ebola's Lessons," *Foreign Affairs*, September/October, 2015, paragraph 22–23, https://www.foreignaffairs.com/articles/west-africa/2015-08-18/ebola-s-lessons?campaign=Garrett.

2. Miatta Zenabu Gbanya, quoted in Garrett, "How the WHO Mishandled the Crisis," paragraph 25.

3. Garrett, "Ebola's Lessons," paragraph 20.

4. Ibid., paragraph 20.

5. Jared Jones, "Ebola, Emerging: The Limitations of Culturalist Discourses in Epidemiology," *Journal of Global Health* 1, no. 1 (Spring, 2011): 1–6, 1.

6. James G. Hodge Jr., Gregory Measer, and Asha M. Agrawal, "'Top Ten' Issues in Public Health Legal Preparedness and Ebola," *American Bar Association Health Resource* 10, no. 3 (November, 2014): paragraph 3, http://www.americanbar.org/publications/aba_health_esource/2014-2015/november/top10.html.

7. Ibid., paragraph 2.

8. See, for example, U.S. Committee on Health, Education, Labor & Pensions Staff, *Joint Full Committee Hearing: Ebola in West Africa: A Global Challenge and Public*

Health Threat, U.S. Committee on Health, Education, Labor & Pensions, September 16, 2014, http://www.help.senate.gov/hearings/ebola-in-west-africa-a-global-challenge-and-public-health-threat.

9. Kent Brantly, quoted by NPR, "Dr. Kent Brantly, "Ebola Survivor Gives Testimony On the Hill," NPR, last modified September 16, 2014, paragraphs 2–3, http://www.npr.org/sections/goatsandsoda/2014/09/16/349012693/dr-kent-brantly-ebola-survivor-gives-testimony-on-the-hill.

10. Ibid., paragraph 4.

11. Ibid., paragraphs 5–6.

12. For a critique of Rudyard Kipling's assumptions, see John A. Stotesbury, "Rudyard Kipling and His Imperial Verse: Critical Dilemmas," *Hungarian Journal of English and American Studies* 1, no. 2 (1995): 37–46.

13. For some intriguing essays on some of heroic figures that populated the geographic imaginaries of so many British and other European imperialists, see David Arnold, *Imperial Medicine and Indigenous Societies* (New York: Manchester University Press, 1988).

14. For a critique of the Mill notion of non-intervention, see Michael W. Doyle, "A Few Words on Mill, Walzer, and Noninterventionism," *Ethics & International Affairs* 23, no. 4 (December, 2009): 349–369.

15. Dana L. Cloud, "The Null Persona: Race and the Rhetoric of Silence in the Uprising of '34," *Rhetoric & Public Affairs* 2, no. 2 (Summer, 1999): 177–209, 177.

16. Philip Wander, "The Third Persona: An Ideological Turn in Rhetorical Theory," *Central States Speech Journal* 35 (1984): 197–216.

17. See, for example, Raymie E. McKerrow, "Space and Time in the Postmodern Polity," *Western Journal of Communication* 63, no. 2 (1999): 271–290.

18. Michel Foucault, "Nietzsche, Genealogy, History," in *The Foucault Reader*, ed. P. Rabinow (Harmondsworth: Penguin, 1984), 87–90. Foucault once explained what he meant by genealogy, and how it differed from more positivistic, essentialist, or foundational ways of viewing medical histories or knowledge:

> And this is what I call genealogy, that is, a form of history which can account for the constitution of knowledges, discourses, domains of objects, etc., without having to make reference to a subject which is either transcendental in relation to a field of events or runs into its sameness throughout the course of history.

Michel Foucault, "Truth and Power," in *Power/Knowledge: Selected Interviews and Other Writings, 1971–1977*, ed. C. Gordon, trans. C. Gordon, L. Marshall, J. Mepham, and K. Soper (Hemel Hemptstead: Harvester Wheatsheaf, 1980), 117. Elsewhere in his discussion of truth effects instead of some static, unalloyed medical "truth" and normality or deviance he talks of the "will to truth." See Michel Foucault, *The History of Sexuality, Vol. 1: The Will to Knowledge*, trans. R. Hurley (London: Penguin, 1998), 79.

19. Garrett, "Ebola's Lessons," paragraph 24.

20. Ibid., paragraph 64.

21. Although contract tracing is not a highly visible job that grabs the headlines of Western mainstream newspapers, knowledgeable public health experts know that this activity is crucial for stopping an Ebola outbreak. Before 2014 most Ebola outbreaks were said to have "burned themselves" out after a few months of

tracking down a few dozen potential EVD victims, but the scope of the problem changes when you are trying to track down suspected patients in three different countries. Moreover, the earlier African Ebola outbreaks, like the 1995 Congo epidemic, happened in rural areas, while the West African governments had to face the panic that came when EVD appeared in urban centers like Monrovia, Liberia.

22. Cláre Ní Chonghaile, "Ebola Effort Needs Another $1 billion Despite Decline in Cases in West Africa, Says U.N.," *The Guardian*, last modified January 22, 2015, paragraph 2, http://www.theguardian.com/global-development/2015/jan/22/ebola-un-funding-1bn-decline-west-africa.

23. Garrett, "Ebola's Lessons," paragraph 64.

24. Michael Bronner, "Treating Ebola: Conversation with Carissa Guild," *Warscapes*, last modified November 10, 2014, paragraph 2, http://www.warscapes.com/conversations/treating-ebola.

25. Ranu S. Dhillon and J. Daniel Kelly, "Community Trust and the Ebola Endgame," *The New England Journal of Medicine* 373 (July, 2015): 787–789.

26. Ibid., 788.

27. David N. Livingstone, "Race, Space and Moral Climatology: Notes toward a Genealogy," *Journal of Historical Geography* 28, no. 2 (2002): 159–180, 162.

28. See, for example, Kent A. Ono and John M. Sloop, "The Critique of Vernacular Discourse," *Communication Monographs* 62 (March, 1995): 19–46. For an example of a critical rhetorical study that studies how contamination metaphors can be used in salient public debates about issues like immigration, see J. David Cisneros, "Contaminated Communities: The Metaphor of "Immigrant as Pollutant" in Media Representations of Immigration," *Rhetoric & Public Affairs* 11, no. 4 (2008): 569–602.

29. Livingstone, "Race, Space and Moral Climatology," 162.

30. Dhillon and Kelly, "Community Trust," 788.

31. Michael Bronner, "Treating Ebola," paragraph 1.

32. Amrai Coen and Malte Henk, "How the Virus Came into the World," *Zeit Online*, last modified November 28, 2014, paragraph 2, http://www.zeit.de/feature/ebola-afrika-virus.

33. Carissa Guild, quoted in Bronner, "Treating Ebola," paragraphs 2–4

34. Ibid., paragraph 25.

35. Ibid., paragraph 25.

36. Ibid., paragraph 33.

37. Daniel Cooney, Vincent Wong, and Yaneer Bar-Yam, *Beyond Contract Tracing: Community-Based Early Detection for Ebola Response* (Cambridge: New England Complex Systems Institute, 2015), 2. One of the purposes of the Cooney, Wong, and Bar-Yam study on contact tracing is to argue that the difficulties associated with this approach should lead others to consider more "community-based monitoring" and limiting travel so that you can reduce "inter-community contagion" (p. 2).

38. Carissa Guild, quoted in Bronner, "Treating Ebola," paragraphs 33–34.

39. Ibid., paragraphs 33–43.

40. Coen and Henk, "How the Virus Came into the World," paragraph 83.

41. Kai Kupferschmidt, "On the Trail of Contagion," *Science* 347, I6218 (January 9, 2015): 120–121, 120.

42. Daniel Cooney, Vincent Wong, and Yaneer Bar-Yam, *Beyond Contract Tracing*, 2.

43. Titilola T. Obilade, "The Political Economy of the Ebola Virus Disease (EVD); Taking Individual and Community Ownership in the Prevention and Control of EVD," *Healthcare* 3 (2015): 36–49, 37.

44. Alexander S. Kekulé, "Learning from Ebola Virus: How to Prevent Future Epidemics," *Viruses* 7 (2015): 3789–3797, 3790–3791.

45. Hans Rosling, quoted in Garrett, "Ebola's Lessons," paragraph 50.

46. See, for example, Centers for Disease Control, "Facts about Bushmeat and Ebola," CDC, [September, 2014], http://www.cdc.gov/vhf/ebola/pdf/bushmeat-and-ebola.pdf; Melissa Hogenboom, "Ebola: Is Bushmeat behind the Outbreak?" BBC, last modified October 19, 2014, http://www.bbc.com/news/health-29604204.

47. CDC, "Questions and Answers: Estimating the Future Numbers of Cases in the Ebola Epidemic—Liberia and Sierra Leone," CDC, last modified November 19, 2014, http://www.cdc.gov/vhf/ebola/outbreaks/2014-west-africa/qa-mmwr-estimating-future-cases.html.

48. Kekulé, "Learning from Ebola Virus," 3793.

49. Arlene C. Chua et al., "The Case for Improved Diagnostic Tools To Control Ebola Virus Disease in West Africa and How to Get There," *PLOS Neglected Tropical Diseases* (June 11, 2015): 1–6.

50. *Al Jazeera*, "Liberian Nurses Threaten Strike over Ebola Pay," *Al Jazeera*, last modified October 12, 2014, paragraphs 1–2, http://www.al-jazeera.com/news/africa/2014/10/liberia-nurses-threaten-strike-over-ebola-pay-20141012134754218261.html.

51. Tolbert Nyenswah, quoted in *Al Jazeera*, "Liberian Nurses Threaten Strike," paragraph 7.

52. *Al Jazeera*, "Liberian Nurses Threaten Strike," paragraph 8.

53. *Al Jazeera*, "Strike over Ebola Pay Hits Liberia Hospitals," *Al Jazeera*, last modified October 13, 2014, http://www.aljazeera.com/news/africa/2014/10/strike-over-ebola-pay-hits-liberia-hospitals-20141013135015206664.html.

54. BBC News, "Ebola Crisis: Sierra Leone Health Workers Strike, BBC News, last modified November 12, http://www.bbc.com/news/world-africa-30019895.

55. Kupferschmidt, "On the Trail of Contagion,"121.

56. Adam Bjork, quoted in Jon Cohen, "Exit Interview: CDC Epidemiologist Sees Hope for Controlling Ebola in Southeastern Liberia," *Science*, last modified October 8, 2014, paragraphs 2–3, http://news.sciencemag.org/africa/2014/10/exit-interview-cdc-epidemiologist-sees-hope-controlling-ebola-southeastern-liberia.

57. Cohen, "Exit Interview," paragraph 6.

58. Bjork, quoted in Cohen, "Exit Interview," paragraph 11.

59. Ibid., paragraph 12.

60. Laurie Garrett, "Liberia Is Stiffing Its Contact Tracers as Ebola Epidemic Continues," *Foreign Policy*, November 11, 2014, paragraph 1, http://foreignpolicy.com/2014/11/11/liberia-is-stiffing-its-contact-tracers-as-ebola-epidemic-continues/.

61. Ibid., paragraph 3.

62. Ibid., paragraph 5.

63. Ibid., paragraph 6.

64. Obilade, "The Political Economy," 44.

65. John Kirby, quoted in Ralph Ellis, "U.S. Bringing Home Almost All Troops Sent to Africa in Ebola Crisis," CNN.com, last modified February 27, 2015, http://www.cnn.com/2015/02/10/us/ebola-u-s-troops-africa/.

66. Kupferschmidt, "On the Trail of Contagion," 120.

67. Ibid., 121.

68. For general overviews of the role that contact tracers play in trying to detect and stop the spread of EVD, see Cooney, Wong, and Bar-Yam, *Beyond Contact Tracing*; Associated Press, "Ebola Outbreak: Sierra Leone Officials Going Door to Door," CBS News, last modified December 17, 2014, http://www.cbsnews.com/news/ebola-outbreak-sierra-leone-officials-going-door-to-door; World Health Organization, "Liberia Succeeds in Fighting Ebola with Local, Sector response," *WHO*, April 2015, http://who.int/features/2015/ebola-sector-approach/en/.

69. Chua et al., "The Case for Improved Diagnostic Tools," 2. See Almea Matonock et al., "Ebola Virus Diseases among Health Care Workers Not Working in Ebola Treatment Units-Liberia, June-August, 2014," *Morbidity and Mortality Weekly* 634 (46) (November 21, 2014): 1077–1081; World Health Organization, "Interim Infection Prevention and Control Guidance for Care of Patients with Suspected or Confirmed Filovirus Haemorrhagic Fever in Health-Care Settings, with Focus on Ebola," *WHO*, December, 2014, http://apps.who.int/iris/bitstream/10665/130596/1/WHO_HIS_SDS_2014.4_eng.pdf?ua=1&ua=1&ua=1.

70. Tom Frieden, "Rapid Detection and Response Are Essential to Stopping Ebola," *The Huffington Post*, last modified February 18, 2015, http://www.huffingtonpost.com/tom-frieden-md-mph/rapid-detection-and-respo_b_6705258.html.

71. Daniel Cooney, Vincent Wong, and Yaneer Bar-Yam, *Beyond Contract Tracing*, 2.

72. For a critique of this supposed exotic behavior, and the problematic nature of prepackaged, universalist Western messages that are not tailored to the needs of communities living in Guinea, Liberia, or Sierra Leone, see Clare Chandler et al., "Ebola: Limitations of Correcting Misinformation," *The Lancet* 384 (April 4, 2015): 1275–1276, 1275.

73. See *GovTrack Insider*, "H.R. 483 (113th Congress): National Nurse Act of 2013," *GovTrack Insider*, n.d., https://www.govtrack.us/congress/bills/113/hr485. This was legislation sponsored by Representative Eddie Johnson that was introduced on February 4, 2013, in a previous sessions of Congress, that was not enacted.

74. Theresa Brown, "Ebola Will Elevate Respect for Nurses," CNN.com, last modified October 23, 2014, paragraph 11, http://www.cnn.com/2014/10/23/opinion/brown-ebola-nurses/.

4

The Saga of Kaci Hickox and the Nature, Scope, and Limits of Human Rights Discourses in Ebola Contexts

For decades, in many Anglo-American or continental law school classes or bioethics seminars, when faculty or students wanted to discuss the clash that sometimes existed between the individual rights principles and extensive state powers of Western communities they often used case studies that focused on periods of declared national emergencies or public necessities. Instructors would often refer to one or several canonical cases that tested the sentimentality of those who are supposed to be guided by objective legal science and not develop answers that were based on their own emotive, knee-jerk, subjective reactions to what are often called "hard cases." For example, professors could point to the old 1920s' eugenical rhetorics that were exemplified by the jurisprudential work of Oliver Wendell Holmes Jr., a jurist who believed in the importance of expansive state powers in order to reduce the numbers of "feebleminded" who lived in America. This famous (or infamous) Civil War veteran commented on precedential nature of the conscription powers of states that allowed for the use of bayonets if need be to get troops to the front during wartime,[1] and he juxtaposed that awesome federal power with the supposedly lesser power that the state of Virginia possessed when it sought to sterilize problematic individuals like Carrie Buck.[2] In another seminal case the Irish immigrant Mary Mallon, stigmatized as the asymptomatic "carrier" known as "Typhoid Mary" by the American presses, appeared in countless classrooms and academic discussions about the nexus that existed between bacteriological theory, stigma, individual recalcitrance, and state powers during times of epidemics.[3]

In this particular chapter I am inviting readers to temporarily shift their gaze away from West African lands and *dispositifs* so that we can see how Anglo-American communities talked and wrote about the balancing of rights and interests once Ebola traveled to Western shores. As I argue in more detail below, many legal commentators in the United States or the United Kingdom did not mind defending positions that allowed for quarantining, cordons, or travel restrictions overseas, but not everyone was comfortable with imposing those same restrictions when they were discussed in American or European contexts.

From a critical legal vantage point, the advent of talk of "emerging" infectious diseases has complicated the ways that we think of those formalistic or positivist balancing texts.[4] Learning the conventional "rules of law" principles in these situations often allows us to see the forms and contours of the typical arguments that are used in public health contexts, but this type of formalistic pedagogy does not help us that much when critical scholars try to get at the motivations of those who have to fill in those argumentative forms with *substantive, ideological, and cultural materials*. As Kit Yee Chan and Daniel Redipath noted in 2003, oftentimes the types of stories that were told about infectious disease carriers assumed that the construction of disease risk involved matters of scientific misunderstanding and not contestation. Confronting EVD became some "knowable, calculable and preventable" problem in dominant social science and public health discourses, and professionals granted awesome state powers wanted to make sure that threatening humans understood their individual responsibilities in dangerous situations. This, Chan and Redipath argued, highlighted the professional responsibility of those who were supposed to manage these diseased carriers, but it often hid the "socio-structure" origins of some of these high-risk behaviors.[5] All citizens, and not just doctors, nurses, lawyers and judges, need to be agonizing over the questions of how best to deal with everything from mandatory quarantining to individual health inspections when they confront infectious disease contexts.

In this particular chapter, I provide readers with critical investigations of the legal and cultural rhetorics that have been used in heated contests about what to do with Ebola "travelers."[6] More specifically, I use the critical interrogation of materials from judicial trials and press coverage of a nurse by the name of Kaci Hickox as an entrée point for discussing the ideological and cultural nature of the answers that are given by various Western social agents who are asked to respond to these questions:

- Given the horrific nature of EVD, doesn't it make sense that U.S. federal and state public health officials apply the "precautionary" principle and demand the mandatory quarantining of all returning travelers from Ebola ravaged regions?

- With all of the scientific uncertainty, fear, and anxiety that swirls around Ebola, can U.S. or U.K. officials really trust nurses and doctors to "self-monitor" in ways that privilege their alleged "civil rights"?
- In situations where elite executive, legislative, and judicial social agents *disagree* about how to balance individual rights with compelling state interests during times of emergency, who should be the "deciders" in Ebola outbreak contexts?
- What are policy makers and empowered health officials at federal and state levels supposed to do in situations where hegemonic communities are demanding that draconian actions be taken that are not allegedly supported by the Ebola "science" that is circulated by elite organizations like the CDC or Doctors Without Borders?
- Are there times when an entire "class" of people—in this case doctors and nurses returning from West Africa—can be deprived of liberty for twenty-one days in the name of public health necessities?
- Who decides whether the state or federal quarantining of an asymptomatic individual can be labeled as "arbitrary, oppressive, and unreasonable"?

These are difficult questions that have no ready answers, even in situations where communities were dealing with rhetorical situations where only a few Ebola patients walked through U.S. hospital doors in 2014.

During the fall of 2014 another important legal or bioethical "precedent" would be set that would trigger these types of queries when a Maine nurse, Kaci Hickox, became the first public test case for a mandatory Ebola quarantine in the United States.[7] Hickox had spent some time working in West Africa, and she had helped with the treatment of West African Ebola patients. The mass-mediate coverage of her "heroism," as well as her alleged abuse at the hands of several governors, created conundrums for elite and public audiences who felt that she should have been thanked for her courage and sacrifices. Instead, Kaci Hickox walked into a prefigured world where for weeks American audiences were bombarded with warnings about the dangers that confronted Western populations when Ebola contagion "might" be spread by travelers who landed on U.S., U.K., or Spanish shores. Both the horrific nature of Ebola, and the rarity of its appearance in the United States, became factors that impacted Hickox's reception when she landed in New Jersey.

Luck would have it that Hickox, a former Doctors Without Borders nurse, was landing at a Newark airport *the day after* the state of New Jersey instituted its new policy of mandatory quarantine.[8] She would be detained for seven hours at the Newark airport after returning from Sierra Leone, and she was then placed in an isolation tent.[9] For the next several weeks mesmerized audiences watched and listened as journalists reported on how she quarreled with public health officials in New Jersey and Maine about the proper steps that should be followed before quarantining those who returned from West Africa. Americans got to listen in as her friend, Ted Wibur, explained that New Jersey governor Chris Christie had "messed with the wrong redhead."[10]

In the same way that Carrie Buck would become an iconic figure in eugenical *dispositifs,* and Mary Mallon's ghostly presence haunted those who wanted to stigmatize asymptomatic "diseased" carriers, Hickox would come to symbolize those knowledgeable, and yet combative health workers who refused to bow down to the will of the state. In Ebola contexts micro-arguments about personalities became entangled in broader public and legal debates about the nature, scope, and limits of state powers during exigent times.

Even before Hickox garnered public attention in America, there had had been hints that ideological fights like these were brewing. Months earlier, populations in Sierra Leone, Liberia, and Guinea were hearing similar arguments about restrictions on travel that came from neighboring African nations. Yet Kaci Hickox saw her conflict through narrower lens, and by late 2014 and early 2015 she was acting as a spokesperson for the rights of returning U.S. public health care workers.

The advent of the Hickox cases in New Jersey and New York contexts meant that legal and scientific fragments in these Ebola *dispositifs* were configured and reconfigured as her supporters and her detractors talked and wrote about the wisdom, and the constitutional legality, of allowing her to "self-monitor" herself so that she would not have to suffer because of the coercive powers of several states. The mass-mediate coverage of Kaci Hickox's trials and tribulations was also coming along during a period when the White House and some states were having heated disagreements about federalism, the nature of Ebola transmission, and the legality of mandatory quarantines, and these debates had everything to do with conflicting Ebola *epistemes,* competing neoliberal ideologies, institutional powers, and the rhetorical status of the arguers. This was not going to be a situation where lawyers and judges simply used formalistic, deductive balancing of rights and interests to "settle" matters by finding the right legal formula. The lawyers and judges involved in this Ebola disputation circulated competing interpretations of constitutional law and administrative health regulations as they verbally sparred over the meaning and significance of the legal histories that covered quarantining in America. Many participants soon discovered that the archives were filled with competing and contradictory images of the legality of all types of quarantining, that were influenced by a host of cultural and ethnic perceptions regarding the dangers that were posed by the "other" who allegedly needed quarantining.

Hickox did not mention these conflictual histories, but she eventually did have to hire lawyers who had to cope with the residual traces of these quarantine contests. Her lawyers used all types of positivist and formalistic reasoning as they critiqued the decisionism of a few governors and state public health authorities who tried to control Hickox's behavior and mobility. However, it was often the journalistic commentary, and the public wrangling about Ebola epidemiology, stigma, selfishness, and so on, that influenced the trajectory of this disputation. At times it appeared as though Hickox tried to magnify her own social agency as she talked about how much she knew about Ebola and how little the governors knew about infectious diseases, but in many ways her positions simply reflected and refracted *select* cultural and scientific *dispositifs* that had been circulating in U.S. venues for generations.

This would not be the first, nor the last time, that ideological arguments, cultural expectations, and societal views regarding restrictive public health measures would influence the interpretations of both the epidemiological and the legal features of these rhetorical situations. Eugenia Tognotti, writing in *Emerging Infectious Diseases*, explained how conflicting views regarding the spreading of disease—through water, air, personal, contact, and so forth—impacted how a region or a nation might accept or reject particular quarantining or cordoning measures. Tognotti outlined some of this polysemy in 2013 when she noted that

> the cultural and social context differed from that in previous centuries. For example, the increasing use of quarantine and isolation conflicted with the affirmation of citizens' rights and growing sentiments of personal freedom fostered by the French Revolution of 1789. In England, liberal reformers contested both quarantine and compulsory vaccination against smallpox. Social and political tensions created an explosive mixture, culminating in popular rebellions and uprisings, a phenomenon that affected numerous European countries. In the Italian states, in which revolutionary groups had taken the cause of unification and republicanism, cholera epidemics provided a justification (i.e., the enforcement of sanitary measures) for increasing police power.[11]

Would America, the land of liberty, have citizens who refused to allow governors to take away Hickox's freedoms? Or would the United States also call for increased police powers?

Interestingly enough, although Hickox's lawyers talked to the press about her due process rights and other criminal or tort topics, she herself often tried to characterize her confinement as a battle between scientific enlightenment and scientific illiteracy. One detects some smugness and *jouissance* as she waged running battles with governors and public health officials over how to treat traveling doctors and nurses. She constantly argued that those who knew anything about Ebola would accept her interpretation of the self-monitoring program that was once put in place by the U.S. Centers for Disease Control and Prevention (CDC).[12]

Many observers who tuned in to the mediated coverage of these events seemed to be shocked by Hickox's brazenness, and her unwillingness to listen to the supposedly sage advice that was coming from others who supported the governors of New Jersey or Maine. When she wouldn't budge, this led to a polarization of Anglo-American public opinion and it pitted those who wanted to quarantine only those who showed signs of having Ebola symbols against those who wanted to quarantine *anyone* who came back home after working with Ebola patients.[13] "I was terrified of the people who were trying to take my rights and what they would do to other healthcare workers," Hickox later argued, and she worried that "they were not held accountable for their actions."[14]

Many of Hickox's defenders would later contend that those who quarantined her did so in the name of "politics" instead of "science."[15] However, I share Professor Sara Bergstresser's opinion that these galvanizing cases involved more than just legal cautionary tales that make us choose between utopian discussions of the primacy of civil rights or dystopic calls for more police state power to enforce restrictive, and mandatory, quarantines. As Professor Bergstresser eloquently explained,

> The polarizing discourse surrounding Ms. Hickox and her case exemplifies the damaging dynamic of mistrust in health and scientific institutions that pervades the United States. Those who champion her case as a fight for rationality present the image of a valiant and heroic victim of injustice. On the other hand, many general public perceptions focus on an image of someone who appears flagrantly unconcerned for the health and safety of her neighbors. This dichotomization has spawned a larger political discourse that imagines the case as a parable of risk and insecurity versus civil rights and rationality, with a pervasive focus on scolding and blame. All of these narratives are caricatures.[16]

These may have been caricatures, but they were also persuasive *dispositifs* that provided us with perceptual clues regarding how American elites and publics wanted to deal with future "emerging" disease contexts.

By the time that readers reach the end of this chapter, I hope that they will see that the Kaci Hickox cases involved the circulation of ambiguous and equivocal materials that provided support for *multiple scientific interpretations*.[17] Moreover, during these heated legal and cultural debates journalists would themselves become participants in this disputation as they talked or wrote about how quarantine precedents supported either Hickox's or the states' cases. This would be another example of a situation that supported Michel Foucault's claims regarding the contested nature of epidemic knowledge in health contexts.[18]

A critical legal rhetorical approach to Hickox's cases reveals how she became a potent mass-mediated condensation symbol for myriad Ebola fears and anxieties. More than a few observers who watched the media coverage of Kaci Hickox's struggles were convinced that both governor Chris Christie of New Jersey and governor Andrew Cuomo of New York were trying to curry favor with worried citizens during election time as they announced the quarantining of those who returned from helping fight Ebola in Guinea, Liberia, and Sierra Leone, and Hickox was credited by some for seeing through this politicizing of Ebola. "Hickox," noted one legal scholar, "sounded more like a seasoned politico than a nurse," and this researcher quipped that the New Jersey governor seemed to be acting out of an "abundance of politics" instead of an abundance of caution.[19]

Did Hickox's cases resolve these situations in ways that would provide lessons for future health workers who travel abroad during Ebola crises? Did the mass-mediate commentaries about her situation provide us with any hints of how empowered American communities were willing to argue about the limits of the coercive powers of the state? Did the circulation of CDC texts about Ebola transmission influence the reception of Hickox's own commentaries?

In order to help answer those types of questions, I want to begin by providing a brief critical analysis of some early American quarantining cases before I look at the ideological positions of those who supported New Jersey's quarantining efforts.

A BRIEF GENEALOGICAL OVERVIEW OF SOME AMERICAN QUARANTINE HISTORIES

As soon as the case of Kaci Hickox was carried in mainstream newspaper outlets and discussed in the blogosphere academics, lawyers, and others went rummaging through the public health archives to find historical examples that might support their ideological positions on the question of whether the state could force her to submit to mandatory quarantines.[20] As Eugene Kontorovich explained,

> While the Supreme Court has long held quarantines to be constitutional, it has not ruled directly on the scope of permissible quarantines. However, in the famous case of *Jacobson v. Massachusetts*, the Court did uphold a blanket mandatory vaccination law, under which resisters were put in jail. The principle here is the same as with quarantine—that one's normal rights to bodily integrity are suspended by a general and serious public need, especially of

an epidemiological variety. Still, in part because quarantines have rarely been imposed since World War II, there is relatively little direct precedent on their permissible scope and circumstances.[21]

Professor Kontorovich, using a blend of "policy" and formalistic types of argumentation, went on to tell readers of *The Washington Post* that most twentieth-century cases had to do with the deaths of those who succumbed to tuberculosis and smallpox, diseases that he characterized as less lethal than Ebola. Citing the examples of conscription, quarantine, and jury duty, he argued that there were just a few times when the state could deprive someone of their liberties *without any showing of problems with personal conduct or any criminal wrongdoing.* He was convinced that his "brief review of the cases" illustrated how Hickox or the ACLU were going to have a difficult time challenging this state power "without a clear showing of medical unreasonableness, or discriminatory application."[22] While Kontorovich could find some successful challenges to the *conditions* that became a part of quarantines he could not find any cases where a quarantine had been lifted on the basis of due process violations.

For those who are looking for historical analogies that might be used to justify the positions of advocates who wanted to make sure that Hickox had to obey the laws of states like New Jersey, they could always cite the 1963 case of *U.S. ex rel Siegel v. Shinnick*,[23] that was decided in the Eastern District of New York. In that particular case the plaintiff was complaining about how the state was trying to confine her after her return from a "smallpox infected area" abroad, in spite of the fact that there was little evidence of her having any direct exposure or symptoms. The court in that case upheld the state quarantining, noting,

> [The] judgment required is that of a public health officer and not of a lawyer used to insist on positive evidence to support action; their task is to measure risk to the public and to seek for what can reassure and, not finding it, to proceed reasonably to make the public health secure. They deal in a terrible context and the consequences of mistaken indulgence can be irretrievably tragic. To supercede their judgment there must be a reliable showing of error.[24]

Doesn't this look like a variant of the cultural fragment that I have been commenting on since chapter 1, having to do with applications of that vaunted "precautionary" principle?

Even if jurists don't use some variant of the precautionary principle in their discussion of quarantining, the deck is often stacked against those individuals who come to courts complaining about false imprisonment as they seek damages for alleged uncivil behavior. Take the case of Mary Craton who in 1911 was bothered by the fact that New York health officials were quarantining her for fifteen days because she lived in a house that was close to someone who contracted smallpox.[25]

In sum, the common conventional legal wisdom seemed to be that as long as public health officials provided some reasonable, health-related rationalization for quarantining or other isolation practices that are imposed during epidemics, then it looked as though many jurists would uphold state restrictions. In theory, they would use formalistic arguments about how they did not want to become "judicial activists" and how they would not second-guess the opinions of public health elites. From an argumentative standpoint the burden of proof would be placed on plaintiffs in civil cases, and defendants in criminal cases, to show that there is no rational scientific basis for making the decision that was reached by the quarantining official. All of this hides the power relationships, and the cultural dynamics of this historical decisionism.

This, as readers might imagine, is easier said than done. If we return to Hickox's case one might be wondering just why New Jersey was in such a hurry to change their quarantine laws, and why were these laws were changed just before she came back from Sierra Leone?

Some of these legal changes were probably triggered when authorities were having to deal with an earlier Ebola case that came to the attention of public health officials and jurists when Craig Spencer, a New York doctor, contracted Ebola. Spencer's mass-mediated journey began when he entered the country through JFK International Airport on October 17, 2014.[26] At first this affable and bright doctor—who also worked for Doctors Without Borders—looked like the poster child for "self-quarantining," an example of how the self-reporting of fevers aid in the containment of EVD. He became the darling of many nurses and doctors who treated him, and he was supposed to have been self-quarantined in his Harlem apartment. The idea here was that if he behaved, then he could avoid having to deal with the coercive powers of New York.

However, within a matter of days after Spencer started all of this self-quarantining, countless media outlets carried stories of his alleged misbehavior, and they followed him and reported on how Spencer was traveling in subways or was seen in bowling alleys in Brooklyn. Investigators who were supposed to keep tabs on his activities only learned of his transgressions after they tracked down his subway pass and his credit card receipts. One U.K. commenter, who sent in a response to an English newspaper article on Spencer, remarked that "instead of Typhoid Mary" we "now have Ebola Craig." This "insider" complained that now millions of dollars were going to have to be spent because of "his self-righteous smugness."[27] Once again the personal had become political.

From a critical legal vantage point a populist metanarrative was crafted in Anglo-American circles *before* Hickox ever set foot in that Newark airport. Readers had been debating about the need for their states and other institutions to respond to these supposedly lax public health standards, and the convergence of worries about West African mortality rates and tales of self-righteous American individuals made for a perfect storm.

HEIGHTENED AMERICAN FEARS
OF EBOLA AND THE ARGUMENTATIVE
SUPPORT FOR NEW JERSEY'S MANDATORY
QUARANTINING OF KACI HICKOX

As noted above, Hickox perhaps first entered these mediascapes when she landed at Newark Liberty International Airport, and all of this started with something that by now was fairly routine—a forehead scan. On that particular late October day, Hickox's forehead scan seemed to indicate that she had a temperature of 101. Hickox later explained to reporters that she had been upset and flushed when her temperature was being taken, and that a later reading with an oral thermometer showed that she actually recorded a normal temperature, 98.6.[28] Ironically, some of the very same instrumentalities, and Ebola calculus, that had become a part of her life overseas were now being transported and (re)used by empowered American authorities to rationalize Hickox's isolation and confinement.

Government officials for the state of New Jersey disagreed with Hickox's personal assessment of her condition, and she was photographed and interviewed while she was quarantined in a tent outside of one of the New Jersey hospitals.[29] Each day a member of some New Jersey medical staff would come to her tent and they would take her vital signs, and every six hours they would clean the portable toilet that had been placed in her tent.

Sometimes these New Jersey staff members avoiding having to go through the same daily routine by asking Hickox to take her own temperature, blood pressure, and heart rate. She apparently took some solace from the fact that she held on to a cell phone, and this meant that she could contact lawyers. Two of them, Norman Siegel and Steven Hyman, eventually insisted that they meet with her while she was quarantined in the tent, and journalists followed them as they talked through the plastic window one Sunday evening.[30] Subsequent blood tests also found no sign of the Ebola virus in Hickox's system.[31] Would all of this mean that the Ebola "science," or the "rule of law," supported Hickox's position?

This, of course, often depends on who has the power and who gets to interpret that raw data and who gets to interpret the motives of those who put her in that tent. At the same time, those "active monitoring" state rules can be contested, and like many individuals who become celebrities, Kaci Hickox found a way of using modern technology and social media outlets to let the world know about her plight. On October 25, 2014, a story that she wrote appeared in *The Dallas Morning News*. It was titled "Her Story: UTA Grad Isolated at New Jersey Hospital in Ebola Quarantine."[32]

The resonance of these personal self-interest stories, as well as the circulation of photographs showing Hickox in the tent, created a rhetorical situation where the governor of New Jersey had to defend his state's quarantine law as well as its specific application in this particular case. In a rambling, and perhaps incoherent statement, Governor Christie explained the rationale behind his action: "If people are symptomatic they go into the hospital. If they live in New Jersey, they get quarantined at home. If they don't, and they're not symptomatic, then we set up quarantine for them outside of state. But if they are symptomatic, they're going to the hospital."[33] Regardless of her health status, it seemed the state was in biopolitical control of Hickox.

Perhaps the governor's Kafkaesque statement was meant to cover all of the hypothetical scientific bases, but it may have produced more heat than light. Was the New Jersey governor talking about *voluntary decisions* to go to hospitals or homes, or was he talking about using mandatory state powers to force the hospitalization of Ebola suspects? Was New Jersey going to pay for the quarantining that might take place *outside* of that state, and which social agents did the setting up of the quarantines? What "they" is the governor referencing? Was he talking about quarantining all returning doctors and nurses from West Africa, or just those whose temperatures rose to a particular level?

To be fair to Governor Christie, before he arranged for Kaci Hickox to be placed in a tent without a shower or a TV, Hickox had been tested by the CDC and some medical officials had given her an Ebola test. That was an expensive test, Christie reasoned, so there must have been some specific reason why medical elites thought she might be symptomatic as well. As far as Christie was concerned, if Hickox had been inconvenienced by his actions, in the same way that those who are late for planes get angry, then so be it. She was supposed to understand that public officials had their own obligations, including the protection of New Jersey publics.

For at least four days Hickox's every move was scrutinized as countless newspapers and television programs asked viewers to weigh in and given their opinions on whether an "asymptomatic" individual, who tested negative for Ebola, could nevertheless be quarantined involuntarily in the name of public necessities. Famous leaders, like UN Secretary-General Ki-Moon, warned against any "unnecessary" restrictions on health care workers, and he argued that their efforts were key in trying to stop the spread of EVD in West Africa. "They are extraordinary people who are giving of themselves," and "they are risking their own lives," he told members of the press in Vienna.[34] This type of consequentialist argument implied that Hickox had become a potent signifier, who was fighting the rights of those who joined Doctors Without Borders or other organizations in the name of medical humanitarianism.

Make no mistake, Governor Christie had plenty of supporters, in the United States and elsewhere, but several pundits were intrigued by the combativeness of this "liberal" nurse who had the temerity to criticize Governor Christie's quarantine policies at the same time that she hired a legal team.

As readers might imagine, many public officials, legal scholars, bioethicists, and others around the world who were interested in what lawyers call "hard cases," or "penumbral," cases where fascinated by what looked like an American extension of the earlier transcontinental debates that had taken place when West African nations imposed their own cordons and quarantines. Now that Ebola, and the fear of Ebola, had migrated to America, would their governmental officials, health experts, and populations react in a similar fashion when they faced challenges from someone like Kaci Hickox?

Governors across the United States stayed in contact with each other, and public health officials in places like Dallas, New York, and Newark rationalized their own potential imposition of quarantines and related measures. Governor Christie, for example, when he released Hickox, tried to show that his policy was not as onerous as everyone thought. Christie reasoned that while Hickox was living in that tent, she did not show symptoms for twenty-four hours, and that this was why she was allowed to make plans to return to her home in Maine. During that same interview Christie then added more controversial commentary:

> And she tested negative for Ebola. So there was no reason to keep her. The reason she was put in the hospital in the first place was because she was running a high fever and was symptomatic.[35]

New Jersey's governor was perhaps trying to show that he was familiar with Ebola terminology.

Some of Christie's statements set off a firestorm of protests as nurses, public health workers, and doctors opined that a powerful politician did not seem to understand what "symptomatic" even meant. Elite science writers and others who tracked the Hickox case argued that state governors and their subordinates seemed to be making decisions that were based on some vague notion of public health "common sense." Governor Christie often admitted during press conferences that he was not a doctor, but he perhaps had a good grasp of what many of his own constituents wanted him to do in the name of communal interests.

Governor Paul R. LePage of Maine, perhaps realizing that he needed to get ready for the media spotlight that was coming his way when Hickox returned home, remarked that he was aware of the good work that health workers were doing in Africa. However, he went on to note that he also had to keep in mind the fact that officials in his state "must be vigilant in our duty to protect the health and safety of all Mainers, as well as anyone who may come in contact with someone who has been exposed to Ebola."[36] These types of populist statements made it appear as though Maine's governor was balancing individual civil liberties with state public necessities.

Hickox would later travel in a black SUV to her home in Fort Kent, Maine, but before she left that New Jersey tent, folks in her hometown were interviewed about how they felt about her return. The town that she lived in, after all, was very small, and it only had one hospital, and one of the residents explained that if "anyone has any type of emergency, that's where they'll go."[37] It was clear that although some in her home town would thank her for her services abroad, that did not mean that they didn't have to worry about her living in their midst. The State of Maine was eventually going to ask for a type of quarantine that would require Hickox to stay at least three feet away from any non-exposed person.[38]

When she was released by the officials in New Jersey and allowed to return to home state of Maine, would the reception be any warmer?

KACI HICKOX'S LEGAL AND PUBLIC BATTLES WITH MAINE OFFICIALS AND THE GROWING INTEREST IN HER "SCIENCE" AND HER LIBERTIES

When Kaci Hickox arrived in Maine she indicated that she was thankful to be home, but she later explained that this sense of euphoria was quickly dashed when the director of the Maine's CDC explained to her that "Maine was requiring home quarantines for all healthcare workers returning from Ebola-affected areas, regardless of their health status or exposure assessment."[39] Given the legal precedents that I mentioned above, and the American legal histories on quarantines, it should not surprise readers that there were probably no shortage of Maine, New England, or American legal cases that could be cited to justify this treatment of even asymptomatic individuals.

The Maine Department of Health and Human Service's Center for Disease Control and Prevention announced that its policy would be that those who were returning would have to be quarantined for the traditional twenty-one-day observation period.[40] Maine officials told the press, even before Hickox's return, that they hoped that these policies would be agreed upon when Ms. Hickox returned from New Jersey. Hickox later implied that it was not coincidental that the Maine CDC protocol was dated October 27, the very day she had arrived in the state.[41]

As many critical legal scholars have pointed out, law often involves performances and a host of visual displays,[42] and after Hickox and her partner arrived home, they woke up to find a state trooper's vehicle parked across the street from their home.[43] The state trooper, according to Maine's Governor LePage, was there for Hickox's own protection.[44] Others were convinced that the state troopers were there to remind Hickox of the inherent power of the state during potential emergencies.

While some states, in the name of public safety, health, and welfare allow a health official to enact mandatory quarantines through the publication of a public health order, Maine was one of those other states that required more than that. Maine required a court order before anyone could take that type of action. As soon as Hickox and her partner planned a bike ride, this seemed to have forced the hand of Maine's Department of Health and Human Services. While police cruisers followed the biking couple, other Maine civil servants petitioned for a court order to try and enforce Hickox's home quarantine.[45]

Once again the media spotlight put on display the ways that Hickox, and her supporters, were trying to use the court of public opinion to prepare for the seemingly inevitable courtroom clashes that were about to occur. Maine's Department of Health and Human Services was able to obtain a temporary court order for her home quarantine, but Hickox's legal team—which included Norman Siegel, Steve Hyman, and her local counsel, David Soley—were able to challenge the temporary order on the ground that she was not a public health threat.[46] On October 31, 2014, Judge Charles LaVerdiere, the chief judge of the Maine District Court, reversed his temporary order, and journalists reported that he found that Hickox "currently does not show symptoms of Ebola and is therefore not infectious."[47] *Slate*'s Josh Voorhees said that this was "more or less the argument that the public health community and the White House had been making for weeks."[48]

Judge LaVerdiere's ruling was hailed by many as a great victory of civil libertarians, but a closer, more critical reading of his texts shows that he was not directly challenging the state of Maine's imposition of mandatory quarantines. Nor was Judge LaVerdiere implying that Hickox, on her own, could unilaterally decide whether or not she would comply with other state procedures. For example, his order indicated that Hickox had to submit to daily monitoring for Ebola symptoms, and she did have to tell state public health officials about any plans that she might have for interstate travel.

Judge LaVerdiere did, however, side with those who worried that irrational fears were motivating the push for more restrictive quarantines in Ebola contexts. He ruled that given the importance of Hickox's due process rights, the state had the burden of showing that she was a public health threat, and it was his opinion that they had not met that burden. Judge LaVerdiere opined that Maine had not provided clear and convincing evidence that limiting Hickox's movements through home quarantine was "necessary" to protect other individuals "from the dangers of infection."[49] While LaVerdiere ordered that Hickox had to continue to follow some direct, active monitoring protocols, he commented on some of the speculation that he believed was fueling these petitions. He noted that "the court is fully aware of the misconceptions, misinformation, bad science and bad information being spread from shore to shore in our country with respect to Ebola," and he asked that Hickox keep in mind that people were fearful.[50] *The New York Times* reported that within hours of Judge LaVerdiere's decision, the state troopers were no longer parking outside of the nurse's home.[51]

Hickox tried to frame LaVerdiere's decision as a damaging and decisive judicial critique of Maine's CDC policies, and she told NBC's *Meet the Press* that this showed that "all the scientific, medical, and public health community agree with me, and I'm really glad that the judge also agreed."[52] This homogenization of all of "science" or "public health" hid the contested nature of much of this Ebola disputation in American contexts.

Hickox may have publicly argued that the "public health community" was solidly behind her, but she may have also sensed that many Americans disagreed with her interpretations of Ebola pathogenesis and the limits that needed to be placed on the powers of state officials. She would later write that in spite of the available medical science and normative public health principles that were out there, she was afraid that "most Americans do not understand the rigorous scientific and legal model that should be applied when considering a public health action as extreme as quarantine."[53] Here one finds no detailed critique of the earlier smallpox and other cases that had allowed for state quarantines without those "rigorous" models that she was referencing. In myriad ways, she seemed to be implying that progressives like herself, by traveling overseas to fight Ebola, had gained a type of frontline situational awareness that others could not appreciate.

This monolithic way of conceptualizing both science and law, that assumed that there was one right method or one right answer that came from applying those methods, ironically created a type of essentialist Ebola commentary that was as dogmatic as some of the critiques that she was trying to interrogate.

Hickox may have been confident there were some rigorous scientific and legalistic models out there that would operate in predictable fashions in order to protect her rights, but many other social agents were not so sure. In many ways the evolutionary nature of her confrontations with the governors of New Jersey and Maine highlighted the contested and ambiguous nature of Ebola sciences.

While the CDC in Atlanta, the ACLU, and the United Nations secretary general all attacked Governor Christie's twenty-one-day mandatory quarantine policy that would impact the lives of all health care workers who were exposed to Ebola, there were some famous scientists and researchers who said *he wasn't going far enough*. Bruce Beutler, who won the 2011 Nobel Prize in Physiology or Medicine, complained that not enough research had been carried out on these matters that demonstrated conclusively that *asymptomatic healthcare workers couldn't transmit Ebola*. "It could be people develop significant *viremia* [where viruses get into the bloodstream and gain access to the rest of the body]," argued Beutler, and then they "are able to transmit the disease before they have a fever, even."[54] Beutler pointed to recent studies that showed that 13 percent of the time those who get Ebola don't report having fevers,[55] and in order to be safe Beutler wanted to go further than Governor Christie and demand that suspected Ebola victims be quarantined in *hospitals, not their homes*. After all, staying in a home with family members made no sense to Dr. Beutler, and he was also bothered by the imperative to maintain open borders, no matter what. He complained that many observers who were following the Hickox situation wanted to "err on the side of total individual freedom rather than the side of public health."[56]

Was it possible that Beutler's reasoned scientific analysis buttressed and supported the ideological positions of many Americans when they conversed about Ebola transmission? Even if they did not use the phrase "precautionary principle," was it possible that the vast major of U.S. citizens agreed with Beutler, to the extent that they would argue that there was no reason to allow talk of civil liberties to get in the way of efficacious disease control?

Many Americans, who sided with the governors, were infuriated when they found out that the State of Maine, in early November, had reached a legal settlement with Hickox that allowed her to travel freely in public—as long as she monitored her health closely and reported any Ebola symptoms. Eric Saunders, one of Hickox's attorneys, understood that it was hard to deny all of the "fear and safety concerns," but he argued that at the same time, "we have to bear in mind what the law and the science says."[57]

Again, Hickox's lawyers were using that same mantra, and they were circulating the same *dispositifs,* that assumed the existence of some objective, arhetorical, and neutral "law" or "science" that would protect the rights of citizens.

We may never know how many shared these fighting faiths in 2014, but what we do know is that many conservative outlets did not view Kaci Hickox as some selfless heroine. Ian Tuttle of the *National Review*, for example, indicated that he felt she had become a "selfish hero," someone who had no excuse for "her petulance." He admitted that she deserved plaudits for going over to Sierra Leone, where some 1,200 had died by the time she got into the debate with Governor Christie, but for Tuttle her arrogance showed that human beings did indeed "contain multitudes."[58] He was especially miffed by what he viewed as some of her contradictory actions when she went on the *Today* show and told Matt Lauer, "If the restrictions placed on me by the State of Maine are not lifted by Thursday morning, I will go to court to fight for my freedom."

Tuttle's chronology of what happened in New Jersey during the tent incident took into account the fact that perceptions mattered. He could not understand why, when you looked through a "plastic window" and saw her "look rather more Sing Sing than merely sanitizary" she would be allowed to go on her way back to Fort Kent, Maine, after having tested negative for Ebola.[59]

Tuttle also argued that liberals or civil libertarians were misrepresenting the nature and scope of the supposed infringement of Hickox's rights. The more that you thought about what the state was asking her to do, Tuttle argued, the more difficult it became to think of "*de facto*" house arrest as some major abrogation of her rights. Having to endure "21 days of it—lavishly funded—to be followed by perfect liberty assuming no problems, seems a minimal sacrifice to ask of those who put themselves voluntarily in danger."[60] In a thanatopical comment that seemed as though it came out of Preston's *The Hot Zone*, Tuttle claimed that "when it comes to a disease that liquefies your internal organs and pushes blood out of your eyeballs" the dictum "better safe than sorry" seemed to be something to which everyone could agree.[61] Once again we get a dose of that omnipresent precautionary principle.

Moderates and liberals used other arguments about contested sciences as they critiqued both the CDC Ebola protocols and the media coverage of the Hickox case. Robert Gatter, for example, made the interesting point that it seemed as though the CDC was keeping track of some of these scientific debates about the reasonableness of Kaci Hickox's actions. He noted how on its guidance webpage, in the Frequently Asked Questions (FAQs) section, the CDC apparently tried to clarify matters by noting that "there is no evidence indicating that Ebola virus is spread by coughing or sneezing." This, as Gatter notes, is different from "saying definitively that the virus *cannot* be spread that way."[62]

Was Gatter implying that the epistemic absence of evidence supported the notion of Ebola airborne transmission? If so, did this mean that conservatives were not the only ones who wanted to avoid taking chances?

I will have more to say about this near the end of this chapter, but at this point I want to point out that Hickox's interventions in this dispute did not end with the reportage of Judge LaVerdiere's opinions.

RHETORICAL ANALYSES OF SOME OF KACI HICKOX'S OWN VISUAL AND TEXTUAL STRATEGIZING

Kaci Hickox may not have had total control over the mass-mediated framing of her confrontations with New Jersey and New York governors, but over time she apparently decided to adopt the subject position of an empowered celebrity who needed to help ensure the protection of other public health workers in America who might be placed in similar predicaments. After the circulation of Judge LaVerdiere's decisions she would give many interviews, and she would write several articles on these topics.

In a number of ways, her written and spoken commentaries could be symbolically linked to the visual images that circulated during, and after, her confrontations with the governors. One iconic photograph of Kaci Hickox shows her peering through some plastic while she stayed in the tent that was erected in a parking lot of the Newark hospital. A second, that many readers may have seen, shows her riding her bike with her partner.[63] Those who adopt perspectival approaches could reasonably argue that these two images appear to be contrasting, and yet related, pictorials that supported some of Hickox's contentions. The first image showed her suffering from what the *New York Post* called "Ebola nurse's quarantine Hell,"[64] and this could be used to magnify New Jersey's transgressive infringement on her rights. The second photo could be read as a liberating image, one that signaled that she was willing to enjoy the freedom that she had earned after standing up to public health officials and their superiors.

Interestingly enough, in a law review article that she wrote for the *Journal of Health and Biomedical Law*, Kaci Hickox has left us with textual materials that provide some hints of how she wanted to remember the heroines and heroes who worked as health care workers in West Africa. In her critique of Governor Paul LePage of Maine she said,

> I often wonder, what would have happened if he had instead met me on my journey from New Jersey at the Maine state line and gave me a big hug to welcome me home? How would Americans have reacted if Governor LePage

chose to model what an evidence-based, compassionate reaction to returning Ebola healthcare workers looked like? Instead, Maine implemented a policy requiring all healthcare workers returning from Ebola-affected areas to home-quarantine. He made accusatory statements to manipulate the public saying about me, "I don't trust her."[65]

The hugs that were given to individuals like Nina Pham could therefore be linked to the science that was "evidenced-based."

Many of Hickox's defenders would argue that these images, along with a court order from a Maine magistrate that rejected a petition for a mandatory quarantine order, seemed to show that she had helped the cause of "science" and the rights of "asymptomatic" carriers, but Gatter has recently made the astute observation that all of this debate about Ebola transmission may have had some unintended consequences. On the day before the State of Maine filed its petition for a quarantine order, the CDC came out with the Interim U.S. Guidance for Monitoring and Movement of Persons with Potential Ebola Virus Exposure.[66] That interim guidance recommended that state and local health agencies needed to monitor, and perhaps quarantine in some cases, "even asymptomatic individuals" who may have been exposed directly to the Ebola virus.[67] The interim report, that was assembled after the world had heard the stories about Craig Spencer, Nina Pham, and Amber Vinson, provided a theoretical framework that would help local, state, and other public health authorities make decisions about what to do about Ebola monitoring, and potential restriction of mobility, of those individuals who could be placed into one of four categories. These interim report categories included those who (1) may have been exposed to Ebola, but had not, or hadn't yet, shown any symptoms, (2) those who presented low risk, (3) those who presented "some" risk, or (4) those who presented "high" risk.[68]

Where would one have placed Hickox, and would this placement have survived public, medical, and legal scrutiny? The CDC Interim Guidance used a reference table to note that asymptomatic clinical criteria still indicated "some risk,"[69] and all of this was signaling that state and local health care workers, and their supervisors, needed to look out for more than just those who were symptomatic. In some ways this can be read as a little more cautious than the Maine court order that rejected the State of Maine's petition based on the idea that Hickox was symptom free. Did this mean that the CDC was no longer endorsing the position that only those who were symptomatic posed any risk to the public safety, health, and welfare? If so, then Hickox, and her lawyers, were citing older materials that no longer represented the latest CDC wisdom. The degree of contact with Ebola victims, rather than the symptoms of the health workers, seemed to determine where one would be placed within the interim report categorization scheme.

Hickox, who once used the CDC critiques of mandatory quarantining of travelers to her advantage, would later find ways of interrogating the modified CDC guidelines. By November of 2014 she had turned into an adamant activist for the rights of those public health workers who were stigmatized after working with Ebola patients. She would ask that transatlantic communities stop calling her "the Ebola nurse."[70] At the same time she reminded readers that she had tested negative for Ebola during the first night that she stayed in New Jersey, and by November 17 she could openly celebrate the fact that she was way past the incubation period.

In Hickox's November chronicling of her ordeals, she was said to have been quarantined by "overzealous politicians" after she had volunteered to treat people affected by Ebola in West Africa. My "liberty, my interests and consequently my civil rights," she claimed, "were ignored because some ambitious governors" saw that they had the opportunity to use an "age-old political tactic: fear."[71]

The former occupant of that New Jersey hospital tent went on the offensive in 2015, and she wrote essays that made it appear as if she was an expert on Ebola epidemiology and legal science. Her experiences in the tent, combined with her work in Sierra Leone, provided her with the credibility that she needed as she wrote about the importance of protecting health care workers' rights. For example, in her essay in the *Journal of Health & Biomedical Law*, she indicated that she spoke to representatives of the New Jersey and Maine Health Departments, and she chronicled how she had "explained" the legal and scientific "principles time and time again."[72] She had to constantly reiterate the point that she should not be quarantined if she did not pose a risk to the public. This was then tethered to the argument that there was little rational reason for her to have to stay in her home if she was not ill, and this all meant that she could not spread EVD. At the same time that Hickox was conjuring up horrifying pictures of historical abuses of quarantines, she told her readers that American officials seemed to be taking some of these extreme measures because they were thinking about Ebola in the same ways that previous generations had thought about measles or influenza.

Hickox's Ebola rhetorics positioned her as one of the protagonists who had to fight public health antagonists who were clueless about Ebola. Hickox, for example, averred that when she first posed these types of questions to officials who worked for New Jersey or Maine health departments, they usually had one of two kinds of responses. They either argued that superiors made those decisions, or they claimed that she needed to know that they were trying to allay the fears of the public.[73]

Critical scholars who study these types of fragments from Kaci Hickox's remarks would notice the selective, rhetorical nature of this type of argumentation. First of all, she appears to be trying to establish her own expertise and her own credibility as she comments on the contemporary state of Ebola "science." Second, her commentaries on how she talks to these representatives of the New Jersey and Maine health departments makes it appear as though she has some special access to empowered decision makers, transforming her into an empowered educator who has to be reckoned with. Third, her commentary indicates that she does not factor in the possibility that her science could be wrong. In other words, the "science" that she views as so ironclad, foundational, and unassailable may be contingent, ambiguous, contested, and changing.

One strategy that Hickox uses focuses attention on the ways that her own case can be linked to the cases of Dr. Craig Spencer[74] and nurses Nina Pham and Amber Vinson. Together, she reasons, these cases all show that there was little likelihood that any of these individuals would infect others.[75] However, what she fails to emphasize are the unique features of each case, and she ignores all of the uncertainties that were swirled around many of these cases. After all, Pham contracted Ebola from Thomas Eric Duncan, and yet even Pham has admitted at times that she does not know *how* she contracted the disease.

While I share Hickox's assessment that Spencer, Pham, and Vinson were all diagnosed with Ebola and yet none of them transmitted Ebola to their households, this does not mean that we can automatically be dismissive of the opinions of others by characterizing them as being motivated solely by fear or ignorance.

CONCLUSION

Critical legal scholars may never know exactly how many Americans shared the views of Governor Chris Christie or someone like Bruce Beutler, but there is plenty of data that supports the conclusion that more than a few were willing to restrict Hickox's constitutional rights. Over the last few years, Hickox has been called someone with a "repulsive sense of entitlement"[76] and a menace, and I have little doubt that with the passage of time she will join the medical pantheon that already includes the likes of Mary Mallon and Carrie Buck.

In the short term, critics might conclude that Ms. Hickox's court victories would help ensure that health care workers would not be deterred from volunteering for overseas duties. However, if we focus on long-term impacts, one wonders just how much consciousness-raising can take place in contexts where polling data shows that some 80 percent of those polled are in favor of mandatory quarantines for travelers who return from places like West Africa that are battling EVD.[77] I share Wendy Parmet's assessment that down the road we are going to get some precedent from an appellate court that will have a different result from the one that Kaci Hickox got from Judge LaVerdiere.[78]

At the same time, what I will call the Kaci Hickox saga reminds us of the negotiated and ideological nature of Ebola sciences in key legal contests. Kaci Hickox, and many others who agree with her lines of reasoning, may write about the need for some stable "evidence-based scientific discourse,"[79] and they may continue to factor in the existence of some monolithic Ebola "science" that can be separated from "politics." However, this chapter has highlighted the ways that particular *dispositifs* are deployed by those who want to avoid the imposition of some twenty-one-day mandatory quarantining period. Hickox may have conjured up an image of stable and dependable CDC guidelines that would protect her rights, but some students of the law, like Robert Gatter, have noticed *that the CDC has circulated contradictory texts*. While Gatter seems to share Hickox's faith in some unitary "science" that shows that only those who touch the blood or bodily fluids of a person who is sick will get Ebola, he makes the point that the changing CDC guidelines can appear to provide "irrational" guidance when they suggest that asymptomatic individuals also constitute threats.[80] Gatter was willing to go so far as to argue that after "almost forty years of experience," and after following some twenty-five thousand cases in Africa and elsewhere, this probably showed that asymptomatic individuals "incubating Ebola do *not* pose a risk of transmission to others" (emphasis in the original).[81] All of this talk of probability would not resonate with those who wanted their governors to perhaps think in *possibilistic*, not probabilistic ways.

President Obama may have helped produce iconic White House images of him hugging nurses like Nina Pham, but his own critiques of mandatory quarantines did not stand in the way of Pentagon officials who securitized and militarized Ebola to the point where they wanted to take no chances with returning travelers from West Africa. On October 29, 2014, the secretary of defense "signed an order that validated a recommendation from the Joint Chiefs of Staff to place all U.S. military service members returning from Ebola response efforts in West Africa into a 21-day controlled monitoring regimen," which will "apply to all military services that are contributing personnel to the fight against Ebola at its source."[82] This meant that while civilian organizations like the CDC were opposed to this mandatory quarantining, the military took a very different approach to the problem. The military seemed to be following populist ways of implementing variants of the precautionary principle.

Moreover, it is very possible that some of Kaci Hickox's supporters misinterpreted Judge LaVerdiere's reasoning in his court orders, and they may not have realized that he was not agreeing with her assessment that she could monitor herself. This judge anticipated that she would have to comply with Maine's "active monitoring" policies. Granted, he thanked her for her service overseas, and part of his opinion did read as though he was adopting her position on how asymptomatic individuals did not risk infecting others, but he was still requiring that she work with Maine health authorities. Those health authorities would be the ones who would be given the mission of making sure that that Hickox was still asymptomatic. In other words, before the twenty-one-day period of time had passed, even Judge LaVerdiere was going to allow the state to impose some restrictions on her mobility.[83]

When all was said and done, the State of Virginia was allowed to sterilize Carrie Buck, and Mary Mallon died in isolation on a New York Island.[84] In all likelihood, Professor Kontorovich is right, the odds are that most U.S. courts would not question the state's right to quarantine individuals, even in cases where "carriers" are asymptomatic.

I want to end this chapter with a counterfactual for readers to think about. Just imagine how many Anglo-Americans would have responded to Hickox's lamentations if U.S. citizens had watched a half a dozen more EVD patients enter local hospitals. Given Ebola fears, it is possible that there would have been far fewer supporters of Hickox's positions.

NOTES

1. The defense of state power for conscription during times of war appears in the *Selective Draft Law Cases*, 245 U.S. 366 (1918).

2. For critiques of Holmes's views on state power and public health, see Mary L. Dudziak, "Oliver Wendell Holmes, Jr. as a Eugenic Reformer: Rhetoric in the Writing of Constitutional Law," *Iowa Law Review* 71 (1985): 833–868; Paul A. Lombardo, "Facing Carrie Buck," *The Hastings Center Report* 33, no. 2 (March/April, 2003): 14–17. DOI: 10.2307/3528148.

3. For studies that investigate the symbolic importance of "Typhoid Mary," see Judith Walzer Leavitt, "Typhoid Mary Strikes Back: Bacteriological Theory and Practice in Early Twentieth-Century Public Health," *ISIS 83*, no. 4 (December, 1992): 608–629; Kit Yee Chan and Daniel D. Reidpath, "'Typhoid Mary' and 'HIV Jane': Responsibility, Agency and Disease Prevention," *Reproductive Health Matters* 11, no. 22 (November 2003): 40–50. doi:10.1016/S0968–8080(03)02291–2. Some commentators who read essays about Hickox made explicit comparisons between "Typhoid Mary" and the "Ebola Nurse." Blossiekins, for example, noted how the usage of the phrase "Ebola Nurse" depersonalized Hickox and made it easier to

clamor for confinement. For this reason, she argued "'Ebola nurse' has the same ring as 'Typhoid Mary.'" Blossiekins, one of the "Featured Comments" after Kaci Hickox, "Stop Calling Me 'The Ebola Nurse,'" *The Guardian*, last modified November 17, 2014, http://www.theguardian.com/commentisfree/2014/nov/17/stop-calling-me-ebola-nurse-kaci-hickox.

4. For an example of another critical legal rhetorical project that tries to go beyond traditional ways of thinking about the "rule of law" in salient social controversies that extends some of my previous work on critical legal rhetorics, see Lolita Buckner Inniss, "A Critical Legal Rhetoric Approach to *In Re African-American Slave Descendants Litigation*," *St. John's Journal of Legal Commentary* 24 (2009): 649–696.

5. Chan and Reidpath, "'Typhoid Mary' and 'HIV Jane,'" 40–50.

6. For related examples of how critical legal scholars can use some critical genealogical approaches in the study of criminal law, see Christine Schwöbel, ed., *Critical Approaches to International Criminal Law* (New York: Routledge, 2014).

7. Lawrence Gostin has argued that the Hickox case appears to be the first time where some governmental institution was trying to impose a quarantine *on a class of people*—doctors who have been exposed to EVD—rather than some individuated case-by-case basis according to symptoms. Yoni Bashan, Melanie Grayce West, and Heather Haddon, "Nurse Detained in New Jersey for Ebola, Calls Conditions 'Really Inhumane,'" *The Wall Street Journal*, last modified October 26, 2014, http://www.wsj.com/articles/nurse-detained-in-new-jersey-for-ebola-calls-conditions-really-inhumane-1414352575.

8. Sam Frizell, "First Ebola Worker Quarantined under New Policy Tests Negative," *Time*, October 25, 2014, http://time.com/3538834/ebola-quarantine-new-york/. Some of these controversies were probably triggered just a few days before Kaci Hickox received all of this attention, when authorities had to deal with the case of Craig Spencer, someone who did come down with Ebola. Spencer's mass-mediated journey began when he entered the country through JFK International Airport on October 17, 2014. Sydney Lupkin, "New Jersey, New York, Illinois, Toughen Ebola Quarantine Rules after Doctor Case," ABC News, October 24, 2014, http://abcnews.go.com/Health/york-doctorebola-quarantine/story?id=26431431.

9. Gail Sullivan, "Why Kaci Hickox Might Lose a Legal Battle against Ebola Quarantine," *The Washington Post*, last modified October 30, 2014, paragraph 3, http://www.washingtonpost.com/news/morning-mix/wp/2014/10/30/why-kaci-hickox-may-lose-a-legal-battle-against-ebola-quarantine/.

10. Wilbur, quoted in Gail Sullivan, "Gov. Christie's Ebola Quarantine Messed with the 'Wrong Redhead,'" *The Washington Post*, last modified October 27, 2014, paragraph 4, http://www.washingtonpost.com/news/morning-mix/wp/2014/10/27/gov-christies-ebola-quarantine-messed-with-the-wrong-redhead/

11. Eugenia Tognotti, "Lessons from the History of Quarantine, From Plague to Influenza A," *Emerging Infectious Disease* 19, no. 2 (February, 2013): 256.

12. Michael McCarthy, "Maine Judge Refuses to Quarantine Nurse Who Cared for Ebola Patients," *British Medical Journal* 349 (November 3, 2014): g6606.

13. The CDC guidelines that were passed on October 27, 2014, contained what I consider to be ambiguous language that seemed to indicate that those doctors,

nurses, or other public health care workers who had worked with Ebola patients overseas were at "some risk" of infection, even if they were without symptoms. That would trigger the need for a public health care worker to check for fear or other symptoms for the twenty-one days after the last potential exposure to EVD. Some have interpreted this to mean that there could be less restrictive ways of monitoring. See Michael McCarthy, "Maine Judge Refuses," g6606; Michael McCarthy, "CDC Rejects Mandatory Quarantine for Travelers Arriving from Ebola Stricken Nations," *British Medical Journal* 349 (2014): g6499.

14. Kaci Hickox, "Caught between Civil Liberties and Public Safety Fears: Personal Reflections from a Healthcare Provider Treating Ebola," *Journal of Health & Biomedical Law* 11 (2015): 9–23, 10.

15. For typical examples of those who talked about this monolithic and foundational "science," see Josh Voorhees, "Main Judge Sides with Science, Rejects State's Attempt to Quarantine Kaci Hickox," *The Slate*, last modified October 31, 2014, http://www.slate.com/blogs/the_slatest/2014/10/31/kaci_hickox_maine_court_decision_judge_charles_laverdiere_rejects_gov_paul.html.

16. Sara M. Bergstresser, "Health Communication, Public Mistrust, and the Politics of 'Rationality,'" *The American Journal of Bioethics* 14, no. 4 (2015): 57–59, doi: 10.1080/15265161.2015.1009570.

17. As I explain in more detail below, I share Michelle Meyer's assessment that a close reading of some of the texts and contexts that are involved in the *Maine DHHS v. Hickox* case shows that it is not always clear just whose "science" was the winner in all of this disputation. Michelle N. Meyer, "Will the Real Evidence-Based Ebola Policy Please Stand Up? Several Takeaways from *Maine DHHS v. Hickox*," last modified, November 6, 2014, http://www.thefacultylounge.org/2014/11/will-the-real-evidence-based-ebola-policy-please-stand-up-seven-take-aways-from-main-dhhs-v-hickox.html.

18. For a similar Foucauldian study that looks at some of the informal norms and other contests that impact that way that we view Ebola and other health care matters in African contexts see Jean-Germain Gross, *Healthcare Policy in Africa: Institutions and Politics from Colonialism to the Present* (Lanham, MD: Rowman & Littlefield, 2015).

19. Robert Gatter, "Ebola Quarantine, and Flawed CDC Policy," *University of Miami Business Law Review* (2015): 375–397, 376.

20. For some fine traditional histories of quarantine that can be found in scientific venues, see Eugenia Tognotti, "Lessons from the History of Quarantine, From Plague to Influenza A," *Emerging Infectious Disease* 19, no. 2 (February, 2013): 254–259.

21. Eugene Kontorovich, "Constitutional Challenge to Quarantine Unlikely to Succeed," *The Washington Post*, October 27, 2014, paragraphs 3–4, https://www.washingtonpost.com/news/volokh-conspiracy/wp/2014/10/27/constitutional-challenge-to-quarantine-unlikely-to-succeed/. The vaccination case that Professor Kontorovich is referencing is *Jacobson v. Massachusetts*, 197 U.S. 11 (1905).

22. Kontorovich, "Constitutional Challenge," paragraphs 5–6.

23. *U.S. ex rel. Siegel v. Shinnick*, 219 F. Supp 789 (E.D. NY 1963).

24. Kontorovich, "Constitutional Challenge," paragraph 5.

25. *Crayton v. Larabee*, 110 N. Rep. 355, 220 N.Y. 493 (N.Y. Ct. of App. 1917). I thank Gail Sullivan of the *Washington Post* for calling this case to our attention. Sullivan, "Why Kaci Hickox Might Lose."

26. Sydney Lupkin, "New Jersey, New York, Illinois, Toughen Ebola Quarantine Rules after Doctor Case," ABC News (October 24, 2014), http://abcnews.go.com/Health/york-doctorebola-quarantine/story?id=26431431.

27. "Insider," comment after Kieran Corcoran, "'Craig and I Are OK,'": Fiancée of New York Ebola Doctor Speaks Out—As She and Two Friends Prepare to Be Released from Quarantine Today," *The Daily Mail*, last modified October 25, 2014, http://www.dailymail.co.uk/news/article-2807623/Fianc-e-New-York-Ebola-doctor-Craig-Spencer-speaks-two-friends-released-hospital-quarantined-home-instead.html.

28. Robbins, Barbaro, and Santora, "Unapologetic, Christie Frees," paragraph 10. See also Matt Arco, "Christie Defends Ebola Quarantine Announcement, Saying He's Trying to Protect N.J. Residents," NJ.com, last modified, Oct. 26, 2014, http://www.nj.com/politics/index.ssf/2014/10/christie_defends_ebola_quarantine_announcement.html.

29. Liz Robbins, Michael Barbaro, and Marc Santora, "Unapologetic, Christie Frees Nurse from Ebola Quarantine," *The New York Times*, last modified October 27, 2014, http://www.nytimes.com/2014/10/28/nyregion/nurse-in-newark-to-be-allowed-to-finish-ebola-quarantine-at-home-christie-says.html?_r=0.

30. Hickox, "Caught between Civil Liberties," 13.

31. Michael McCarthy, "Nurse Says She Will Fight Ebola Quarantine," *British Medical Journal* 349 (2014): g6555.

32. Kaci Hickox, "Her Story: UTA Grad Isolated at New Jersey Hospital in Ebola Quarantine," *The Dallas Morning News*, last modified October 25, 2014, http://www.dallasnews.com/ebola/headlines/20141025–uta-grad-isolated-at-new-jersey-hospital-as-part-of-ebola-quarantine.ece.

33. Christie, quoted in Robbins, Barbaro, and Santora, "Unapologetic, Christie Frees," paragraph 11. For video showing Christie talking about how Hickox was obviously "ill," see Matt Arco, "Ebola: Timeline of Events, Actions by Chris Christie," NJ.com, last modified October 27, 2014, http://www.nj.com/politics/index.ssf/2014/10/ebola_timeline_of_events_actions_by_chris_christie.html. In her law review article, Hickox indicated that she thought that this remark disregarded her right to privacy to her own medical information. Hickox, "Caught between Civil Liberties," 11.

34. Ban Ki-Moon, quoted in Sherwood and Jenkins, "Maine Settles Quarantine Lawsuit," paragraphs 9–10.

35. Christie, quoted in Robbins, Barbaro, and Santora, "Unapologetic, Christie Frees," paragraph 9.

36. Governor LePage, quoted in *Fox News*, "New Fight over Ebola Quarantine Looms as Nurse Returns to Maine," Fox News, last modified, October 28, 2014, http://www.foxnews.com/politics/2014/10/28/new-debate-over-ebola-quarantine-looms-as-nurse-returns-to-maine/.

37. Robbins, Barbaro, and Santora, "Unapologetic, Christie Frees," paragraph 6.

38. Robert Gatter, "Ebola, Quarantine, and Flawed CDC Policy," 376. Elsewhere in the same essay Gatter went on to argue, "As applied here, there is no doubt that prohibiting an asymptomatic individual from traveling, working, being in public places, or otherwise coming within three feet of another person imposes a substantial physical restraint on that individual to the point of consti-

tuting confinement. In other words, such a prohibition deprives the individual of a fundamental liberty interest. Thus, the state would be required to prove that such a physical restraint is narrowly tailored to serve the state's compelling interest in protecting the public from the spread of Ebola" (388).

39. Hickox, "Caught between Civil Liberties," 14.

40. On October 28, 2014, the Department of Health and Human Services Commissioner of Maine described new protocols under which the department will address Ebola: "Any traveler from West Africa who comes to Maine will be monitored for at least 21 days after the last possible exposure to Ebola. This is consistent with federal guidelines. This monitoring includes daily check-ins with a state epidemiologist for any signs of a fever or other Ebola related symptoms. If any symptoms develop, they will receive immediate medical care. We have instituted additional protocols for ensuring that those individuals with a higher level of risk do not unnecessarily make contact with the public. These protocols include voluntary, in-home quarantine for someone who was known to have had direct contact with an Ebola patient."

41. Hickox, "Caught between Civil Liberties," 14.

42. See, for example, Lindsay Pérez Huber and Daniel G. Solorzano, "Visualizing Everyday Racism: Critical Race Theory, Visual Micro-aggressions, and the Historical Imagery of Mexican Banditry," *Qualitative Inquiry* 21, no. 3 (2015): 223–238, doi: 10.1177/1077800414562899; Inniss, "A Critical Legal Rhetoric Approach," 649–696.

43. For readers who might be wondering, Kaci Hickox's partner was Theodore Michael Wilbur, and he faced his own hurdles when he was trying to get through nursing school. Wilbur had been a nursing student at the University of Maine at Fort Kent, but officials there warned of the "hysteria" that followed in the wake of Hickox's return. These officials allegedly asked Wilbur to stay away from campus. Scott Dolan, "Ebola Nurse Kaci Hickox Moving to Southern Maine," *Press Herald*, last modified November 10, 2014, paragraphs 4–5, http://www.pressherald. com/2014/11/10/ebola-nurse-moving-to-southern-maine/. The two apparently decided to move from Maine to Oregon.

44. Stephanie Gosk and Erin McClam, "Kaci Hickox, Nurse in Ebola Quarantine Standoff, Goes for a Bike Ride," NBC News, last modified Oct. 30, 2014, http://www.nbcnews.com/storyline/ebola-virus-outbreak/kaci-hickox-nurse-ebola-quarantine-standoff-goes-bike-ride-n237421 (reporting on Governor LePage's response to Hickox's arrival to Maine).

45. See Maine Revised Statute, Title 22, § 812 (2014) (requiring treatment for individual deemed by court to be a public health threat); Verified Petition for Public Health Order at 5–6, *Mayhew v. Hickox*, No. CV-2014-36 (Oct. 30, 2014) (outlining State's case for monitoring).

46. Hickox, "Caught between Civil Liberties," 15.

47. Judge Charles LaVerdiere quoted in Gregg Gonsalves and Peter Staley, "Panic, Paranoia, and Public Health—The AIDS Epidemic's Lessons for Ebola," *The New England Journal of Medicine* 371 (December 18, 2014): 2348–2349, 2349.

48. Josh Voorhees, "Main Judge Sides with Science," paragraph 1.

49. Order Pending Hearing at 3, *Mayhew v. Hickox*, No. CV-2014-36 (Oct. 31, 2014) (allowing general monitoring but restricting State's ability to home quarantine).

50. McCarthy "Main Judge Refuses," g6606.

51. Jess Bidgood and Dave Philipps, "Judge in Maine Eases Restrictions on Nurse," *The New York Times*, last modified October 31, 2014, http://www.ny times.com/2014/11/01/us/ebola-maine-nurse-kaci-hickox.html?_r=0.

52. Hickox, quoted in McCarthy "Main Judge Refuses," g6606.

53. Hickox, "Caught between Civil Liberties," 15.

54. Bruce Beutler, quoted in Chaude Brodesser-Akner, "Christie's Controversial Ebola Quarantine Now Embraced by Nobel Prize–Winning Doctor," NJ.com, last modified October 28, 2014, paragraph 5, http://www.nj.com/politics/index. ssf/2014/10/christies_quarantine_policy_attacked_by_aclu_cdc_and_even_the_ un_is_embraced_by_2011_nobel_prize_win.html.

55. For examples of the contentious nature of "fevers" being a sign for EVD, see David Willman, "Ebola Research: Fever Not a Surefire Sign of Infection," *Los Angeles Times*, last modified October 12, 2014, http://www.latimes.com/nation/ la-na-1012-ebola-fever-20141012-story.html#page=1. Contrast this with those who claim that fever always precedes the contagion stage for EVD. Jeffrey M. Drazen et al., "Ebola and Quarantine," *The New England Journal of Medicine* 371 (November 20, 2014): 2029–2030.

56. Beutler, quoted in Chaude Brodesser-Akner, "Christie's Controversial Ebola Quarantine," paragraph 25.

57. Eric Saunders, quoted in Dave Sherwood and Colleen Jenkins, "Maine Settles Quarantine Lawsuit with Nurse Who Worked with Ebola Patients in West Africa," *Scientific American*, November 3, 2014, paragraph 7, http://www.scienti- ficamerican.com/article/nurse-kaci-hickox-and-state-of-maine-settle-quarantine- lawsuit/.

58. Ian Tuttle, "Kaci Hickox, Selfish Hero," *The National Review*, October 28, 2014, paragraphs 1–2, http://www.nationalreview.com/article/391415/kaci- hickox-selfish-hero-ian-tuttle.

59. Ibid., paragraph 3.

60. Ibid., paragraph 6.

61. Ibid., paragraph 6.

62. Gatter, "Ebola Quarantine, and Flawed CDC Policy," 395.

63. CBS News, "Nurse Defies Ebola Quarantine in Maine, Rides Bike," CBS News, last modified, Oct. 30, 2014, http://www.cbsnews.com/news/ebola- nurse-kaci-hickox-defies-quarantine-in-maine-goes-on-bike-ride/.

64. Frank Rosario and Joe Tacopino, "Ebola Nurse's Quarantine Hell," *The New York Post*, last modified October 27, 2014, http://nypost.com/2014/10/27/ebola- nurse-gets-prison-treatment-in-quarantine-hell/.

65. Hickox, "Caught between Civil Liberties," 11–12. For the comment on lack of trust on the part of the Maine Governor, see Robert F. Bukaty, "Judge Rejects Ebola Quarantine for Nurse Kaci Hickox," *The Boston Globe*, last modified October 31, 2014, http://www.bostonglobe.com/metro/2014/10/31/maine-asking- court-limit-movements-nurse-kaci-hickox/9tGSogqyPYlu3Vq7WjG84L/story. html (reporting court outcome and Governor LePage's reaction). For a discussion of the passage of the Maine laws on Ebola isolation and quarantining, see Maine Government Staff, "Maine's Laws—Ebola Protocol for Travelers from Liberia, Sierra Leone and Guinea," *Maine Centers for Disease Control and Prevention*, last

modified October 27, 2014, http://www.maine.gov/dhhs/mecdc/infectious-disease/epi/zoonotic/ebola/documents/Maine-Ebola-Protocols-October-27.pdf (establishing Maine Ebola monitoring protocols); Maine Government Staff, "Ebola," Maine Division for Infectious Disease, 215, http://www.maine.gov/dhhs/mecdc/infectious-disease/epi/zoonotic/ebola/.

66. CDC, *Interim U.S. Guidance for Monitoring and Movement of Persons with Potential Ebola Virus Exposure*, CDC, December 24, 2014, last modified May 13, 2015, http://www.cdc.gov/vhf/ebola/exposure/monitoring-and-movement-of-persons-with-exposure.html. CDC Ebola guidance has been updated and amended by CDC since its initial publication.

67. "Ebola, Quarantine, and Flawed CDC Policy," 377.

68. David S. Addington, "Ebola: Dallas and New York City Experiences Drive Governments to Change Practices," *The Heritage Foundation Backgrounder* 2974, October 30, 2014, http://www.heritage.org/research/reports/2014/10/ebola-dallas-and-new-york-city-experiences-drive-governments-to-change-practices, p. 4.

69. CDC, Interim U.S. Guidance, (Dec. 24, 2014 version), 9; Gatter, "Ebola, Quarantine," 377. For Hickox's own critique of this same passage that mentions "some risk" to go along with "high risk," see Hickox, "Caught between Civil Liberties," 19. She argued that the use of the term "risk" was confusing to members of the general public, and that this ambiguity contributed to the failure to "offer a standardized, scientific approach" that she believed was warranted. Hickox liked what she viewed as the "evidence-based guidelines" of the European Centre for Disease Prevention and Control (ECDC), which left out the word risk when it discussed individual exposure assessments. European Center for Disease Prevention and Control, "Infection Prevention and Control Measure for Ebola Virus Disease Public Health Management of Healthcare Workers Returning from Ebola-affected Areas," European Center for Disease and Prevention Control, last modified Nov. 7, 2014), 6, http://ecdc.europa.eu/en/publications/Publications/management-healthcare-workers-returning-Ebola-affected-areas.pdf.

70. Kaci Hickox, "Stop Calling Me 'The Ebola Nurse,'" *The Guardian*, last modified November 17, 2014, http://www.theguardian.com/commentisfree/2014/nov/17/stop-calling-me-ebola-nurse-kaci-hickox; Dan Kedmey, "Kaci Hickox: 'Stop Calling Me the 'Ebola Nurse'—Now!'" Time.com, November 17, 2014, http://time.com/3588930/kaci-hickox-ebola-nurse/.

71. Hickox, "Stop Calling Me 'The Ebola Nurse,'" paragraphs 1–3.

72. Hickox, "Caught between Civil Liberties," 16.

73. Ibid., 16.

74. Another interesting point here is that these doctors and nurses did not always agree about the soundness of the science, or the correctness of the protocols, that were used in these Ebola contexts. While Craig Spencer used his case to argue that the protocols worked, Nina Pham's lawsuit alleged that there were some problems with the protocols that she had to deal with at the Dallas Presbyterian Hospital. Compare Lauren Gambino, "Craig Spencer, Declared Free of Ebola, Says He Is a "Living Example" of How Virus Protocols Worked," *The Guardian*, last modified November 11, 2014, http://www.theguardian.com/us-news/2014/nov/11/no-ebola-america-craig-spencer-leaves-hospital.

75. Hickox, "Caught between Civil Liberties," 17.

76. Tuttle, "Kaci Hickox, Selfish Hero," paragraph 9.

77. Sarah Dutton, Jennifer De Pinto, Anthony Salvanto, and Fred Backus, "Do Americans Believe There Should be a Quarantine to Deal with Ebola," CBSnews.com, last modified October 29, 2014, http://www.cbsnews.com/news/do-americans-believe-there-should-be-a-quarantine-to-deal-with-ebola/.

78. Wendy Parmet, quoted in Voorhees, "Main Judge Sides with Science," paragraph 6.

79. Frederick M. Burkle Jr., and Dan Hanfling, "Political Leadership in the Time of Crises: *Primum non Nocere*," *PLOS Currents*, May 29, 2015, doi: 10.1371/currents.dis.fd8aaf6707cd5dd252e33c771d08b949.

80. Gatter, "Ebola Quarantine," 378. Gatter says that these contradictory messages by the CDC are "unfathomable" because these are supposed to be experts who should be aware that they "lacked a basis in the science of Ebola transmission," (378), but I can think of a number of reasons why we have been bequeathed these contradictory texts. First of all, there are many individuals who work for the CDC, and the texts could have been prepared by several different individuals. Moreover, given the contested nature of Ebola pathogenesis and transmission, not everyone is going to be on the same page, especially those who believe the "precautionary principle" that I discussed elsewhere in the book. Third, this revised statement may have been written in order to either respond to updates in empirical research, or, more cynically, to avoid potential legal liability. On the next page of his essay Gatter himself raises some plausible reasons for these contradictory fragments, including "the political pressure to stop the rising tide of fear, or perhaps the CDC silently suspected that this strain of the virus was more easily transmissible than earlier strains with which experts had experience" (p. 379). Later he even mentions the possibility that fear of embarrassment, of making another mistake, may also have been part of the rhetorical context that allowed for this type of contradiction (pp. 389–390).

81. Gatter, "Ebola Quarantine," 396,

82. U.S. Department of Defense Staff, "Statement from Pentagon Press Secretary Rear Admiral John Kirby on Controlled Monitoring for Personnel Returning from Operation United Assistance," U.S. Department of Defense, last modified Oct. 29, 2014, http://www.defense.gov/Releases/Release.aspx?ReleaseID=17007.

83. See Michelle Meyer's excellent parsing of the words of the four levels of risk that appeared in the CDC guidelines after October 27, 2014, as well as her critique of what the Maine CDC guidelines were trying to accomplish. Meyer, "Will the Real Evidence-Based Ebola Policy." The judge in Hickox's case was not trying to overturn the "some risk" portions of the guidelines, and as Meyer's argues, because of human psychology it made sense for Maine to try to require "direct active monitoring" instead of Hickox's own monitoring because human beings often deceive themselves about the meanings of fevers, and so on.

84. The commentary on Ebola has obviously also helped revive interest in the Mary Mallon case. See, for example, Jennifer Latson, "Refusing Quarantine: Why Typhoid Mary Did It," *Time*, last modified November 11, 2014, http://time.com/3563182/typhoid-mary/.

5

+

The IMF, the World Bank, and Debates about the Role of Political Economy in Ebola Outbreak Contexts

In other chapters of this book I will focus attention on some of the scientific, cultural, military, and legal features of the debates that we have had about the 2013–2015 West African outbreak, and in this chapter, I complement those analyses with critical cultural readings of the economic dimensions of this Ebola epidemic. One of my goals, as usual, is to underscore the contested, the partial, and the contingent nature of the various *dispositifs* that circulated during this period in various venues, and I am interested in explicating the ideological roles that financing and budgeting played in the decisions that were made regarding everything from the concentration on "mobile" emergency care to the assiduous avoidance of any discussions of long-development public health projects in Liberia, Guinea, and Sierra Leone. Although they were often overlooked, there were a host of financial reasons why rhetors in these conversations wanted to talk about the efficacy of swift, but temporary, foreign medical and military interventionism. Moreover, there were monetary reasons why so many wanted to talk about the importance of following established protocols for surveillance and warning systems for EVD instead of conversing about the tens of billions that might be needed by West Africans who were trying to rebuild their health care infrastructures. "When you're three steps removed from war or a coup," noted Columbia political science professor Chris Blattman, "and you don't have a functioning police or justice system, building a fine public health system is not your first investment."[1] While many cultural critics might dispute Blattman's characterization of West African nations as failed states that did not have functioning judiciaries or policing communities, he was nevertheless getting at the *perceptual* difficulties that manifested themselves when Ebola emerged in the aftermath of decades of diamond and other resource wars or conflicts. Long before the advent of this latest Ebola crisis, leaders like Charles Taylor were said to have acted in ways that perpetuated the violence and led to even more exploitation of impoverished populations in places like Liberia.[2]

As I noted in chapter 2, organizations like MSF prided themselves on having helped "end" or "contain" the 2013–2015 Ebola outbreak in West Africa, but there were many other parties who were involved in the provision of unilateral, bilateral, or multi-lateral aid to the region. This did not go unnoticed, and not everyone was sure about the supposed beneficence that came from this type of aid. For example, why didn't the world prioritize *pan-African solutions* to West African problems, where regional powers like South Africa or Nigeria led medical humanitarian initiatives in the war against Ebola? Was it possible that the belated, but massive help from "the North" served as a type of "moral hazard?" Ibrahim Abdullah, writing in October 18, 2014, had this to say about some of the intended or unintended consequences of some of this interventionism:

> Is it coincidence that the so-called Ebola humanitarian crisis . . . is unfolding on the upper Guinea coast . . . ? This dependence, now bilateral; now multilateral; continues to shape relations between Africa and the West as the neoliberal economic machine becomes the only framework within which solutions are sought.[3]

Many of those in the global South thus resented how the major financing decisions during this Ebola crisis were being made by empowered members of the North, who had their own biases, their own interests, and their own paradigmatic ways of viewing the economic dimensions of this particular Ebola outbreak.

Many critical cultural scholars and critical legal researchers have profited from the work of writers like Michel Foucault and Ann Stoler,[4] and in this particular chapter, I invite readers to extend their work so that we can unpack the critical genealogical dimensions of all of this talk of dependence and financial support during public health crises in West Africa. Given the fact that organizations like the IMF or the World Bank had already established relationships with many of the nations in this region before the advent of the latest Ebola outbreak, it makes sense that we follow Stoler's suggestion that when we want to track the traces left by those in power we look at the longue durée of the *epistemes* and the *dispositifs* that impacted how many global observers wrote and talked about rhetorical features of geopolitical terrains. This is especially important in West African contexts, because, as Morten Boas explains, during chaotic times people and communities strive desperately to find some means of "control" in their lives during times of "war, conflict, and violence," and this affective dimension of personal struggles should not be lost as we use our critical "frames of power, patronage, patrimonialism," marginalization, "vulnerability and poverty."[5]

In this chapter, I will be touching on many of these topics as a I talk about global flows of capital, *realpolitik* state concerns, and structural constraints, but my major goal will be to use some of the materials from these West African economic histories and archives in ways that allow me to explain how well-intention defenders of contemporary banking policies can justify the decisions that they have made during Ebola outbreaks. Given the horrors of EVD epidemics many of us often wonder why other nation-states, philanthropists, NGOs, and banking institutions didn't automatically throw money at this problem, and I am convinced that we can't understand the hesitancy to do this without an understanding of some of the prior histories and antecedent rhetorics that circulated about West Africa generations before the 2013–2015 Ebola outbreak.

COLONIAL AND DECOLONIZATION WORRIES ABOUT THE FINANCIAL COSTS OF WEST AFRICAN EPIDEMICS

There is little disagreement that poverty, economic dislocation, and post-conflict struggles played a key role in hindering the efforts of health care workers in Guinea, Liberia, and Sierra Leone when they tried to contain the Ebola epidemic, but this negotiated consensus breaks down once social scientists, humanists, decision makers, and others start to specify the exact histories and historiographies that contributed to these difficulties. Did all of these West African struggles begin as early as the nineteenth century, when coastal regions of Sierra Leone were characterized by Westerners as the "White Man's Grave?"[6] Would it be the colonial and imperial "tropical" disease policies that were put in place later, for the containment of malaria and smallpox, which would provide the prefigurative economic *dispositifs* that would influence today's economic rationing or triage schemes?[7]

A critical review of some key historical ruptures in time, when the colonized and the colonizers had to cope with other infectious diseases in West Africa, reminds us of the eternal recurrence of the linkages that can be made by those who connect public health problems with costly outside interventionism. For example, in 1899 Ronald Ross, who left the Indian Medical Service so that he could study mosquito-malarial relationships, would be appointed a lecturer in the newly established Liverpool School of Tropical Medicine. After spending a few months of residency in that school, he decided that he needed to plan an expedition to Freetown, in the British colony of Sierra Leone, so that he could work on "showing exactly how the disease could be prevented in topical countries."[8] A very cautious colonial office listened to his schemes about how to get rid of some one hundred breeding pools for mosquitoes in Freetown, and they were not always sure that this was the best way to "diminish the risk from malaria to health and life" of "Government Officials."[9] As Stephen Frankel and John Western explain, given the fact that some parts of the British Empire "had never been highly profitable and where much money might be spent with little promise of return," many new projects in this region were viewed as too expensive and "schemes to increase profitability continually proposed."[10]

In the ideal British imagination, the West African colonies were supposed to be self-supporting, and proper medical equipment was a scarce colonial resource. The colonial surgeon in Sierra Leone complained that budgetary problems created a situation where there was "not even a trustworthy microscope at the Colonial Hospital."[11] The British built bungalows and railways in the region, but they often viewed the costs of taking care of those in the colonial services—that had to factor in everything from furloughs to paying for segregated quarters—as a burden on imperial leger sheets. One English judge, who visited West Africa had this to say about the economic conundrums that were posed by malaria in that region:

> The Fever Demon has compelled us to double, aye, often to treble, our executive staff in our West African possessions. It has caused civilization and trade alike to stagnate over side areas; it has retarded the opening up of vast tracts of rich and fertile country; and has cost the Empire many millions of pounds sterling to hold in even partial check.[12]

For centuries British administrators, travelers to the region, military leaders, and others had written about the challenges that confronted those who were willing to tackle the challenges posed by this "White Man's Grave," and in theory as soon as progressive medicine arrived on the scene places like Sierra Leone were supposed to become profitable colonies.

Perhaps, for those readers who do not want us to travel that far back in time, and who don't like to apportion blame, we may need to follow the tales of economic privations, and struggles, which circulated in Liberia, Guinea, and Sierra Leone following decolonization. If that is too far for us to go back, then perhaps a more popular, neoliberal way of talking about the political economy woes of this region would highlight how twenty-first-century planners responded to some of the twentieth-century devastation in the region as state leaders worked with representatives of the

IMF and the World Bank to try and rebuild some of the infrastructures of countries like Liberia and Sierra Leone. In these post-conflict debates, would we see discourses about "failed" states that looked like the old colonial rhetorics of the "White Man's Grave," and stingy budgetary spending, or would the passage of time mean that we could anticipate the formation of different *dispositifs*?

POST-CONFLICT ECONOMIC PLANNING, TALK OF "STRUCTURAL ADJUSTMENTS," AND NEOLIBERAL PLANS FOR REBUILDING WEST AFRICAN ECONOMIES

In order for us to understand what critics like Ibrahim Abdullah were complaining about when they referenced the problems of "dependence" on foreign economic aid, we need to have some understanding of the contexts behind some of the criticisms that have been leveled at organizations like the World Bank and the IMF. As I note in more detail below, the personnel who work for these organizations often configure themselves as some of the *rescuers* who have helped with the gradual rebuilding of countries like Liberia, Guinea, and Sierra Leone, but their detractors characterize them as stingy villains who have little understanding of the health needs of West African populations who have to cope with endemic and epidemic diseases.

Whether we think of these World Bank or IMF planners as sinners or saints often depends on how we react to the rhetorics of what are called "structural adjustment" schemes. In theory, instead of just handing over aid without strings to impoverished Western African populations these banking planners worked on finding cost-efficient ways to overcome the hurdles that were supposedly presented in the aftermath of the "civil wars" that were fought by child soldiers and many others during the 1990s. Instead of simply exacerbating the postwar situation by working with corrupt African officials global financial institutions talked of tightening purse strings and teaching West Africans about fiscal responsibility. Grammars that were filled with commentaries on austerity, accountability, and profitability were used to explain how the adoption of Western financial schemes might provide the incremental means for gradually lifting these African nations out of poverty, and this in turn was supposed to bring peace and stability to the region. At the same time, the adoption of fiscal management plans from the West helped impoverished nations build, maintain, and support the public health care infrastructures that had been destroyed during previous decades. James Pfeiffer and Rachel

Chapman, two University of Washington anthropologists who studied public health issues in Mozambique, explain that the ideographic phrase "structural adjustment" became popular within global economic circles during the early 1980s. This was a period when international financial institutions like the World Bank and the International Monetary Fund were trying to promote an ideology of "market fundamentalism" that they claimed constituted the very "core of neoliberalism."[13]

Neoliberal rhetorics that were produced during these periods assumed that many in the Global South wanted to emulate the successes of the Global North. Yet in order for any of this to work, impoverished nations needed to quit talking and writing about neocolonial schemes and put aside their neo-Marxist critiques so that they could embrace some capitalist ideologies. Those who understood the basic tenets of neoliberal economic planning understood the importance of using instruments like global and regional trade compacts, embargoes, and even occasional military intervention to set things right, and those who listened to these Western suggestions argued that there would be times when structural adjustment programs (SAPs) would be needed to help with country-specific planning. Pfeiffer and Chapman go on to explain:

> The primary tenets of neoliberalism—promotion of free markets, privatization, small government, and economic deregulation—have been operationalized at country level through concerted, formulaic, and strategically harmonized action by the IMF and World Bank through SAPs. The advent of structural adjustment came on the heels of colonialism and independence in much of the developing world, especially Africa, and signaled a definitive shift in the relationship of the West to its former colonies; a shift characterized by novel tools of extraction and new strategies of abandonment.[14]

Pfeiffer and Chapman were clearly no fans of these structural adjustments, and they argued that the "stories that anthropologists tell from the field overwhelming speak to a new intensity of immiseration produced by adjustment programs that have ravaged public sector services for the poor."[15] They complained that as international financing institutions moved away from Keynesian principles of government interventionism and toward more free-market approaches that were espoused by the monetarists who worked at places like the University of Chicago school of economics, African countries had to cope with Western policies that were based on trickle-down theories of progress and poverty reformation.[16]

Harsh critics of IMF or World Bank policies argued that all of this neoliberal planning benefited the West but not the rest. For example, Pfeiffer and Chapman, writing in 2010, argued that three decades of structural adjustment had led to a failed experiment where African landscapes were marred by structural violence that created the political conditions that set the stage for the denial of human rights. By extending Paul Farmer's arguments about how economic rights were also human rights, they argued for a more "robust public sector" that would be formed when critics of structural adjustment got together and *stopped the systematic dismantling* of the public health, education, agriculture, water, and safety nets that they felt led to excessive mortality and morbidity.[17] "In practical terms," argued Pfeiffer and Chapman, "the struggle for public health in the structural adjustment era" is "the struggle to preserve, renew, and revitalize the idea and role of the public sphere."[18]

Those observers who agreed with these types of critiques tried to provide readers and planners with a plethora of evidence of how structural adjustments were failing to help most of the economies of the world. One attempt to concretize some of these assertions, which tried to provide empirical evidence of the supposed obstructionism that comes from these austerity plans of the IMF or the World Bank, appeared in the work of Richard Rowden, the author of *The Deadly Ideas of Capitalism: How the IMF has Undermined Public Health and the Fight against AIDS.*[19] Another book, Paul Farmer's *AIDS and Accusation*, showed the adverse impact of some well-intentioned development projects in places like Haiti, where the Duvalier regime built a dam that displaced peasant farmers while increasing HIV risk. On the last pages of his book, which used cultural critiques to explain the role that ideology and economics were playing in global configures of Haiti and HIV/AIDs, Farmer argued,

> For AIDS in Haiti is about proximity rather than distance. AIDS in Haiti is a tale of ties to the United States, rather than to Africa; it is a story of unemployment rates greater than 70 percent. AIDS in Haiti has far more to do with the pursuit of trade and tourism in a dirt-poor country.[20]

More than two decades later Farmer and several co-authors would argue that the Ebola epidemic had "placed this failure in stark relief, exposing the pathology of chronic neglect amid broad global inequalities."[21]

Yet in many ways these critics of the IMF and World Bank policies were fighting an uphill battle, because it is often very difficult for researchers to disaggregate causes when multiple factors converge during particularly volatile times. After all, the neoliberal ideologies that focus on "failed states" can be used to explain the economic features of civil wars that others might link to military, political, or social unrest. In "Globalization, State Failure, and Collective Violence: The Case of Sierra Leone," Earl Conteh-Morgan argues that some of today's resistance to IMF or World Bank policies can be traced back to the early pre–Civil War government policies of President Siaka Stevens.[22] Conteh-Morgan argued that while the international political systems were often characterized as being based on "cleavages (East/West, North/South, and so forth), it appears that globalization may have produced a more rigidly bifurcated system of intensifying global integration and cooperation." This involved the "fragmentation" and "conflictual" situations that plagued the poorer countries.[23] He argued that the infatuation in the empowered countries with what he called "transnational hegemonic power" manifested itself in the ways that decisions, actions, and "impositions" of the World Trade Organization, World Bank, and IMF used neoliberal organizing principles that had "a significant negative impact on individuals, groups, or communities within the nations of the developing world."[24]

Earl Conteh-Morgan provided his readers with several historical and contemporary examples of the allegedly pernicious impact of these policies. For example, he commented on how some of the neoliberal ideas about the need for legitimacy, and contemporary consolidations of power, could be linked to a time when the government of Sierra Leone was viewed as a "mere replica of the British colonial administration." This meant that the British colonial government in Sierra Leone tried to "enforce policies of fiscal austerity as a way of minimizing the cost of ruling the country."[25] This contextualization of one key economic aspect of this West African nation's colonial legacy could then be used to illustrate some of the political and historical origins of some of the ideologies that led to the structural adjustment policies of the 1980s.

Interestingly enough, Earl Conteh-Morgan did not deny that African corruption played a key role in some of the devastation and civil wars that Sierra Leone would experience in the post-independence years. For example, he wrote that by the end of the 1970s the euphoria and revolutionary spirits that was tied to independence had given way to feelings of disenchantment as post-colonial Sierra Leone dealt with "neopatrimonialism," "clientism," "neopotism" and corruption. Neopatrimonialism referred to the ways that the elite intellectual leaders and others tried to mimic the behavior of their former colonizers, while clientelism had to do with the reciprocity that existed between the ruling elite and their supports.[26]

Conteh-Morgan showed how all of these various "–isms" impacted the ways that the government of President Stevens reacted to some of the first Structural Adjustment Programs that were negotiated with Sierra Leone, and he explained how in the beginning many West Africans in that country were worried that these plans would hurt rice producers as well as the sale of petroleum products. Later on, when the World Bank recommended that state employment be reduced by one third, and when some of these World Bank/IMF policies were adopted by the Momoh regime, the price of rice, the staple diet of the country, rose by almost 180 percent and the cost of petrol rose as well. All of this, Conteh-Morgan argued, helped the state of soldiers' dissatisfaction with salaries, and this exacerbated, rather than alleviated, Sierra Leone's economic woes.[27]

Sadly, Conteh-Morgan's 2006 discussion of how all of this impacted Sierra Leone's health care may help explain why that nation had such difficulties coping with the Ebola outbreak that it faced in 2014–2015. He outlined in his essay how the IMF structural adjustment policies and other austerity measures that were imposed on the people of Sierra Leone resulted in drastic cuts in health care delivery services. The combined effect of the "oil shocks, the adverse impact on foreign trade created a situation where by the early 1990s Sierra Leone was characterized as one of the countries with the worst quality of life, where the infant mortality rate was 160 per 100 live births, and the life expectancy was only 40 years for both sexes. "Prior to the implement of cost recovery programs," argued Conteh-Morgan, "medical services and drugs were provided almost free of charge," but with the adoption of austerity measures prices rose and the public could not to pay for either drugs or hospital care.[28] Many of the people living in Sierra Leone, he claimed, were convinced that all of these economic hardships later produced rebellions and civil wars.

While cultural critics and legal scholars need to be wary of accepting at face value this commentary on what looks like an idyllic world of free medical services before all of this austerity, Conteh-Morgan's work does remind us of the lingering impact of colonial, imperial, and decolonizing financial *epistemes*. The governments and populations of West Africa who tried to rebuild their lives after decades of conflict may have had to confront even more challenges when they had to deal with those in the global North who were trying to rescue them from their economic woes. In 2011 the Deputy Minister of Health for Planning Research, and Development in Liberia, Tornorlah Varpilah, wrote a co-authored essay where he and his colleagues explained what President Ellen Johnson Sirleaf's administration was trying to do about the fact that so members of that nation's health workforce were leaving the country.[29] They explained how a fourteen-year civil war (1989–2003) had left Liberia's health care system in shambles, and how most of the health care professionals who were living in that region had either fled or had died during the fighting. To give readers a vivid picture of the impact of the war, Varpilah and his co-authors offered the staggering statistic that in 1988 there had been around 3,500 persons working in the public health sector in Liberia, but ten years later there were only about 1,400 persons left, with only 89 physicians and 329 nurses.[30]

Even before she officially took office, President Ellen Johnson Sirleaf had put together a 2005 plan for emergency human resources (HR), but Varpilah and his colleagues had to admit that Liberia was still dependent on foreign medical humanitarianism. In one section of their paper they explain,

> By 1990 most medical specialists had left Liberia, leaving only general prac-
> titioners. From 1989 to 2003, civil war resulted in a severely fragmented and
> incapacitated health system. As concessionaires and high-level workers left,
> non-governmental organization (NGO) emergency aid organizations began
> to arrive. The first to enter was Médecins Sans Frontières (MSF) in 1989. This
> began an NGO-centric health care system in which health facilities were
> dependent on external aid to function. By 2003, Liberia had 420 facilities (12
> public hospitals, 32 public health centers, 189 public clinics, 10 private hospi-
> tals, 10 private health centers, 167 private clinics), 45% of which were being
> managed by NGOs and faith-based organizations (FBOs).[31]

Given these scenarios, we can readily understand some of the resentment that had been building up before the arrival of the latest Ebola outbreak. In a host of ways, well-intentioned medical interventionism was con-tributing to a cycle of dependence, which in turn catalyzed new debates about the political economies of long-term and short-term health plans. After the 2003 signing of the Comprehensive Peace Agreement in Ghana, more than $80 million in international aid flowed into Liberia, but the exodus of elite medical professionals meant that six years later that nation was still having to deal with "ruined infrastructure, limited funding, lack of faculty and training capacity, overcrowded classes, outdated curricula, insufficient resources and no regulation."[32]

Varpilah and his co-authors also noted how some of the negotiated limits that had been set by the Liberian government in its dealing with global financial institutions meant that payments to health care workers were consistently delayed. These problems were compounded by the lack of incentives for health workers who could have been deployed to under-served rural locations. All of these salary problems, along with a lack of any national government benefits package, resulted in a further migration of skilled staff in Liberia to NGO health facilities.[33]

At this point in their chronicling of Liberia's historical health woes, Varpilah and his co-authors explained that they tried to draw some les-sons from some other African health systems, and they worked with the Department of Ministry to incrementally raise some salaries, but part of the strings that were attached to debt relief plans negotiated with the IMF meant that Liberians had to accept an employment ban in the public sector. The World Bank Heavily Indebted Poor Country Initiative (HIPC) was revised in 2007 to allow for a moderate increase in the minimum wage but the low salaries still made it difficult for the Liberian govern-ment to compete when they were looking for qualified civil servants. The Liberians managed to get by through the use of temporary donor gap-filling efforts that raised some $20 million to help with the salaries of doctors, pharmacists, and other health workers.[34]

As one of Liberia's leading health planners, Varpilah had to be circumspect in the way that he discussed IMF and World Bank austerity measures, but at one point in their essay Virpilah and his co-authors were quite candid that Liberians had their own ideas about how to combat their health problems. "Many of the standard international strategies to improve health resources such as continuing education, supervision and incentive payment" did not work in Liberian contexts, they argued, because they "do not consider Liberia's specific challenges."[35]

Yet as readers might imagine, others defended IMF or World Bank practices, and they were the social agents who were convinced that structural adjustments had nothing to do with lack of Ebola preparedness.

DEFENDING THE IMF AND WORLD BANK
AND THE FUNDING OF EBOLA RELIEF EFFORTS

Defenders of the World Bank or the IMF responded to these lamentations in two different, and diametrically opposed ways. While some supporters of fiscal austerity and structural adjustment plans wanted *to magnify* the contributions that were provided by global financial planners others wanted to avoid this ideological quagmire by going in the other direction and *minimizing* the power of these same institutions.[36] For example it could be argued that these global, foreign financial institutions have little do with West African resource conflicts, revolutions, famines, or the decisions that are made by regional or local governmental powers. Banking personnel or their defenders could argue that the IMF does not have "direct influence," and that health "ministry officials do not routinely meet IMF missions to discuss the conditions of bailouts."[37] While one approach embraced the politicized nature of this funding, the other sought to dissociate IMF policies from state political decisionism.

Those who took this latter approach could configure the IMF and the World Bank as global public servants, communities who relied on economic experts who helped impoverished nations learn the lessons that come from studying basic economic theories and practices. If that meant having to learn about austerity measures and the exodus of some doctors and nurses, then so be it. Those who adopt this position can argue that the unanticipated appearance of a "natural" phenomenon, like Ebola, has nothing to do with the financial concerns or expertise of large international money lenders.

In the same way that WHO leaders were attacked for their belated interventionism, IMF employees had to explain why their financial planning had not interfered with Ebola fighting efforts. The December 2014

announcement that the IMF was going to help with debt relief supported
the efforts of those who chose to magnify the economic power of external financial institutions. For example, the deputy director for the IMF
fiscal Affairs Department, Sanjeev Gupta, wrote about how critics were
wrong to cite statistics that showed that health expenditures in West
Africa *had gone down* after they received support from the International
Monetary Fund. He argued that if you looked at the cumulative data
provided by the World Bank you would find that the "health outcomes"
in sub-Saharan Africa, including Liberia, Guinea, and Sierra Leone, had
improved over the last decade.[38] At the same time, he pointed out that
according to IMF estimates, in the three years before the Ebola outbreak
health spending had increased 0.7 percentage points in Guinea, in Liberia
by 1.6 percentage points, and in Sierra Leone by 0.24 percentage points.[39]
Furthermore, he argued that it was a myth to believe that the IMF still
required caps on the public sector wage bills in West Africa.[40]

Using these types of statistics Sanjeev Gupta painted a fairly rosy picture of a West Africa that had been steadily inching forward, a region
that was making economic progress, before the advent of the latest Ebola
outbreak. No doubt the fourteen-year civil war had a devastating effect
on the social structures, and "the arrival of Ebola put severe pressure on
already fragile infrastructure and health care systems," but Gupta argued
that this did not mean that the IMF hadn't mobilized quickly and or
hadn't offered urgent assistance to these needy nations. After all, he could
point out that in 2014 the IMF "made available" another $130 million so
that Liberia, Guinea, and Sierra Leone could fight Ebola.[41]

As soon as critics started to complain about the inordinate power
and the unwarranted interference of the World Bank or the IMF, many
economists, political scientists, financial planners, and others defended
the polices of the "North." For example, some participants in this debate,
who had confidence in their credentials, reminded the readers of their
essays of the continued importance of taking into account the economic
facets of this epidemic. Chris Blattman, for example, tried to argue that
critics of organizations like the World Bank or the IMF simply did not understand the governmentalities of "these places," their "local politics," or
the difficulties associated with dealing with "weak states."[42] He accused
these detractors of doing "research from afar," and he lamented the fact
that they were "ignoring politics." Blattman was convinced that his own
research showed that countries like Liberia and Sierra Leone were "actually awash with more outside money than ever before," and he implied
that the absence of fiscally responsible measures would lead to even more
waste of needed capital.[43]

These types of neoliberal critiques did not dwell on the economic histories behind these exploitations or the creative destruction that might

have contributed to formation of these supposed "failed states" in the first place. Note, for example, how Blattman tried to divert the attention of readers of *The Washington Post* away from the social agency of the IMF and toward a variety of external factors that had to do with localized geopolitical conditions and the motivations of bureaucrats in West Africa. After "decades of war and political instability," argued Blattman, the "real problem is that they don't have the people or the public organizations capable of spending more money well," even if they wanted to.[44] As far as Blattman was concerned, the nations of West Africa were "lining the pockets of supporters" while they also prioritized the building of roads and power lines.[45] For like-minded economists and other pundits, this mixing and matching of irrational and rational decision making was something that was missed by detractors who bashed the IMF.

There are of course a number of hidden, conservative premises that were operating in these neoliberal ways of viewing the role that Western financial institutions could play in helping the West Africans. This type of *dispositif* assumed that the IMF was supervised by beneficent Westerners who had no interest in resource dispossession. Scenarios like Blattman's assumed that Africans were the ones who played the major roles in the dystopic wars and other conflicts of the 1980s and 1990s. This made it appear as if economic instability in the region existed before, or apart from, any interference from the West.

At the same time these neoliberal *dispositifs* resonated with many economists and bankers in the West because they allowed these decision makers to assume that those in the "North" were the ones who could rescue the West Africans who suffered from the ravages of Ebola and other diseases. In theory, empowered countries outside of African had the right economic roadmaps for recovery, the right people, and the right organizations that would set things right. In another portion of his *Washington Post* piece, Blattman explains that because of firsthand experience he knew what it was like to work in a "weak state," and his analysis contained personal asides as he commented on how his previous work on unnamed programs in Liberia nearly "broke" him. This all adds to his ethos as he argued that this situational awareness provided him with needed, and rare, insight into how some of these countries had actually experienced only about a decade of real stability. A "lot that we take for granted in other countries," even in other poor countries, explained an exasperated Blattman, simply do not work in places like Liberia.[46]

What was really bothering Blattman were the assertions that appeared in an article in *The Lancet*, which was written by some researchers at the London School of Hygiene and Tropical Medicine. In an essay authored by Alexander Kentikelenis, Lawrence King, Martin McKee, and David Stuckler, the authors applauded the fact that in December of 2014 the

International Monetary Fund had finally announced that almost $430 million in funding was going to set aside to fight Ebola in West Africa. However, they qualified this praise by raising the question of whether decades of earlier IMF policies had "enabled the crisis to arise in the first place."[47] In his summary of the work of Kenitkelenis and his colleagues Blattman claimed that their basic argument was that the IMF was just giving "lip service" to social services, and that the IMF's "insistence on financial austerity" was starving the health systems of West African countries.[48]

Given the fact that more than 11,300 people have died from EVD since this most recent Ebola outbreak in West Africa,[49] it is obvious that this is not just a disciplinary squabble between professors from three leading British universities and a political economist who once worked in Liberia. Nor are their arguments just about the particular fiscal policies that were made by the IMF during one month in late 2014. The disputes that we are witnessing between these writers is a twenty-first-century permutation of an ancient quarrel, which reprises the old colonial and imperial debates about how to best expend scarce world resources. In the same way that British imperialists once defended the selective funding of tropical disease programs in the "White Man's graveyard" contemporaries now argued about the strategic deployment of international debt repayment or increased medical humanitarianism in the form of more social spending. Like usual, these financial positions were often linked to broader ideological assumptions that were being made about the needs of Westerners as well as the needs of the recipients of this beneficence.

At the same time that global audiences were hearing about the possible containment of the Ebola outbreak, some of the detractors of IMF and World Bank policies were circulating narratives about the pernicious nature of outside financial interference. Just a few months before Liberia announced that it was "free" of Ebola, Alexander Kentikelenis, Lawrence King, and Martin McKee were busy responding to those who defended the IMF's practices in West African contexts. They argued that political scientists like Chris Blattman, who thought that the "IMF is irrelevant to the discussions of health policies in poor countries," were making mistakes when they ignored the large body of research that showed some of the varied effects that IMF programs had on tuberculosis, HIV, and other health programs. IMF policies, they averred in January of 2015, "exacerbated the problems of state capacity" during post-conflict periods.[50]

Instead of praising those at the IMF who sent more money flows in the direction of West African nations, Kentikelenis, King, and McKee argued that you needed to keep any eye on the actual impact of these efforts. After all, what good could come of this if austerity measures remained in place, to the point where little of this monetary flow translated into additional government health expenditures? How much of this financial help, asked Kentikelenis, King, and McKee, turned into health aid displacement?

Notwithstanding the release of the December 2014 expenditures, these skeptics argued that the "impact of the IMF" over the years has been to place Guinea and Liberia, and then Sierra Leone, under "IMF tutelage."[51] This type of argumentative language sounded as if West Africa was still the "Gold Coast" of yesteryear, a place in the Global "South" that was under the economic thumb of those in the North who thought that they knew better.

In many ways those who participated in these debates about the positive or negative impacts of IMF policies were producing economic *dispositifs* that resembled the more graphic Ebola apocalyptic rhetorics, but this time the antagonists were those financiers who were promoting problematic Western policies. This is one of the reasons why, when Kentikelenis, King, and McKee mention the "collateral damage" from IMF conditionalities on public spending, or why when they talk about adverse impacts despite "the rhetoric of the IMF to the contrary," we get pictures in our heads of a thanatopolitical world of chaos that was brought on by misleading lending policies. As Professor Dionne explains, there may be times when rural Africans may not be that interested in Western priorities or fiscal planning, when they have their own ideas regarding public health prioritization. She noted how they may want to prioritize spending that goes toward improved public health or sanitation projects that help with tuberculosis or diarrheal diseases that are prevalent in sub-Sahara Africa.[52]

Readers can of course anticipate that neoliberals can respond that fiscally irresponsible West Africans should not have the dominant say in how to prioritize the fiscal policies that might guide future economic planning in the region. For example, in a follow-up essay to his previous article in *The Washington Post*, the indefatigable Chris Blattman, on January 7, 2015, asked millions of readers this question: "Who Has Responsibility for Ebola? The IMF, the West, or Unpleasant Accounting?"[53] Blattman, like many defenders of international financial institutions, tried to distance himself from any discussion of the slave trade, colonialism, ecological devastation, and so forth. While he thought it was useful to keep this familiar "history" in mind, he really wanted to focus most of his attention on IMF's "current policies."[54] From a critical cultural vantage point one could argue this allows him to strategically focus on the social agency of the West Africans while treating those in the North as innocent parties who have to react to chaotic "African" activities.

Blattman, in his 2015 essay, argued that the notion that "austerity kills" was not something unique to West African relationships with the IMF, and he was convinced that this was the type of rhetoric that was used by many of those who "hold the IMF and their ilk responsible" for the lack of social spending in this region.[55] What bothered him, as a political scientist, were all of the apparent inferential leaps that were being made by detractors who were intent on connecting the dots that could then be used to place blame at the doorsteps of the global financial institutions. In one portion of his 2015 essay he remarked,

> There are a lot of assumptions you have to make to connect IMF policies to something like Ebola. A whole string of them runs through a simple chain from more money to health outcomes, something like this: *If* the government had more money, and *if* it chose to spend it on health, and *if* it chose to spend it on health investments that would help respond to this particular kind of health crisis, and *if* more inputs resulted in better health care and systems (meaning something else isn't holding back good public service delivery), then, yes, more government funding would have helped avert the crisis.[56] [Emphases in the original]

He seemed to be implying that social scientists and other observers needed to accept the evidentiary burden of replacing those "ifs" with actual causal connects.

Yet like many arguers who wanted to focus on economic warrants and evidence, Blattman's supposed objective assessment is filled with implicit *normative* assumptions about economic conditions, governmental relationships, and the spending habits of West Africans. Blattman's sub-claims and overarching narrative were being use to imply that West Africans did not necessarily deserve, or need, more aid. Blattman argued that during the Ebola crisis you had to think like economists, in terms of "trade-offs," and he alleged that this was something that the critics of the IMF were unwilling to do. The skeptics were writing as if places like Liberia had multiple revenue streams, or they were talking as if other countries had an obligation to provide more aid, and he thought that all of this did not take into account the fact that these countries had to be forced into making "hard choices."[57] Instead of viewing the Ebola-ravaged countries as needy, impoverished nations, Blattman portrayed places like Liberia and Sierra Leone as countries that had already spent a lot of money and he asserted that readers would be hard-pressed to find other places in the world that had spent "more money than they did in the last 10 years." This led him to ultimately conclude that this health care mess was really just an "unpleasant accounting" issue that had to be faced by those who were unwilling to learn the hard economic lessons that needed to be taught by the IMF—that poor countries, which had few tax revenues, can only get so much aid, and they needed to be cautious about how they spent it.[58]

The rhetorical beauty of this type of argumentation is that it allows the defenders of international financial institutions to appear as though they are innocent bystanders, *reactive or defensive* parties who are pressured into helping irrational communities who have little ability to control their pocketbooks. Bloggers and writers like Blattman explicitly bracket out colonial histories in a rush to talk about contemporary conditions, and they don't mind treating health care finances as an "accounting" problem that makes it appear as if the West African should shoulder the lion's share of the blame for the lack of Ebola preparedness.

I would go so far as to argue that a critical cultural review of some of this economic discourse may help us understand some of the ideological complexities of the situation, and why we would be naïve to think that everyone simply wanted to handle the West African Ebola crisis by throwing money at it. In one of key segment of his 2015 *Washington Post* essay, Blattman wrote that the "IMF is the messenger, cheerleader, and sometimes the enforcer of this so-called fiscal discipline." Yes, it was true, the IMF could at times be "bossy, undemocratic, often ideological, and sometimes wrong," but wasn't it possible that the other alternatives— "bankruptcy or full scale financial meltdown"—were even worse?[59]

In sum, the defenders of the IMF have their own ways of coming up with dystopic visions of what will happen if you don't listen to the perceived wisdom of international financial institutions during times of perceived crises.[60]

CONCLUSION

In this particular chapter I have argued that the adoption of critical genealogical perspectives that have been advocated by critical cultural or critical legal scholars allows readers to see some of the symbolic and material linkages that can be made between the *epistemes* that circulated in colonial periods and today's economic climate. The arguments that resurfaced in more contemporary debates about the roles that the IMF and the World Bank played before, during, and after the advent of the 2013–2015 West African Ebola outbreak can be thought of as echoes of older arguments that once circulated during a period when West Africa was configured as the "White Man's Grave," a costly place that drained the British empire.

Viewing some of the genealogical origins of these elite and public attacks and defenses of some of these global institutions helps us understand some of the empirical and theoretical difficulties that confronted leaders in Guinea, Sierra Leone, and Liberia who had to watch the exodus of needed doctors, nurses, and other health care workers before the December 2013 "discovery" of Patient Zero. If the critics of IMF and World Bank policies are to be believed, then the structural adjustments that were put in place before this time made it difficult, if not impossible, to provide the financial incentives that were needed to keep together a viable public health care labor force that could contain the Ebola epidemic. We therefore need to understand some of the ideological and political tensions that were represented by the heated conversations that took place between writers like Blattman and Kenitkelenis and his co-authors, so that we can produce informed critiques of the role that the IMF, the World Bank, empowered nation-states in the "North," and even private philanthropists can play when emerging infectious diseases wreak this type of havoc.

One of the reasons that I spent this much time in this chapter parsing the words of these particular disputants is that this debate in *The Washington Post* about the IMF and the responsibilities of the West ideologically drifted into the blogosphere. Lee Crawfurd, for example, an economist, agreed with Blattman and thought it was a mistake to think of the IMF as "some kind of magic money tree."[61] Crawfurd differentiated between the rights of those in the West, who could rail against austerity and still support fiscal discipline, and the rights of those in poor countries who he felt were trying to argue that the IMF should be blamed for not letting them spend more of their "income definitely."[62] This type of argumentative strategy allowed all types of participants in these conversations to avoid having to say very much about Ebola, or the dismantling of public health infrastructures, as they dispassionately discussed abstract neoliberal theories of fiscal responsibility. What all of this hid, of course, was the fact that some in the West did not want to pay for the fiscal sins of "the other" overseas.

By early 2015 an increased number of academics, decision makers, and others were willing to argue that World Bank or IMF policies may have hurt Ebola containment efforts. Adia Benton and Kim Yi Dionne, who were active contributors to both mainstream newspaper debates as well as blogging conversations, cited Blattman's work and then proceeded to refute many of his arguments.[63] Both of these scholars had already written important manuscripts on the geopolitics of HIV/AIDS relief,[64] and they now explained how some global policy priorities and donors' "misaligned funding" were hindering the fight against the spread of Ebola. Powerful "Western agencies like PEFAR, the Global Fund and UNAIDS," they averred, "often organize and fund their priorities with limited insights from the local communities who are their 'intended beneficiaries.'"[65]

Benton and Dionne realized that there were many divergent factors that led to the discovery of Patient Zero and the beginning of the latest Ebola outbreak in West Africa in December of 2013, and they were will willing to say that the IMF was not "wholly to blame" for the epidemic, but they were convinced that the IMF and organizations like that one had played an "important role in creating a political environment in which the epidemic could emerge and become the deadliest on record."[66] Benton and Dionne also placed some of the blame on the shoulders of the governments of Liberia, Guinea, and Sierra Leone, but they also wanted to underscore the "myopia" that they thought was an inherent feature of much of the international funding for health in the region. They elaborated by noting how the IMF put a premium on projects that were "mobile, replicable, and scalable," and that these templates were chosen because they appealed to major donors who thought that they could be implemented everywhere and anywhere by anyone.[67]

Many of the critics of the IMF and World Bank argued that if you just looked at the economic picture through single snapshots of time that traced money flows over months, or paid attention to what happened during a single year, then you missed the *longitudinal impact* of these aid trends and their adverse impact on the poor nations that dealt with endemic and epidemic situations. For example, one group of researchers were adamant that the IMF "legacy of austerity measures" and structural reforms, if viewed through cumulative prisms, allowed one to see the long-term adverse consequences of these restrictions.[68]

NOTES

1. Chris Blattman, quoted in Tom Murphy, "Wonks Disagree over Whether IMF Contributed to Ebola Crisis," Humanosphere, last modified January 14, 2015, paragraph 8, http://www.humanosphere.org/world-politics/2015/01/wonks-disagree-whether-imf-contributed-ebola-crisis/.

2. Neoliberals who talk about how to combat "emerging" infectious diseases have often blamed kleptomaniacs like Charles Taylor and his ilk for making sure that corrupt officials interfered with the mythic economic marketplace that otherwise might have helped these countries.

3. Ibrahim Abdullah, "Ebola: Where We Are, Where We Should Be," Africa Is a Country, last modified October 18, 2014, http://africasacountry.com/2014/10/ebola-where-we-are-where-we-should-be/.

4. See, for example, Ann Laura Stoler, "Colonial Archives and the Arts of Governance," *Archival Science* 2 (2002): 87–109.

5. Morten Boas, *The Politics of Conflict Economies: Miners, Merchants, and Warriors in the African Borderlands* (New York: Routledge, 2015), xv–xvi.

6. See, for example, the classic commentary on these fears that appears in F. Harrison Rankin, *The White Man's Grave: A Visit to Sierra Leone, in 1834* (London: Richard Bently, 1836).

7. For an intriguing discussion of some of the cultural, social, and economic features of anti-malarial campaigns during British imperial periods in Sierra Leone, see Stephen Frankel and John Western, "Pretext or Prophylaxis? Racial Segregation and Malarial Mosquitos in a British Tropical Colony: Sierra Leone," *Annals of the Association of American Geographers* 78, no. 2 (June, 1988): 211–228.

8. Ronald Ross, quoted in Frankel and Western, "Pretext or Prophylaxis," 214.

9. Frankel and Western, "Pretext or Prophylaxis," 214.

10. Ibid., 222.

11. Ibid., 222.

12. C. Braithwaite Wallis, *The Advance of Our West Africa Empire* (1903; New York: Negro Universities, 1969), 263.

13. James Pfeiffer and Rachel Chapman, "Anthropological Perspectives on Structural Adjustment and Public Health," *Annual Review of Anthropology* 39 (2010): 149–165.

14. Pfeiffer and Chapman, "Anthropological Perspectives," 150. Pfeiffer and Chapman are of course not the observers who have noted the colonial, imperial, or neo-colonial dimensions of the current Ebola outbreak in West Africa. Ibrahim Abdullah has opined,

> That an imperial rescue mission had to evolve as the preferred form of Western response to the so-called Ebola crisis begins to undermine the lie about the UN and WHO in providing the necessary wherewithal to make robust intervention a reality. Both the UN and the WHO are dependent on funding from the imperial citadels. Starved of funds they just cannot function. . . . The UNDP, UNIDO, WHO et al [sic] operate, or are in business, because of us; the other; they were not designed for or operate in the West. Similarly organisations like WHO, UNDP, UNIDO serve the interest of those at the imperial citadels through funding and control. Like the UN, WHO could not intervene in a timely manner not only because they have funding problems but precisely because the organisation's haemorrhagic fever department had being dismantled after the SARS scare in 2008/09. Why dismantle a department that exclusively serves a disadvantaged region of the world in an outfit that is supposedly designed as a global institution? (Abdullah, "Ebola: Where We Are," paragraph 6)

15. Pfeiffer and Chapman, "Anthropological Perspectives," 150.

16. See David Harvey, *A Brief History of Neoliberalism* (Oxford: Oxford Univ. Press, 2005).

17. Pfeiffer and Chapman, "Anthropological Perspectives," 158.

18. Ibid., 158.

19. Richard Rowden, *The Deadly Ideas of Neoliberalism: How the IMF Has Undermined Public Health and the Fight against AIDS* (London: Zed Books, 2009).

20. Paul Farmer, *AIDS and Accusation: Haiti and Geography of Blame* (Berkeley: University of California Press, 1992), 264.

21. Andrew S. Boozary, Paul E. Farmer, and Ashish K. Jha, "The Ebola Outbreak: Fragile Health Systems and Quality as a Cure," *The Journal of the American Medical Association* 312, no. 18 (November 12, 2014): 1859–1860, 1859.

22. Earl Conteh-Morgan, Globalization, State Failure, and Collective Violence: The Case of Sierra Leone," *International Journal of Peace Studies* 11, no. 2 (Autumn/Winter, 2006): 87–103, http://www.gmu.edu/programs/icar/ijps/vol11_2/11n2C-M.pdf.

23. Ibid., 87.

24. Ibid., 88.

25. Ibid., 96.

26. Ibid., 96.

27. Ibid., 96–98.

28. Ibid., 99.

29. Tornorlah Varpilah et al., "Rebuilding Human Resources for Health: A Case Study from Liberia," *Human Resources for Health* 9, no. 11 (2011): 1–9, http://www.human-resources-health.com/content/pdf/1478-4491-9-11.pdf. For more on Tornorlah Varpilah's background, see *All Africa* Staff, "Liberia: Deputy Minister of Health Tornorlah," *Allafrica.com*, last modified October 18, 2007, http://allafrica.com/stories/200710181227.html.

30. Varpilah et al., "Rebuilding Human Resources," 1.

31. Ibid., 2. See Government of Liberia: Ministry of Health and Social Welfare and World Health Organization, *Liberia Health Situation Analysis, Final Report* (Geneva: World Health Organization, 2002).

32. Varpilah et al., "Rebuilding Human Resources," 2, 4.

33. Ibid., 3.

34. Ibid., 4.

35. Ibid., 8.

36. For example, a 2004 study by Ricardo Martin and Alex Segura-Ubiergo argued that the countries that were supported by the IMF did not experience any major adverse effect on their public social spending. Ricardo Martin and Alex Segura-Ubiergo, "Social Spending in IMF-Supported Programs," *IEO Background Paper*, 2004, http://econwpa.repec.org/eps/pe/papers/0504/0504011.pdf.

37. Kentikelenis, King, and McKee, "The IMF's Influence on Poor Countries' Health," paragraph 4. This is how these three authors are trying to interpret Blattman's argument about how the IMF has no "real influence." They surmised that he meant that the IMF only had indirect influence.

38. Sanjeev Gupta, "Response to 'The International Monetary Fund and the Ebola Outbreak,'" *The Lancet* 3, no. 2 (January 5, 2015): e78. Another defense of IMF Policies appears in another co-authored essay by Sangeev Gupta. See B. Clements, Sanjeev Gupta, and M. Nozaki, "What Happens to Public Health Spending in IMF-Supported Programs? Another look," Blogimf, last modified December 21, 2014, http://blog-imfdirect.imf.org/2014/12/21/what-happens-to-public-health-spending-in-imf-supported-programs-another-look/.

39. Gupta, "Response to 'The International Monetary Fund,'" e78.

40. See also Jan Kees Martijn and Shamsuddin Tareq, "IMF Moves to Clarify Aid Role," International Monetary Fund, last modified July 20, 2007, http://www.imf.org/external/pubs/ft/survey/so/2007/NEW0720B.htm.

41. Gupta, "Response to 'The International Monetary Fund,'" e78. Gupta cited IMF Survey. "IMF Approves $130 Million for Countries Worst Hit by Ebola," International Monetary Fund, last modified September 26, 2014, http://www.imf.org/external/pubs/ft/survey/so/2014/new092614a.htm.

42. Chris Blattman, for example, in an essay titled "Did the International Monetary Fund Help Make the Ebola Outbreak?," *The Washington Post*, last modified December 30, 2014, http://www.washingtonpost.com/blogs/monkey-cage/wp/2014/12/30/did-the-international-monetary-fund-help-make-the-ebola-crisis/. Blattman is providing just a representative example of this type of discourse,

where researchers are trying to investigate the impact of particular governmental or multilateral initiatives. Note here the work of Peter Nunnenkamp and Hannes Öhler, "Throwing Foreign Aid at HIV/AIDS in Developing Countries: Missing the Target?" *World Development* 39, no. 10 (2011): 1704–1723.

43. Blattman, "Did the International Monetary Fund," paragraphs 5–6.

44. Ibid., paragraph 7.

45. Ibid., paragraph 7.

46. Ibid., paragraph 8.

47. Alexander Kenitkelenis, Lawrence King, Martin McKee, and David Stuckler, "The International Monetary Fund and the Ebola Crisis," *The Lancet* 3 (February 2015) e69–e70, e69. Kentikelenis and his co-authors also provided a detailed, point-by-point refutation of Blattman's *Washington Post* essay in that same venue. Alexander Kentikelenis, Lawrence King, and Martin McKee, "The IMF's Influence on Poor Countries' Health System—And Ebola, Explained," *The Washington Post*, last modified January 6, 2015, http://www.washingtonpost.com/blogs/monkey-cage/wp/2015/01/06/the-imfs-influence-on-poor-countries-health-systems-and-ebola-explained/. Their response included citations to a wealth of previous studies on the impact that IMF policies had on various public health care programs around the world. See, for example, David Stuckler, Lawrence P. King, and Sanjay Basu, "International Monetary Fund Programs and Tuberculosis Outcome in Post-Communist Countries," *PLoS Medicine* 5 (July 2008): 1079–1090; Doris A. Oberdabernig," Revisiting the Effects of IMF Programs On Poverty and Inequality," *World Development* 46 (June, 2013): 113–142.

48. Blattman, "Did the International Monetary Fund," paragraph 4. Actually Kenitkelenis, King, and McKee were talking about a series of interrelated problems, including limitations on what health professionals in West Africa could be paid, the encouragement of reduction in government spending that came from IMF external pressures, and impact this had on a decentralized health care system.

49. *The Economist*, "The Toll of a Tragedy," *The Economist*, last modified August 27, 2015, http://www.economist.com/blogs/graphicdetail/2015/08/ebola-graphics.

50. Alexander Kentikelenis, Lawrence King, and Martin McKee, "The IMF's Influence on Poor Countries' Health," paragraphs 2–3.

51. Ibid., paragraph 4.

52. Kim Yi Dionne, "Local Demand for a Global Intervention: Policy Priorities in the Time of AIDS, *World Development* 40, no. 12 (December 1, 2012): 2468–2477, 2474. doi:10.1016/j.worlddev.2012.05.016.

53. Chris Blattman, "Who has Responsibility for Ebola? The IMF, the West, or Unpleasant Accounting?" *The Washington Post*, last modified January 7, 2015, http://www.washingtonpost.com/blogs/monkey-cage/wp/2015/01/07/who-has-responsibility-for-ebola-the-imf-the-west-or-unpleasant-accounting/.

54. Ibid., paragraph 2.

55. Ibid., paragraph 6.

56. Ibid., paragraph 7.

57. Ibid., paragraphs 10–13.

58. Ibid., paragraph 14.

59. Ibid., paragraph 14.

60. Like those who attacked him, Blattman had his own preferred reading lists. One of the texts that he suggested that readers of *The Washington Post* get their hands on was Nicolas Van de Walle, *African Economies and the Politics of Permanent Crisis, 1979–1999* (New York: Cambridge University Press, 2001).

61. Lee Crawfurd, "The IMF and Ebola," RovingBandit.com, last modified January 7, 2015, paragraph 3, http://www.rovingbandit.com/2015/01/the-imf-and-ebola.html.

62. Crawfurd, "The IMF and Ebola," paragraph 4.

63. Adia Benton and Kim Yi Dionne, "5 Things You Should Read before Saying the IMF is Blameless in the 2014 Ebola Outbreak," *The Washington Post,* last modified January 5, 2015, http://www.washingtonpost.com/blogs/monkey-cage/wp/2015/01/05/5-things-you-should-read-before-saying-the-imf-is-blameless-in-the-2014-ebola-outbreak/.

64. Adia Benton, *HIV Exceptionalism: Development through Disease in Sierra Leone* (Minneapolis: University of Minnesota Press, 2015); Dionne, "Local Demand for a Global Intervention."

65. Benton and Dionne, "5 Things You Should Read," paragraph 10.

66. Ibid., paragraph 11.

67. Ibid., paragraphs 10–11.

68. Kentikelenis, King, and McKee, "The IMF's Influence on Poor Countries' Health," paragraph 4.

6

Anticipating the Ebola Apocalypse and American Mediascapes

Government authorities, public health officials, and journalists who talk and write about the spread of infectious diseases have a difficult time drawing that mythic line that is supposed to exist between providing citizens with adequate warnings and creating moral panic.[1] As Laurie Garrett would write in February of 2015, it seems as though "humans always overreact" during disease outbreaks because they each have "social and political ramifications that go far beyond anything that sound reasonable" as we try to handle "the interaction of our species with a particular set of microbes."[2] The stories that are still told about the U.S. governmental response to the outbreak of "Spanish flu" in 1918, for example, remind us that responsible social agents sometimes made the mistake of *not sounding* needed alarms. Critics of American policies during that period later complained that the public had not been adequately warned before bodies started piling up during a global pandemic that killed millions.[3]

At other times governmental officials, and members of the media, don't err on the side of caution, and instead of allaying fears they anger communities when they are accused of hyping threats, such as the infamous 1976 swine flu "debacle."[4] All of this becomes incredibly complicated in public health contexts when so many stakeholders—pharmaceutical companies, government officials, public health employees, doctors, nurses, and others—become participants in cultural and legal debates about what to do in "emerging" infectious disease contexts.

This particular chapter draws from the work of Arjun Appadurai and his discussion of "global cultural" flows like "mediascapes" and "ideoscapes" so that I can put on display the ways that films, popular books, and media displays circulate Ebola *dispositifs* that reflected and refracted what American audiences *wanted to see and wanted to hear* about disease prevention and containment.[5] While many mass media scholars are surely right to point out that the media uses particular epistemic or axiological "frames" to help set the agenda during salient controversies, they often do so in ways that are circumscribed and informed by audience expectations.

Journalists and other social agents involved in the production of me-diascapes co-produce these Ebola rhetorics, and they do so in dynamic and recursive ways. For example, both media outlets and public audiences are involved in the decisions that are made to grant, or to withhold, scientific legitimacy in public health contexts. They get to decide who are the contending, and the pretending, "Ebola experts." These decisions, in turn, impact the ways that communities view clarion calls that a particular event constitutes a "crisis," as well as the ways that populations evaluate potential solutions to perceived crises. Stephen Collier and Andrew Lakoff recently commented on how both the manufacturing of crisis, as well the production of solutions, were all parts of what they called a "vital systems security" diagram "of power."[6]

The heuristic value of applying some of Appadurai's conceptual apparatus in studies of global exchange of information, *epistemes*, and other figurations for critical cultural scholars comes from the ways that this approach allows us to apply post-structural, post-colonial, or post-modernist ideas as we study some of these Ebola *dispositifs*. As I argued back in chapter 1, rather than thinking of contemporary debates about Ebola as matters that can be improved by the preservation of some arhetorical, unvarnished and transparent *a priori* monolithic "truths" about Ebola, this stance invites researchers to study the negotiated Foucauldian "truth effects" that take into account the rhetorical production of those perceptual truths.[7]

In Ebola contexts, epidemiological views on EVD pathogenesis, transmission, and containment can be viewed as multilayered parts of what Appadurai would call global "flows" that cross porous borders. From a methodological or perspectival standpoint, this means that critics attend not only to "fact-checking" of some presentist argument that is being made in Ebola debates during press interviews or television broadcasts, but to the sedimented formation of what Appadurai calls an ideoscape.

In this particular chapter, I want unpack the *anticipatory*, often thanato-political apocalyptic outbreak narratives that were produced by several generations of book writers, film makers, and others who claimed that their textual or visual portrayals of EVD or other contagions mirrored historical or contemporaries. I will be arguing that these antecedent rhetorics often set the stage for how Anglo-American and other global audiences would react to the news about the discovery of "Patient Zero" in Guinea in December of 2013. Moreover, the fact that that latest outbreak revived interest in earlier books and movies about Ebola only magnified the persuasive powers of these archival materials.

Certain ideoscapes—especially those that were made up of fragments from neoliberal *dispositifs* on proper health care, mobile relief during emergencies, and the responsibilities of the African "other"—influenced the production and circulation of key twenty-first-century mediascapes. For example, it was taken as a given for decades that those who dealt with "tropical" diseases after the Cold War years had to familiarize themselves with the 1976 "Zaire" Ebola, so that they could see how rural communities in the jungle regions learned about isolation practices. The "rescue" templates that were formed during these earlier times contained ideoscapes that assumed that denizens of Congo or Uganda only needed the interventionist help of a few dozen elite foreigners who worked alongside local health care workers as they made sure that any Ebola epidemic "burned itself out." These representations of the exotic and horrific nature of Ebola, that had little to do with actual health care risks in the West, ensured that mediascapes invented in the global North put on display *possibilistic* scenarios of contagion that mesmerized readers and viewers.

During the first six or seven months of 2014, mainstream media outlets in places like the United States and Europe did occasionally carry stories about Ebola, and they did provide some consciousness raising. However, I will be arguing that the work of writers like Richard Preston and Laurie Garrett, as well as the circulation of movies like *Outbreak* (1995) or *Contagion* (2011), also helped with the co-production of familiar ideoscapes and mediascapes that selectively and strategically contextualized Ebola dangers for Western audiences.[8] The recycling of some of these rhetorical materials may have helped with consciousness raising and some fundraising for organizations like WHO or MSF, but this also had the unintended consequence of encouraged the recirculation of some problematic Ebola representations.

For now, suffice it to say that the fascination with some mediated representations of Ebola ensured that Richard Preston, Laurie Garrett, and even movie producers were sometimes turned into Ebola "experts" at the very time when the Centers for Disease Control and Prevention confirmed the detection of the first "Zaire" Ebola case in the U.S.[9] "Until American doctors treated patients with Ebola were diagnosed with the disease," observed Emily Thomas in early October of 2015, "the current Ebola outbreak has been largely faceless, mainly about statistics and if and when the virus would spread to American soil."[10] Yet as I noted in other chapters, as soon as victims like Thomas Eric Duncan or Nina Pham contracted EVD, interest in Ebola filmic representations and other depictions of infectious diseases spiked.

Some of this facelessness was removed when science journalists, mainstream writers, and authors of alternative press blogs invited their readers and their viewers to pick up those old copies of Preston's *Hot Zone* to help familiarize themselves with current events. Others worried that this was the *last thing* you wanted to do if you wanted to educate yourself about Ebola. As Tara Smith, a writer for Science Blogs would note in October of 2014 for her column on Aetiology,

> I'm still going to criticize *The Hot Zone*, because as a mature infectious disease epidemiologist and a science communicator in the midst of the biggest Ebola outbreak in history, *The Hot Zone* is now one of the banes of my existence. A recent article noted that the book is back on the bestseller list, going as high as #7 on the *New York Times* list recently, and #23 on Amazon. It's sold over 3.5 million copies, and it's reported as "a terrifying true story." Many people have gotten almost all of their Ebola education from just *The Hot Zone* (as they've told me over, and over, and over in the comments to this blog and other sites).[11]

I don't think this will be the last time that we see supposedly "true" or factual representations of Ebola crises used for didactic purposes.

I would argue in this part of my book that if a critical legal scholar or a critical cultural researcher studies some of the mass-mediated reportage of Ebola that circulated between 1976 and 2012, and if they then compare these representations of infectious diseases with the ones that circulated between 2014 and 2015, they will find that the ideoscapes and mediascapes that floated around during these periods were remarkably similar, and that these uncanny, and repetitive arguments worked to decontextualize some of these outbreaks. Oftentimes the books and the movies that circulated before and during this latest Ebola outbreak served as rhetorical vehicles for Ebola *dispositifs* that were produced with little input from Africans or others who were actually "on the spot" fighting Ebola overseas.[12]

What I am arguing here is that the ideoscapes and mediascapes that were popularized during these periods were co-produced by small, but influential groups who lived far away from the EVD "frontlines," and yet their arguments gained traction in Western outlets because they reflected the hegemonic expectations of their viewers and readers. For example, if late twentieth-century or early twenty-first-century audiences expected to see "airborne" Ebola transmissions scenarios, then they were not going to be disappointed. If they wanted to see how Ebola was a complex zoonotic disease, then these influential rhetors could provide visualizations or texts that put on display the transmission of EVD from bats[13] or monkeys to humans. They got to see that "jumping" from species to species.

In other words, even the most detailed of scientific commentaries on Ebola that appear in movies—that may take on the guise of apolitical, innocent, and objective truth telling—need to be thought of as just parts of larger ideoscapes or mediascapes. As Collier and Lakoff explained in 2015, our contemporary ideas regarding "vital systems" vulnerability have been influenced by "anticipatory" and often "rancorous debates" about catastrophic events.[14]

With this in mind, I want to begin by explaining how some earlier Ebola ideoscapes and mediascapes circulated in popular books that were later used to help evidence the credentials of key Ebola "experts."

VIRAL RESCUE TALES, LAURIE GARRETT, AND THE MASS-MEDIATED CRAFTING OF EBOLA EXPERTS

If cultural critics review several decades of media coverage of Ebola *dispositifs* they can't help but notice that some of the same names keep reappearing as Western audiences seek guidance on how they, and their governments, can best respond to the occasional Ebola outbreak. Peter Piot, David Heymann, and Richard Preston are some of the most popular of these figures. Piot was involved with the 1976 outbreak, while David Heymann was there in 1995, when the Congo experienced another epidemic. All three would be interviewed by science reporters or newspaper writers, but it could be argued that it is Laurie Garrett who often receives the lion's share of attention when journalists need to interview "the" key Ebola personality.

Garrett graduated with a degree in immunology from U.C. Berkeley, and since the publication of *The Coming Plague* she has lectured in front of diverse audiences. Moreover, her essays are critiqued in both traditional and alternative press news outlets. Cultural anthropologists and other academics in the blogosphere often express ambivalence when they read her work, but she is the type of affable person that interviewers like to approach when they want to hear about how those in the Global North lavish too much attention on heart disease and cancer and not enough on emerging infectious diseases.

Garrett's work resonates with both elite and lay audiences and she garnered even more attention after becoming the senior fellow for global health at the Council on Foreign Relations. During the fall of 2014, when she was telling audiences that the Ebola epidemic was "doubling every 10 to 20 days," and when she surmised that we didn't have a lot of time because we were racing against the clock,[15] people listened. She was also one of the interviewees who applauded President Obama's decision to send U.S. troops overseas in the name of military humanitarianism.

Interestingly enough, Garrett often adopts the subject position of an expert scientific journalist who is bothered by sensationalist news coverage of Ebola. For example, in an article that appeared in the *Tulsa World*, Garrett both entertained and informed her readers when she explained in September of 2014,

> World, you still just don't get it. . . . The Ebola epidemic . . . will not be conquered with principles of global solidarity and earnest appeals. It will not be stopped with dribbling funds, dozens of volunteer health workers, and barriers across national borders. . . . The WHO doesn't have a giant SWAT team of disease-fighting soldiers ready to swoop into a beleaguered area. . . . In reality, the WHO begs airlines for tickets in coach, pleads with drug companies and protective gear manufacturers for free handouts, and has only the expertise on hand that governments are prepared to payroll and donate.[16]

Note several points here. First of all, notice how Garrett is responding to the belated efforts of WHO, one of the topics that I discussed in chapter 2. At the same time, she is commenting on the austerity measures and the neoliberal trickle-down economic policies that were discussed in the previous chapter on economic argumentation in public health contexts. She belittles the "dribbling funds" that are given grudgingly during Ebola epidemics. Readers, who in an age filled with talk about the "global war on terrorism," can of course guess where she may have gotten that idea of referencing some giant "SWAT team."

The neoliberal ideoscape that Garrett invited her readers to build was a pragmatic one, where organizations like Doctors Without Borders would work with the UN, the U.S. military, and anyone else who was willing to admit that the politicization of WHO had led to its demise. This, in theory, was no time to believe in sentimental humanitarianism and stick by dogmatic universalizing principles, because people in West Africa were dying. Garrett was imploring those in "the North" to do more than circulate what scientists might call "mere rhetoric." She was providing them with a healthy dose of reality.

We should not forget that Garrett was also an empowered scientific journalist who may have had her own motivations and agenda. Lisa Lynch has published what I consider to be a brilliant rhetorical decoding of some of Garrett's earlier work, and she contends that Garrett's pandemic narratives allow readers to see both the impact of the environmental changes that contributed to the catastrophic spread of contagions as well as the adverse effects of global capitalism that helped impoverish Africa. Here, Lynch explains, one does not find that usual "Western teleological narrative of progress" in a review of emerging infectious diseases, but instead works like *The Coming Plague* explain how "colonialism, re-source exploitation, slavery and cultural destruction" had their effect.[17]

Lynch gives Garrett credit for mentioning all of this economic destruc-tion, but she goes on to note that Garrett's static ways of writing about African cultures before modernity borders on primitivism, and Lynch worries that these particular pandemic *rhetorics* leave no room for admit-ting that African communities have "produced their own epistemologies, politics, and social structures *through contact* and *over time*" [emphasis in the original].[18] Near the end of *The Coming Plague*, Garrett argues that the survival of African cultures in the face of contagions like Ebola will depend on the creation of some "rational global village that affords the microbes few opportunities," but as Lynch opined, this particular "viral apocalypse" narrative seemed to be too dystopic.[19]

I would extend some of Lynch's critiques and argue that part of Gar-rett's appeal for U.S. audiences stems from the ways that she writes as if she is always *anticipating* and thinking ahead; this helps Americans conceptualize how they can best prepare themselves for that next viral apocalypse. Her many interviews create the impression that she is dispel-ling popular myths and media misimpressions, but her own biopolitics and thanatopolitics simply produce other, competing mythic figurations.

Garrett's metanarratives usually begin with plotlines that put on display belated preparedness, and she uses these to advocate for cost-effective, strategic, mobile, and modernist foreign interventionism. For Garrett, the problem for those who suffer from EVD in West Africa is not just the cuts in programs, the corruption of African leaders, or even the poverty of the African continent: It is the waste, the misplaced priorities, the weakness of WHO, and the lack of the adequate preparedness strate-gies that get in the way of Ebola eradication.

Over the years more general news coverage of Ebola, combined with Garrett's adroit usages of her skills, has contributed to a rhetorical situ-ation where Garrett's commentaries about infectious diseases appear on YouTube, Twitter, Council of Foreign Relations websites, and countless newspaper postings.

To be fair to Garrett, I need to note here that she was one of the few commentators—especially between March and July of 2014—who talked incessantly about problematic conditions in Sierra Leone, Guinea, and Liberia at a time when many other journalists ignored or marginalized the uncontrolled spread of Ebola. I am convinced that there is little to no question that her rhetorical power, and her views on contested epide-miological and political positions, may have resonated with millions who shared her neoliberal views.

In a host of ways, the revival of interest in the latest Ebola outbreak also provided opportunities for image events that allowed Americans to incrementally get used to the idea that many scientists, science journalists, and others had anticipating the need for President Obama's Ebola military "surge" during the fall of 2014. It is no coincidence that this was also a time when Garrett would be interviewed by dozens and dozens of news outlets who sought out her informed opinion.

These informed opinions were not produced in a vacuum. Garrett's *The Coming Plague*, and all of her works that had been produced since the 1990s, took into account the cumulative morbidity and mortality rates of the previous dozen Ebola outbreaks in places like Zaire (now the Democratic Republic of the Congo), Sudan, Uganda, and elsewhere. In each of those early cases a flare-up had occurred in rural areas that witnessed the arrival of Ebola "hunters," who then worked with local public health officials to put out those earlier outbreaks. All total, effective containment had meant that less than five hundred lives had been lost. Garrett's earlier Cassandra-like warnings of impending doom must have sounded at times like moral panic instead of edification, but this would not be the case with the latest West African outbreak.

Now, in the second decade of the twenty-first century, it seemed as though the past had become prologue for Garrett and many of her readers. She continually shared with her followers what she had learned about historical isolation strategies, quarantines, and cordons. One of the best illustrations of how these earlier experiences provided Garrett with even more scientific ethos can be found in the ways that she frequently talked and wrote in 2014 about the time that she spent in Kikwit, Zaire, in 1995. In April of 2014—some five months before most mainstream newspapers provided extensive coverage or returning nurses and doctors—Garrett was telling reporters that MSF was right when they called this outbreak "unprecedented," and she reminisced about the difficulties that were posed by those who lived in Zaire during their earlier outbreak. She recalled how those historical Ebola fighters in 1995 had all wished that they had Land Rovers to navigate difficult terrains.[20] Tales of equipment shortages thus become a part of these Ebola ideoscapes.

Long before the desertion of Monrovia streets, Garrett was conjuring up visions of a geopolitical locale that had no streets, no roads, no real airports for those who contracted some infectious diseases, and now, during the latest outbreak, she could reference her earlier work by writing about something that looked like some urban apocalypse. Fear, Garrett argued, was the number one obstacle for those living in places like Conakry or Dakar, because this was the region where there were many diverse religious organizations, cultural communities, and languages that hindered the "conquering" of Ebola.[21]

Although Garrett is perfectly capable of making logical and rational arguments about Ebola pathogenesis, the responsibility of the World

Health Organization, the aftereffects of West African civil wars, and the need for U.S. military interventionism, there are other times when her own sensationalistic fragments take center stage. Note, for example, the graphic nature of her depictions of EVD deaths that were presented during an interview that was taking place near the end of the first stage of the West African intervention:

> Yes, Ebola is an RNA virus, a very small virus that attacks the endothelial linings that maintain the integrity of your blood vessels, blood veins, capillaries, first little microscopic holes through which bits of blood and fluids will leak, but eventually larger and larger holes, until the individual begins to hemorrhage internally, and hemorrhaging blood through tears, from the mouth, from the nose, all over the body, so that they become quite frightening to see. And individuals will get a high fever. They may get blood in the brain, which will lead to even more insane behavior, a kind of deranged look in their eyes, all of which contributes to a great deal of fear.[22]

This, obviously was meant to provide PBS's *NewsHour* with accurate information about Ebola symptoms, but this type of graphic contextualization might be deemed voyeuristic or sensationalist, and it may had contributed to the very fear mongering that Garrett was talking about.

Unlike some of the discourses that were produced by other journalists or chroniclers of Ebola pasts, Garrett's more recent essays are not nihilistic. Garrett's particular permutations of Ebola outbreak *dispositifs* often begin with a chronicling of all of problems that stand in the way of Ebola fighters, but they usually go on to provide solutions that underscore the importance of taking into account resource scarcity, recent epidemiological knowledge, proper governmentality, the development of political will, and reductions of societal misunderstands. For example, in July of 2014 she explained to CNN listeners that there was no question that West Africa was traumatized during this period when even heroic doctors and nurses, like Sheik Umar Khan, were losing their lives in a chaotic fight. She was able to fetch some good from this evil when she argued that all of us needed to keep in mind that this current crisis, that threatened eleven nations in the region, was not so much a "biological" or a "medical" problem but a "political one." This is one of her more uplifting commentaries, where human collective actions continue to be relevant, even in the face of some massive uncertainties.

Garrett is not the type of author who writes about pan-African solutions to Ebola problems that might obviate the need for Western interventionism. Nor is she a radical, socialist, or neo-Marxist critic who views all forms of military interventionism to be unethical hindrances that stand in the way of medical humanitarianism. Instead, what we get from Garrett is a typical neoliberal critique of West African failures that are juxtaposed with Western successes. At one point she told journalists that the "three nations in Ebola's thrall need technical support from outsiders but will not succeed in stopping the virus until each nation's leaders embrace effective governance."[23] Although Garrett did not go into great detail explaining what she meant by "effective" governance, she did provide readers with some hints when she wrote about the need for rapid identification of the sick, the removal of the ailing and deceased from their homes, and the quarantining and "high hygiene measures" that were needed to prevent Ebola transmission to family members as well as health care workers.[24] She once again brought up her early journalistic experience covering the 1995 Kirwit outbreak in Zaire as she proffered these solutions.

As many post-structural, post-colonial, or postmodern critics have observed in their studies of infectious diseases in general, and Ebola in particular, empowered experts who are constantly being interviewed cannot help preaching about the good that comes from changing African behaviors and traditions.[25] In Garrett's case an intertextual review of dozens of her articles, interviews, and other commentaries reveals how most of her articles contain snippets about the plight of indigenous communities who faced economic hardship or grappled with religious or cultural traditions. However, after appearing to sympathize with these African communities she then goes on in other parts of her commentaries to explain how some of those very same communities *have to change* their religious practices or cultural behaviors as a precondition to stopping Ebola.

Garrett is no longer just an immunologist or a scientific journalist when she produces ideoscapes that try to answer a host of political, legal, and bioethical questions. In that same July, 2014 CNN article where she talks about poverty in this region, she also moralizes about the need to see transcendent governance and peace:

> Nobody, in any culture, relishes having their ailing loved ones removed from a family's care, or their bodies hauled off to ignominious mass graves. But the violent reaction to such measures in West Africa is far more extreme than anything that has occurred in other Ebola crises since the virus's first appearance in Zaire in 1976. . . . In these three nations few families have not experienced murders, rapes, torture, maiming, loss of homes and death. Fear, suspicion, poverty, pain and superstition are the norm, the noise that everybody lives with, every minute of their lives. Ebola is simply a new scream heard above that terrible background din. . . . [T]he challenge today in these barely functioning states . . . [is to] bring governance and peace.[26]

It does not take much imagination to decide who has to bring that peace and police so that Africans can experience that new governance.

At other times Laurie Garrett writes as if she was producing a Richard Preston novel that anthropomorphizes the Ebola virus. For example, in

September of 2014, as she wrote about the responsibilities of the World Bank, the IMF, the United States, and other institutions or governments, she also wrote about some of the epidemiological and pathogenic features of EVD. When she was asked about the dangers that might develop if this contagion mutated and went "airborne," she explained that *the virus had already mutated at least 300 times during the last five months.* So far it did not seem to have made any difference in the transmission rates of EVD, but she elaborated by noting:

> I'm less worried about the virus become airborne than I am about it being able to outmaneuver any vaccine we throw at it. My concern is that Ebola is mutating and that, even if we find a vaccine, it may have very limited efficacy because of the virus's capacity to constantly change its code.[27]

It would be difficult to find a more concrete example of the typical arguments that assumed that the biological features of Ebola mutations might, in the future, require more efficacious interventions.

In the next section of this chapter, I want to illustrate how many other social agents were producing mediascapes that often contained evocative fragments that resembled many of Garrett's figurations. Again, these antecedent rhetorics seemed to have framed, and to have anticipated, how we were supposed to conceptualize Ebola problems and solutions.

VISUALIZING EBOLA THREATS, 1976 TO 2012

Interestingly enough, during the 1970s, when many publics and scientific communities thought about infectious diseases, they dwelled on the *successes* of modernity. This was a generation that liked to write and about how vaccines and other medical wonders were helping with the "quasi-eradication in industrialized countries of polio, typhoid, tetanus, and many childhood diseases."[28] The 1976 outbreaks in places like Zaire helped audiences on several continents wake up from their dogmatic slumber as they realized that they had been granted a short reprieve in the enduring battles that had been waged between microbes and humans over the centuries.

During the 1980s and 1990s virologists and other scientists did their best to warn American communities that they simply were not prepared for a major "tropical" disease outbreak. At a plenary sessions of the annual meeting of the American Society of Tropical Disease and Medicine, that was held in Honolulu in December of 1989, Department of Defense leaders and civilian public health administrators talked amongst themselves about the need to prepare for real or hypothetical infectious disease threats. A Yale University virologist famous remarked—"It is not

whether an outbreak will occur, but when!"[29] Several years later, based
on these conversations, Llewellyn Legters and other members of an
Emergency Interagency Working Group dreamed up a scenario of a "hypothetical [global epidemic emergency] in which the causative agent was
an Ebola-like disease."[30] The fictional outbreak would occur in the future,
in 1994, at an imaginary place called "Changa." An audience of some
eight hundred tropical disease experts, including conference attendees
from the CDC, the National Institute of Health, WHO, and elsewhere took
on various personae and roles as they played this "medical war game"
about Changa. In this hypothetical scenario, Changa was described as an
impoverished nation that was already suffering from five years of civil
war that had killed an estimated 200,000 Changans.

Legters and his colleagues used this scenario to describe how the government of Changa was unable to cope with the displaced persons who
were forced to seek asylum, and they used the scenario to illustrate the
unpreparedness of both "Changa" and the West. Others might have been
oblivious to the growing threat posed by "emerging" diseases, but this
was not the case with the virologists and others who in 1989 could "see"
what was happening, and what was going to happen, through ecological
and epidemiological prisms. Possibilistic scenarios that circulated during this convention thus became key rhetorical fragments in other catastrophic, apocalyptic military and civilian *dispositifs*.

These types of published hypothetical scenarios, which appeared in
Stephen Morse's book *Emerging Viruses*, illustrate how virologists and
other public health planners not only anticipated the emergence of a major
outbreak—they could also use their geopolitical imaginations to pinpoint
where it would happen, in West Africa—twenty years before the 2013–2015
Ebola outbreak! Professor Legters, after setting up this scenario about
Changa, was interviewed and asked about tropical disease preparedness,
and he commented on how the "accidental transmission of zoonotic diseases to humans," combined with population pressures, or dislocations of
populations might converge in ways that overwhelmed poor nations. He
lamented the fact that U.S. interest in "tropical infectious diseases waxes
and wanes with our political and military involvement overseas."[31]

The well-publicized 1989 conference scenarios, along with reportage
on the actual outbreaks in the Congo and Uganda, and media coverage of
the Reston "monkey" incident in Virginia, all contributed to a rhetorical
situation where publics and elites alike were imagining what they would
do if pandemics came their way. Richard Preston's *The Hot Zone* was
published at just the right time, and his book was characterized as both
a bio-thriller and a didactic text that would help with Ebola education.

Preston's book dealt with the genesis of viral hemorrhagic fevers, and
he provided readers with a wealth of descriptive—as well as conjec-

tural—information about Ebola and Marburg diseases. The narrative arc of *The Hot Zone* told the story of how some monkeys had been imported into the United States, and how those animals had arrived "infected with a mysterious rain-forest virus thought to be the deadliest ever known."[32] Books like this helped ensure that the evolutionary trajectory of Ebola representations went from "anonymity to notoriety."[33]

By the middle of the 1990s, argues Bill Albertini, both "public health and popular narratives" started to follow a "familiar pattern," where outbreak narratives chronicled the identification of infectious disease threats so that they could aid in the "process of making visible, and thus avoidable or containable, the invisible threat of contagion."[34] In 1995, for example, a British television channel screened the 1995 Hollywood thriller *Outbreak*, a film that followed the activities of a maverick military virologist who worked with his ex-wife as they tried to find a "vaccine to halt the spread of a deadly African virus in California before the military obliterates the town where it has taken hold."[35] Described by some as a "goofy piece"[36] of cinematic representation, *Outbreak* told the story of how Colonel Sam Daniel (Dustin Hoffman) an employee of the U.S Army Medical Research Institute of Infectious Diseases at Fort Detrick, Maryland, worked to develop a cure for a fictional disease caused by the "Motaba virus."

In the same way that audiences today are asked to travel back in time to study what happened in Zaire in 1976 with Peter Piot, moviegoers who watched *Outbreak* watched as Hoffman worked his magic as he fought a corrupt general by the name of Donald McClintock (Donald Sutherland) who had once ordered the annihilation of a camp in Zaire. The plot thickens when Daniels's ex-wife, Roberta "Robby" Keough (Rene Russo) of the CDC, joins Hoffman as they work together to contain the spread of Ebola at the same time that they battle militarists who are trying to weaponize Motaba.[37]

Cinematic representations like this were used to put on display the traditional military humanitarianism versus medical humanitarian tensions, and these versions of the outbreak narratives also underscored the importance of finding vaccines that might help stop the spread of diseases that resembled Ebola.

A critical review of textual and media representations of Ebola during the late 1990s reveals how this might have been a period that witnessed Ebola fatigue, when the media experienced a type of saturation point. During these particular years, Anglo-American audiences were presented with few new books, television programs, or movies about Ebola. Given the fact that Ebola had only killed a few hundreds of people by the late 1990s, while other endemic or epidemic diseases killed many more, researchers and journalists wondered about the voyeuristic and counterproductive nature of Ebola-viewing obsessions. Susan Moeller, for example, in her *Compassion Fatigue*, would write that Ebola was not like AIDS/HIV in that "an epidemic of Ebola seems to last a finite, fairly short period of time," while AIDS involved longer spans of time and had killed at least one and a quarter million people by the time her book was released.[38]

The attacks by Osama Bin Laden's minions helped revive interest in Ebola as a potential bioterrorist agent. By 9/11 securitized rhetorics about the role of globalization in helping terrorist networking were supplemented with commentaries on the detrimental effects of technological shifts, economic dislocation, ecological changes, urbanization, and "a range of cultural productions" that were used to invite viewing audiences to think of a world "without borders, where bodies and spaces intermingled to deadly effect."[39] Moviegoers were now watching all sorts of zombie science fiction movies as well as films with post-apocalyptic infectious disease scenarios.

By 2001 Rebecca Weldon, in her essay, "The Rhetorical Construction of the Predatorial Virus," could opine that Ebola viruses were characterized as microscopic stalkers "of the human race," contagions that "captured the attention of billions around the globe."[40] She noted how many of these alarming descriptions did not "reflect the actual morbidity and threat of this viral hemorrhagic fever to the world at large."[41] Elsewhere she argued that media representations of various illnesses impacted everything from public health care funding to perceptions of treatment options, and she argued that critics needed to analyze Ebola storytelling so that they could do more than just "debunk" these tales.[42] She was interesting in exploring what these popular representations of a "virus as a sentient being, stalking, invading, capable of hunting and capturing prey" said about our culture and the decisions that were made about disease prevention.[43] Weldon concluded that the rhetorical usage of basic common stories, depth of details, the use of authoritative figures, the power of storytelling, the conveyance of latent meanings, and the fact that readers got the sense that *they could* become Ebola victims all were contributing influences that added luster to the aura of the "image of the predator virus."[44]

Over the next decade there would be growing interest in producing books, documentaries, films, and other materials that helped global audiences visualize what some Ebola-type outbreak would be like, but perhaps one of the most famous of these was Steven Soderbergh's 2011 thriller *Contagion*.[45] Alyssa Rosenberg, who was writing just after it was being reported in 2014 that some nine hundred people had died from EVD in West Africa, complained that the lethal spread of "unusually lethal diseases" was echoed by our pandemic-obsessed popular culture," which was "fond" of "killer viruses."[46] She argued that *Contagion* was the "best movie to watch during the current Ebola outbreak" because it was one of those rare films that showed that "real life" was more "disconcerting than almost anything fiction writers could dream up."[47]

Contagion was a big-ticket Hollywood movie, and one viewer characterized it as a film that also served as an "infomercial promoting specific national and international agencies while encouraging specific behaviors from the public."[48] The polysemic and polyvalent nature of the movie allowed audiences to conjure up visions of how they would react if they touched abject objects like glasses, door handles, or even gaming dice from casinos that could become vectors of contagion. This complex movie also invited viewers to think about the motives of the critics of the CDC, the perils of travel from infected regions, the need for martial law, the relationship between morality and disease, and the drastic steps that had to be taken in situations where millions of lives might be at stake.

Matt Damon, Laurence Fishburne, Jude Law, and Gwyneth Paltrow were some of the stars who appeared in Soderbergh's *Contagion*, and more than a few insightful observers thought that it was no coincidence that some of the plotlines in the movie looked as though they were based on what happened during the 2009 H1N1 scare that left many citizens wondering about the competence, and the state of preparedness, of local, regional, and national communities. The H1N1 scare would later be ridiculed as a mass-mediated image event that did little more than market some unnecessary mass vaccination schemes,[49] and many considered it to be an example of biosecurity threat inflation, but the movie *Contagion* was supposedly different in that the existential dangers were "real." The film "conditions the masses to expect martial law," argued one critic, so that they would "throw themselves at the first available vaccine in case of a crisis."[50] The imaginary vaccine in *Contagion* thus served in the movie as a medical magic bullet, a way to immunize surviving millions from both future medical threats as well as governmental coercive practices.

Contagion was a movie that involved the collaboration of screen writer Scott Z. Burns, the composer Cliff Martinez, and the editor Stephen Mirrione, and both the dark aesthetics and the somber music in the film helps moviegoers feel as though they are looking into some existential abyss, where the human race is trying desperately to find a way out of all of this chaotic madness. The incremental nature of the body counts of the dead keeps viewers on the edge of their seats. Are they witnessing their own dismal future, that ends with an infectious disease apocalypse?

Some of the early action in the first portion of *Contagion* revolves around the decisions that are made by a Minnesota executive, Beth Emhoff, who is played by Gwyneth Paltrow. Emhoff takes a company trip to Hong Kong, and film goers are horrified when they have to watch Emhoff succumb to some unknown disease. We become witnesses to Emhoff's bodily transformation as she loses her beauty, and her life, to an unknown viral killer. Mitch, Emhoff's husband (played by Matt Damon) is overcome with grief when he takes his wife to a hospital, hoping to hear the best, only to be told by doctors that she had already died from the mysterious virus. "Nothing moves slowly here," explained Manohla Dargis, because movie goers become vicarious witnesses who observe how this virus "cuts down seemingly everyone who's been within touching, kissing, handshaking, dice-blowing distance of a carrier."[51] We are left to wonder if this transmission involves just human-to-human, or aerial transmission as well.

Soderbergh manages to complicate matters by showing Emhoff having an affair on her trip, and during one scene the camera shifts away from Beth as she takes a call at the airport from her unseen lover so that movie goers can get a glimpse of her wedding ring. Are we supposed to feel sorry for this adultress, and have her transgressions anything to do with her medical situation? Beth becomes a literal and figurative "Typhoid Mary" as she lingers on a jar of shelled peanuts at an airport bar, and her slightest touch turns some materials into abject objects of horror. Even the credit card that she hands the waitress can transmit the unknown virus, and we watch as several people—including a young man in in a Hong Kong market, a Japanese salesperson on the plane, and a model staggering around London—remind us of the transglobal nature of Beth's handy work.[52] Soderbergh's artfully conceived didactic message is clear—a single individual carrying along the virus on a trip can set in motion a pandemic, and today's airlines and global connectedness makes the world smaller, and more dangerous, than we would like to imagine.

Hope, however, springs eternal in *Contagion* because Soderbergh adds some ethical and theological dimensions to a story that will begin with Emhoff infecting a few unfortunate people on several continents and will end with the discovery of a vaccine that saves humanity. Those who are interested in redemption and contrition can interpret the movie as an example of what might happen when transglobal public health communities act in moral, and concerted ways, to overcome incredible obstacles.

The middle portions of *Contagion* focus on the actions of governmental agents and others who are scrambling to find the right biosecurity surveillance and control measures that will help put an end to the outbreak of this pandemic. Ellis Cheever, played by Laurence Fishburne, is the deputy director at the Centers for Disease Control and Prevention in Atlanta, and he tries to assuage the public fears of many. Soderbergh, however, allows us to see some of the contradictions and tensions that are a part of this chaos when Cheever gets into trouble for violating some of his own organization's protocols when he warns some of his loved ones that they need to leave Chicago as soon as they can. Erin Mears, a medical-intelligence specialist (Kate Winslet), is sent out by Cheever into the field to serve as a sentinel for the governmental efforts, and she soon reports back to him about the mounting mortality rates and the rising anxieties of populations.

Years before the government of Liberia cordoned off the borders and placed a quarantine around West Point, Soderbergh's *Contagion* showed what happened when global communities were dealing with the militarization and the securitization of emerging disease threats, and they have to deal with anxious populations clamoring for some time of protection. Scenes in the movie show panic engulfing several countries, as crowds go into stores and into banks, and violence erupts out in countless places.

In *Contagion* workers at the CDC are shown feverishly working away at trying to find that life-saving vaccine. Dr. Ally Hextall (Jennifer Ehle) is the one who slaves away in a CDC lab so that they can try to isolate the virus and develop a serum, and we watch her as she wears the orange nylon protective garb that signals the appearance of deadly viruses. Sadly, that vaccine discovery by Dr. Hextall took six months of development, and by that time viewers realize that the planet has already suffered the loss of millions of lives. While some parts of the movie put on display individual acts of heroism, other portions of *Contagion* are filled with darkness, to the point where some describe it as a clinical, cold, and gruesome movie.

One of the most intriguing characters in *Contagion* is Jude Law's character, Alan Krumwiede, a nefarious San Francisco blogger who markets himself as a post-apocalyptic dispenser of *parrhesia*, who is willing to tell members of the blogosphere what is really going on behind the scenes.[53] Krumwiede signals that he is a member of the alternative press who is enchanted by the potential of the blogosphere, and at one point in the movie he shouts that "print media" is dying. Krumwiede uses his blog— "Truth Serum Now"—to attract millions of delusional viewers who crave the magic bullet, and they allegedly share his distrust of the CDC. In the movie Krumwiede pushes a bizarre holistic cure, called forsythia, that came from a yellow flowering plant that was used in traditional Chinese medicine.[54] The Krumwiede character allows Soderbergh to provide a not-so-veiled critique of those who would argue that internet freedom, and the diffusion of vernacular information, will automatically help contain the spread of viruses as well as misinformation.

Manahola Dargis is certainly on point when she argued in 2011 that Soderbergh's *Contagion* was a "dystopic vision" of a calamitous present that was infected by "fear, paranoia, self-interest, and the denial of science," and she felt that it was "certainly of the moment," even as it evoked the past.[55] David Denby similarly remarked that this was a highly-controlled film of a chaotic problem, a sure-handed and intelligent movie that was a "brief against magical thinking."[56]

Many parts of *Contagion* will resonate with audiences who understand the problems that are posed by the spread of fear and panic during pandemics. In the movie, while government officials are trying to explain Emhoff's death as they try to stop the spread of moral panic, Law's character works to whip up hysteria in the name of truth-seeking and the protection of the Fourth Estate. At the beginning of the movie some may view this character as an obsessive, and yet important symbol for needed investigative journalism, but later on in the movie we learn that he is actually a troublemaking blogger who is trying to make money from his internet celebrity status.

Several scientists have been asked to present their views on the "science' or "realism" in the film, and oftentimes their particular scientific specialty and beliefs regarding emerging infectious diseases seemed to have influenced how these interviewees talked about Soderbergh's *Contagion*. For example, years before he appeared on television screens hugging Nina Pham, the Dallas nurse who came down with Ebola after treating Thomas Eric Duncan, Dr. Anthony Fauci would tell reporters that *Contagion* was "one of the most accurate movies" that he had "seen on infectious disease outbreaks of any type."[57] Bill Hanage, an epidemiologist at Harvard University, opined that some of the early scenes with Beth Emhoff, the executive traveler, were the least plausible parts of the movie. "In reality," he noted, "something that would be that infectious" would stir up "rumblings in local populations."[58] Ghose explained that if you really wanted to learn about the usual pathogenesis of a disease like this, then this would mean that you would keep your eye on the worker at a pig farm who would be a more likely "patient zero" than a jet-setting Western executive from Minnesota.[59]

Interestingly enough, one of the mysterious parts of the movie involves the *question of how* Beth Emhoff got this deadly virus in the first place. Moviegoers are left to infer that she caught it from a chef, who may have gotten it from some animals. Barbara Reynolds, a crisis communication specialist at the CDC in Atlanta, argued that this pictorial representation of the pathway from animals to humans was very realistic, and she told readers that it reminded her of how a bird helped start the infamous 1918 Spanish influenza. She estimated that some 75 percent of the threats that humans face come from animals and insects, and that this type of interaction meant that there was always the potential for "a virus to mutate and be transmitted" to humans.[60]

The fictional virus in *Contagion* is called MEV-1, and it is based on a real pathogen, called Nipah virus, that can indeed kill somewhere between 40 to 90 percent of its victims. Symptoms of Nipah virus include respiratory problems, encephalitis, and seizures, and it has sickened hundreds of individuals living in Bangladesh and Malaysia. However, argues Pramila

Walpita, a virologist who developed a vaccine for Nipah, this particular vaccine has a difficult time transmitting between human to humans.[61] Bill Hanage, who was asked to compare the transmission rate of the real Nipah virus with the fictive MEV-1, said that the movie virus seemed "rather restrained," killing every one out of four people that it infected, and spreading to two people for every person who got the disease. This, he averred, was a very realistic profile of the transmission rates.[62]

At the very end of *Contagion* Soderbergh does a masterful job of clearing up some of the mystery behind the pathogenic origins of the fictional MEV-1 when he shows a bat habitat being razed so that humans can build a factory. All of this industrial deforestation is intended to send a message, and the "popular cultural characterization of Ebola-like viruses place the blame for the spread of disease squarely on the shoulders of globalization and man's careless despoiling of the environment."[63] In many ways this echoed some of the messages that appeared in Dr. Legters discussion of ecological pressures in the "Changa" scenario, and Preston's moralizing in *The Hot Zone*.

Earlier parts of the movie had shown a virus that became a part of a "globe-sprinting pandemic that cuts across borders and through bodies,"[64] but near the end of *Contagion* we got to see a bat fly to a big farm, where a fruit drops from the bat's mouth and then mingles with food that was eaten by some pigs. One of the pigs is then slaughtered in the fancy Hong Kong restaurant where Emhoff shakes hands with the chef, and this allows us to go full circle as we see the ecological chain of all of this zoonoses.[65]

In many ways Soderbergh's *Contagion* is taking advantage of both elite and vernacular interest in zoonoses, or the study of how animal diseases can be transmitted to humans, and Nicholas Fontané and Frédéric Keck have written about how all of this research is tied to our contemporary global "biosecurity" reframes of animal and human surveillance.[66] They argue that in recent years social scientific research into zoonoses has undergone paradigmatic shifts. Researchers have moved away from previous forms of biopolitics that were based on predictive, measured risks that used statistical modeling and toward more catastrophic models that assume that some imminent threats are incalculable. "The emergence of a new pathogen," Fontané and Keck explain, is "perceived to be an event for which health authorities must be prepared, by imagining its yet uncertain consequences for the human population."[67]

Is Soderbergh's *Contagion* serving to fill this perceptual void, and is it providing that imaginative, artistic creation that helps with future preparedness for Ebola and other emerging infectious diseases?

I would argue that part of the attraction of *Contagion*, and the perceived "realism" of the film, comes from the way that Soderbergh's pandemic thriller is able to tap into what audiences expect to see when they flock to their cinemaplex. For example, their notion of a realistic story about an Ebola predator needs to include some allusions to the type of airborne or aerosol science that puts on display the unpredictable, unmanaged, and clinical nature of the most horrific diseases, and that is what they get when they go see *Contagion*.

Soderbergh sutures together fact with fiction as he invites his viewers to think of the dangers that might arise when one innocent cough, or the touch of a martini glass, can help with the pathogenesis of a deadly disease. "Critics and scientists alike," noted Tia Ghose in September of 2011, "touted the movie as a more realistic depiction of disease transmission," because this was not a flick filled with movie stars that turn into "flesh-eating zombies" where some "previously unknown disease does not kill every person it encounters."[68]

One of the most ambiguous, and tension-filled parts of *Contagion* has to do with the race to find a vaccine for the fictional MEV-1. Since isolation practices, quarantines, and even cordons failed to stop the spread of disease in the movie, everyone hopes that the scientific experts can find a precious vaccine. At the beginning of the movie the virus was completely unknown, and scientists managed to culture it in twelve days. Dr Walpita says that all of this was a stretch," because as she notes, we have known about Ebola since at least 1976, and we still don't have any vaccine. Some paramyxovirus that look like the fictional MEV-1 have been studied for more than four decades, but we still don't have any vaccine.[69]

As I note in the final chapter of this book, the race to find an Ebola vaccine is still an on-going adventure.

THE "AFRICANIZATION" OF EBOLA

Laurie Garrett's perceived expertise provided her with a scientific soapbox for lecturing her viewers on the failures of those who inadequately prepared for Ebola outbreaks, and Soderbergh's *Contagion* served as a filmic vehicle for assessing civilian and military responses to horrific pandemics, but these two rhetors were just a few of the many social agents who helped co-produce influential Ebola ideoscapes and mediascapes. Juliet Musabeyezu, Yusuph Mkangara, and Hamma Amanuel, writing for the *Harvard Political Review* in February of 2015, argued that those who studied mainstream media outlets were becoming witnesses to what they called "the Africanization of Ebola."[70] One of the major premises of their diatribe was that "many media outlets and Western anti-Ebola campaigns have perpetuated the devaluating of black lives everywhere by misrepresenting the tens of thousands of "black lives taken by the Ebola virus in Liberia, Sierra Leone, Guinea, and Mali."[71]

The essay by Musabeyezu, Mkangara, and Amanuel proved myriad examples of how contemporary mediascapes "represented Ebola as an 'African disease' that ravaged the lives of faceless and nameless Africans" at the same time that they heralded the "salvation from the West."[72] For example, mainstream media outlets rarely mentioned that the two-year-old toddler who was often configured as "patient zero" during the latest outbreak had a name—Emile Oumouno—and even fewer provided any details of the lives of villagers in Meliandou or the deaths of the Guinean midwife, health care worker, and community doctor who lost their lives in "service to Emile." Western audiences were presented with the names of several of the Western nurses or doctors who returned from West Africa and contracted Ebola (Kent Brantly, etc.) but all of this "imagery of white saviors" often "overshadowed, and rendered invisible the Africans" who worked to stop the spread of EVD in both afflicted countries and elsewhere on the continent.[73] The West seemed unfamiliar with the efforts of Sierra Leonean doctors like Victor Willoughby and Aiah Solomon Konoyeima, Liberian doctor Samuel Brisbane, or Stella Shade Ameyo Adadevoh, who was credited with sacrificing her life in Nigeria as she worked tirelessly fighting Ebola in her country.

African students, scholars, doctors, administrators and others understood some of the motives beyond the public interest stories that allowed American and other Western audiences to identify with the dangers associated with the Ebola outbreak, but this type of selective, and self-serving, consciousness raising was infuriating. Rumbi Mushavi, a first year student at Harvard's medical school, averred that it was really shocking for him to see a "photo spread of the people at the forefront of the Ebola outbreak" that posted pictures of "American or European expatriate doctors, while posting pictures of African gravediggers and janitors."[74] This not only made it appear as if foreigners were doing the bulk of the work during the West African outbreak, it implied that there were power hierarchies and social relationships where the expatriates were the bosses who knew everything about Ebola symptoms, pathogenesis, and control, while the local Africans provided all of the manual labor. Sadly, a review of some of these literatures revealed that even some of the World Health Organization essays that commented on how Nigeria was Ebola free failed to mention the work of Adadevoh and other African workers.[75]

Given the lingering influence of colonial and imperial "tropical disease" *dispositifs*, this was not the first time that some have complained about the "Africanization" of Ebola. Lisa Lynch, writing in 1998, explained how many popular best-sellers that appeared on *The New York Times*' best-seller lists sometimes "found the 'meaning' of epidemic diseased in Anglo-European fantasies about Africa," that were allowed writers to "Africanize the Ebola virus."[76] Several years earlier, Graham Harrison discussed the links between Ebola and structural violence, and complained about celebrities and the media coverage of the "Africanization of poverty."[77]

In some cases those living in the "North" also suffered some of this stigmatization. On October 24, 2014, two brothers, eleven and thirteen, who just returned from Senegal, were greeted at their Bronx intermediate school by classmates who pummeled them verbally by yelling "Ebola."[78] On Fox News, Elizabeth Hasselbeck allegedly advocated the "closing of borders" to ensure that undocumented immigrants didn't sneak across the border and bring contagion with them.

These are just a few of the micro-image events that become a part of our mediascapes during the fall of 2014, and the Ebola images that flowed across the blogosphere played well in front of national and international audiences who may have believed that they needed to prepare for an Ebola apocalypse. As Steven Weinstein would write in November of 2014, by the time some of the "hyperventilating media coverage of the outbreak was in remission," and the news carried less talk of Hazmat suits, the damage had been done.[79]

As Foucault and others have noted there are times when counterhistories can be cobbled together to try and reverse power flows, and Andrè Carrilho was one of the cultural critics who used visual depictions to critique the lack of balanced coverage of the Ebola victims in Western mediascapes. Carrilho's image of two photographers, with masks over their faces as they interview a white Ebola victim in a room while they ignore rows of dozens of black Ebola victims, appears to have been motivated by a desire to comment on the differential treatment of victims, based on ethnicity, nationality, or race. "I think unfortunately, in the Western media," argued Carrilho, "there are first-world diseases and third-world diseases, and the attention devoted to the latter depends on the threat they pose to us, not on a universal measure of human suffering," he said.[80] "A death in Africa, or Asia for that matter," he went on to explain, "should be as tragic as a death in Europe or the USA, and it doesn't seem to be."[81]

These types of visual critiques were used to provide illustrative examples of how absence, as well as presence, could be used to Africanize the Ebola outbreak.

THE CNN COMPARISONS OF EBOLA WITH ISIS

Many pundits who lampooned the efforts of CNN in their coverage that linked Ebola and ISIS often targeted the segment that appeared on October 6, 2014, when CNN's Ashleigh Banfield asked whether the dangerous nature of each required the United States to treat them "with the same kind of" strategy?[82] CNN was lampooned for making for what many regarded as a misleading and silly analogy, but what some of these observers missed were the ways that Banfield was simply taking advantage of an argumentative line that was part of a much denser *dispositif.* By the time she and other CNN interviewers made these parallels between ISIS and Ebola, these arguments had already turned into a meme that circulated on the blogosphere.[83]

Moreover, these comparisons were not just being made by television personalities but by military figures and policy planners who cared about efficacious counterterrorism. For example, on October 1, 2014, CNN presented a piece of televised work on "How to Treat Threats of Ebola and ISIS," that both symbolically and literally brought together the expertise of the U.S. military with the scientific public health knowledge that came from experts on infectious diseases. That piece was co-authored by Stanley McChrystal and Kristina Talbert-Slagle.[84]

Both of these authors had an incredible amount of ethos in their respective technical spheres. Stanley McChrystal, before he was famously sacked for disagreeing with some Obama strategizing in Afghanistan, was the former Commander of U.S. forces in Afghanistan, and he is often credited with building the Joint Special Operations Command (JSOC) counterterrorist systems. These were systems that were supposed to help with the dismantling of Al-Qaeda and Taliban networked threats. By the time that McChrystal wrote this article, he was serving as a senior fellow at the Yale University Jackson Institute for International Affairs.

McChrystal has entered the pantheon of military historical experts who are said to have helped with the massive building up of the CIA, the emphasis on drone war, the turn to countless night raids, and other forms of covert operations. Kristina Talbert-Slagle, his co-author, was the senior scientific officer who worked at the Yale Global Health Leadership Institute. She was also a lecturer at the Yale University of Public Health. In their co-authored piece for CNN, McChrystal and Talbert-Slagle invited their readers to use their imaginations as they conjured up some of the hypothetical and practical links that could be made between the spread of Ebola, a global health threat, and the growing power of ISIS, that they characterized as an "international security crisis by an insurgent group."[85]

The McChrystal and Talbert-Slagle piece was written in a style that mimicked the formulaic templates that were used in both military scientific outlets and medical scientific outlets. In this particular case, as the title of their essay implies, the authors were going to lay out the perceived threats and then they were going to proceed to give advice on "how to treat" a particular disease or problem. They argued that if readers juxtaposed the fact that some 3100 people had already died in West Africa, with the "unknown number of people who died at the hands of members of the Islamic State in Iraq and Syria," then readers would find that the two problems had "much in common."[86] Elsewhere in their essay, they characterized ISIS and Ebola as "opportunistic infections,"[87] thus implying that these were entities with intentionalist characteristics.

The McChrystal and Talbert-Slagle article was coming out during a period when Anglo-American viewers of CNN and other networks were hearing about the case of Thomas Eric Duncan, the Liberian who died in Dallas from Ebola, so it seemed plausible to some when McChrystal and Talbert-Slagle averred that both Ebola and ISIS were "threats that were initially underestimated, even denied, by national and international powers."[88] This of course implied that these two experts were not deluded by false assurances of control, and their global imaginations allowed them to wander as they wrote about how both Ebola and ISIS "persisted" as threats. This persistence meant that those who wanted to treat these threats "now require a complex, multisectoral strategy that includes, political, military, infrastructural, and humanitarian interventions."[89] The use of term "political" creates the impression that civilians will be in control of the military, while the use of the world "humanitarian" in the string citation brushes away any notion that military humanitarianism might be an oxymoron.

Here one finds no discussion of what the few African doctors and nurses were doing in West Africa, or any commentary on the need to support the efforts of NGOs like Doctors Without Borders. The McChrystal and Talbert-Slagle essay provides a grandiose metanarrative on the general responsibilities of Western nations to make up for past failures as they write about the "national immunodeficiency" that contributed to the rise of both ISIS and Ebola.[90]

The militarized and medicalized frames that are used by McChrystal and Talbert-Slagle mention the poverty and the lack of public health infrastructure in West Africa, but these are treated as pieces of information in a much more complex puzzle where Ebola and ISIS are represented as "serious threats to the health of people not only in their own nations, but also to populations around the world."[91] They mention that we have seen this all before, but what they do not mention are the ways that all of this rhetoric echoes that ways that post-9/11 militarists used the language of other nations being "unable" or "unwilling" to control terrorist as a pretext for extraterritorial intervention in places like Yemen or Pakistan. McChrystal and Talbert-Slagle, consciously or unconsciously, were tapping into the vernacular and elite biosecurity rhetorics that had been circulating for decades.[92]

Of course when you use immunization metaphors and circulate your own militarized versions of Ebola outbreak narrative you need to provide your readers with some closure and talk about diagnostics, potential remedies, and militarized cures for those problems, and McChrystal and Talbert-Slagle do not disappoint their readers. They mention how the United States and how other nations in the West need to help the "weakened, vulnerable systems" that need to treat both Ebola and ISIS. Both problems, these co-authors argued, needed to be treated with "state-of-the art, targeted therapy." For example, they explained how the deployment of "targeted approaches in Liberia, Iraq and Syria," by the United States, had "demonstrated strategic leadership in addressing these invasive threats."[93] The melding together of contagion rhetorics with military talk of "targeted" solutions allows readers to think of taking out ISIS and Ebola in the same way that drone strikes in Afghanistan took out the Taliban or the ways that targeted killings in Iraq helped eradicate Al Qaeda terrorist networks.

McChrystal and Talbert-Slagle wrote as if this targeted, calculating military approach was something that would be planned out by Western strategists and would receive a warm reception in West Africa. They wrote about the need to "rebuild the health of national systems" and the importance of regaining the "trust of the population"[94] They should be lauded for at least recognizing that Guinea, Liberia, and Sierra Leone needed sustainable, well-funded, public health infrastructures, but they were obfuscating the ways that military interventionism often interferes with those very systems. In the geographical imaginary vision that they set out in their essay, military intervention is a part of the solution, not the problem with all of this "immunodeficiency," and it is up to the world to avoid denialism, learn for the history of the AIDS epidemic, and intervene as soon as possible in that region.

Writing during the fall of 2014, after more than thirteen years of talk of warfare and overseas adventurism, McChrystal and Talbert-Slagle must have sensed that all of this sounded like mission-creep that just added to the worries of those who already talked about the never-ending war on terrorism. They take this argument head on, at the end of their essay, when they conclude by writing,

> Admittedly, this is not a popular strategy for a war-weary nation, or with the allies with whom we must partner, but in a globally connected world, we may not have a choice. As Ebola and ISIS are teaching us—and as we have learned before from AIDS—treating only the opportunistic infections that take hold in a weakened system does not make the problem go away. Let's learn from experience.[95]

The lessons that would learned from this analogy were supposed to help both Ebola fighters as well as the Coalition troops who fought ISIS forces.

CONCLUSION

What this chapter has emphasized are the ways that book authors and television reporters would become some of the influential social agents who helped produce, and helped circulate, select mediascapes and ideoscapes. The fragments that were crafted before the 2013–2015 West African outbreak provided some of the discursive and the visual materials that went into the production of *dispositifs* that could be used to identity Ebola experts or vilify those Africans who traveled abroad. Natalie Baker and her co-authors complained about a "hyperbolic portrayal" of Ebola in the U.S. media that resulted in what they called a "crisis of misinformation," that was complicated when "non-expert" members of these journalistic outlets who tried to come up with all sources of fantasies about foreign invaders bringing along with them Ebola contagion.[96] In some cases we have seen how even military experts, like Stanley McCrystal, or medical specialists, like Talbert-Slagle, could co-produce antecedent rhetorics that linked together ISIS and Ebola in ways that magnified the dangers of both. The existential pathogenic dangers posed by Ebola in West Africa were real enough, but the linkage to ISIS made it appear as if fighting Ebola was not only a humanitarian *but a counterterrorist imperative* as well.

Some scholars were horrified by some of the media coverage of Ebola that appeared on television screens. Almudena Marí Sáez, Ann Kelly, and Hannah Brown, for example, complained that

> the news media have exploded with unsettling images of doctors in full body protective gear and residents running from police in riot gear attempting to cordon off neighborhoods. Twitter feeds and Facebook pages are rife with apocalyptic scenarios, rumors and blame for the failure to stamp out the spread of the virus. From the perspective of social scientists working in the context of global health delivery and policy, there is much to say about the failures of biosecurity measures, the racist undertones of many media representations, and the histories of violence inscribed in weak health infrastructures and the misrepresented and poorly understood resistance to biomedical practices.[97]

Media outlets that were supposed to be informing Western audiences about Ebola were sensationalizing their coverage in problematic ways. Yet in spite of this, Richard Preston couldn't help pontificating near the end of October 2014 on how readers of *The New Yorker* needed to take seriously the possibility that the Ebola virus could mutate and "could become more contagious even without becoming airborne."[98]

NOTES

1. Although this chapter focuses on Anglo-American media representations, it is obvious that other nations, their governments, and their media representatives have a difficult time reporting on the spread of infectious diseases. For example, in Liberia, just one day after a few journalists reported on how there was an Ebola patient discovered in Monrovia, the Liberian Minister of Information, Culture and Tourism, Lewis Brown, was telling readers of the Liberian Observer that

EVD was in Guinea but not in Liberia. Alvin Worzi, "Ebola Not in Liberia," *Daily Observer* [Liberia], last modified March 27, 2014, http://www.liberianobserver. com/health/%E2%80%98ebola-not-liberia%E2%80%99.

2. Laurie Garrett, quoted in Jessica Taylor, "Fueling the Fear: Global Health Crisis and Mass Media," Multibriefs.com, last modified February 24, 2015, paragraph 2, http://exclusive.multibriefs.com/content/fueling-the-fear-global-health-crisis-and-mass-media/medical-allied-healthcare.

3. John M. Berry, "Pandemics: Avoiding the Mistakes of 1918," *Nature* 459 (May 21, 2009): 324–325.

4. Shari Roan, "Swine Flu 'Debacle' of 1976 is Recalled," *Los Angeles Times*, last modified April 27, 2009, http://articles.latimes.com/2009/apr/27/science/sci-swine-history27/.

5. On global cultural flows, see Arjun Appadurai, "Disjuncture and Difference in the Global Cultural Economy," *Public Culture* 2, no. 2 (1990): 1–24, 9. doi: 10.1215/08992363-2-2-1. Mediascapes and ideoscapes were just two of the five conceptual "scapes" that Arjun Appadurai would theorize about as he studied the flow of information in regional, national, and international contexts. The others three "scapes" that he theorized about were ethnoscapes, technoscapes, and financescapes.

6. Stephen J. Collier and Andrew Lakoff, "Vital Systems Security: Reflexive Biopolitics and the Government of Emergency," *Theory, Culture, & Society* 32, no. 2 (2015): 19–51, 20.

7. For more on these Foucauldian "truth effects," see Thomas Lemke, "Foucault, Governmentality, and Critique," *Rethinking Marxism* 14, no. 3 (2002): 49–64.

8. See, for example, how in October of 2014 Richard Preston was treated as an authority on the evolution of Ebola by *The New York Times*. Alexandra Alter, "Updating a Chronicle of Suffering: Author of *The Hot Zone* Tracks Ebola's Evolution," *The New York Times*, October 19, 2014, http://www.nytimes.com/2014/10/20/books/the-hot-zone-author-tracks-ebolas-evolution.html.

9. Centers for Disease Control and Prevention Staff, "Cases of Ebola Diagnosed in the United States," n.d., CDC.gov, http://www.cdc.gov/vhf/ebola/outbreaks/2014-west-africa/united-states-imported-case.html.

10. Emily Thomas, "This Illustration of Ebola Coverage Shows How Problematic Media Reports Can Be," *The Huffington Post*, last modified October 8, 2014, paragraph 2, http://www.huffingtonpost.com/2014/10/08/ebola-illustration-andre-carrilho_n_5955192.html.

11. Tara C. Smith, "'The Hot Zone,' and the Mythos of Ebola," Scienceblogs, last modified October 21, 2014, paragraph 2, http://scienceblogs.com/aetiology/2014/10/21/the-hot-zone-and-the-mythos-of-ebola/.

12. As I note in other chapters, when journalists from the "North" did choose to interview those who were involved on the "frontlines" in the "South," it was usually some American or British nurse, doctor, or health care worker who was lionized for their "heroism," rescue efforts, or knowledge of Ebola virology or epidemiology, and their suggested opens gained gravitas.

13. A typical scientific discussion of how a bat might have been a part of the EVD transmission chain that began with a two-year-old in Meliandou, Guinea, appears in A. Mari Saéz et al., "Investigating the Zoonotic Origin of the West

African Ebola Epidemic," *EMBO Molecular Medicine* 7, no. 1 (December 30, 2014): 17–23, doi: 10.15252/emmm.201404792.

14. Collier and Lakoff, "Vital Systems Security," 19–20.

15. Judy Woodruff, "As Epidemic Escalates, Can U.S. Aid for Ebola Be Deployed Quickly Enough," *PBS Newshour,* last modified September 16, 2014, paragraph 8, http://www.pbs.org/newshour/bb/epidemic-multiplies-can-u-s-aid-ebola-deployed-quickly-enough/.

16. Laurie Garrett, "Public Health Officials Blew Off Ebola Warning Signs," *Tulsa World,* last modified September 21, 2014, paragraphs 1, 6, http://www.tulsaworld.com/laurie-garrett-public-health-officials-blew-off-ebola-warning-signs/article_18900436-1cad-5915-92c6-9457a06ba0b9.html.

17. Lisa Lynch, "The Neo/bio/colonial Hot Zone: African Viruses, American Fairytales," *International Journal of Cultural Studies* 1, no 2 (1998): 242.

18. Ibid., 243.

19. Ibid., 243–244.

20. Garrett, Judy Woodruff, "Unprecedented Ebola Outbreak Crosses Borders in West Africa," *PBS NewsHour,* last modified April 8, 2014, paragraph 16–17, http://www.pbs.org/newshour/bb/ebola-epidemic-update/.

21. Ibid., paragraphs 17–18.

22. Ibid., paragraph 9. For a very similar and typical Garrett characterization of Ebola horrors, note this fragment that appeared on a CNN webpage: "In the absence of such measures, Ebola will kill upwards of 70% of those it infects, as the virus punches holes in veins, causing massive internal hemorrhaging and bleeding from the eyes, ears, mouth and all other orifices."

Laurie Garrett, "Why an Ebola Epidemic Is Spinning Out of Control," CNN, last modified July, 2014, paragraph 5, http://www.cnn.com/2014/07/24/opinion/garrett-ebola/.

23. Garrett, "Why an Ebola Epidemic Is Spinning Out of Control," paragraph 3.

24. Ibid., paragraph 3.

25. More traditional types of scholarship can also be concerned about the treatment of the "other" during Ebola outbreaks. See, for example, Jason Steinhauer, "Ebola, Colonialism, and the History of International Aid Organizations," Library of Congress Blog, last modified February 3, 2015, http://blogs.loc.gov/kluge/2015/02/ebola-colonialism-history-international-aid-organizations-in-africa/.

26. Ibid., paragraphs 23–24.

27. Danielle Renwick, "Epic Failures Feeding Ebola Crisis," Council on Foreign Affairs, last modified September 18, 2014, paragraph 15, http://www.cfr.org/public-health-threats-and-pandemics/epic-failures-feeding-ebola-crisis/p33465.

28. Daniel K. Sokol, *From Anonymity to Notoriety: Historical Problems Associated with Outbreaks of Emerging Infectious Diseases* (MS, University of Oxford, 2002), 44.

29. Llewellyn J. Legters, Linda H. Brink, and Ernest T. Takafuji, "Are We Prepared for a Viral Outbreak Emergency?" in *Emerging Diseases,* edited by Stephen S. Morse (New York: Oxford University Press, 1993), 269–282, 272.

30. Heather Schell, "Outburst! A Chilling True Story about Emerging-Virus Narratives and Pandemic Social Change," *Configurations* 5, no. 1 (1997): 93–133, 100.

31. Lefters, in Legters, Brink, and Takfuji, "Are We Prepared," 277–279.

32. Karen Herzog, "'Hot Zone' Led Wisconsin Scientist to Ebola Research," *Milwaukee Journal Sentinel*, last modified October 24, 2014, paragraph 2, http://www.startribune.com/hot-zone-led-wisconsin-scientist-to-ebola-research/280363202. Monkeys, and the role that they can play in transmission of viruses to humans, was also the subject of *28 Days Later*, a film that puts on display an epidemic that was traced back to chimpanzees.

33. Daniel K. Sokol, *From Anonymity to Notoriety: Historical Problems Associated with Outbreaks of Emerging Infectious Diseases* (MS, University of Oxford, 2002).

34. Bill Albertini, "Contagion and the Necessary Accident," *Discourse* 30, no. 3 (Fall, 2008): 443–467, 443.

35. London Review of Books, "The Ultimate Predator," *The Guardian*, last modified March 15, 2001, http://www.theguardian.com/science/2001/mar/15/infectiousdiseases.

36. Matt Taylor, "We Asked an Expert if the Ebola Virus Will Kill You," Vice, last modified July 30, 2014, paragraph 2, http://www.vice.com/read/we-asked-an-expert-if-the-ebola-virus-will-kill-you-730.

37. IMDB, "FAQ for Outbreak (1995), IMDB.com, n.d., http://www.imdb.com/title/tt0114069/faq.

38. Susan D. Moeller, *Compassion Fatigue: How the Media Sell Disease, Famine, War and Death* (New York: Routledge, 1999).

39. Bill Albertine, "The Geographies of Contagion," *Rhizomes* 19 (Summer, 2009): paragraph 1, http://www.rhizomes.net/issue19/albertini.html.

40. Rebecca A. Weldon, "The Rhetorical Construction of Predatorial Virus: A Burkian Analysis of Nonfiction Accounts of the Ebola Virus," *Qualitative Health Research* 11, no. 1 (2001): 5–25, 5, doi: 10.1177/104973201129118902.

41. Weldon, "The Rhetorical Construction," 5.

42. Rebecca Weldon, "An 'Urban Legend' of Global Proportions: An Analysis of NonFiction Accounts of Ebola Virus," *Journal of Health Communication: International Perspectives* 6, no. 3 (2001): 281–294, 285, doi: 10.1080/108107301752384451.

43. Ibid., 285.

44. Ibid., 285–292.

45. For examples of press and critical responses to the 2011 movie *Contagion*, see Willa Paskin, "The Ebola Story," *Slate*, last modified October 22, 2014, http://www.slate.com/articles/arts/culturebox/2014/10/narrative_and_ebola_how_our_brains_build_stories_out_of_disaster.html; Chris Jones, "Why We Link Ebola to Fictional Stories Like Contagion," *Chicago Tribune*, last modified October 23, 2014, http://www.chicagotribune.com/entertainment/theater/ct-ebola-link-movies-contagion-column.html; Hilary Lewis, "Updated: It's Worse Than Ebola," *The Hollywood Reporter*, last modified, August 5, 2014, http://www.hollywoodreporter.com/news/ebola-fear-is-real-pandemic-723385.

46. Alyssa Rosenberg, "The Best Movie to Watch during the Current Ebola Outbreak," *The Washington Post*, last modified August 4, 2014, paragraph 1, https://www.washingtonpost.com/news/act-four/wp/2014/08/04/the-best-movie-to-watch-during-the-current-ebola-outbreak/.

47. Ibid., paragraph 1.

48. The Vigilant Citizen, "'Contagion' or How Disaster Movies 'Educate' The Masses," VigilantCitizen.com, last modified March 8, 2012, paragraph 2, http://

vigilantcitizen.com/moviesandtv/contagion-or-how-disaster-movies-educate-the-masses/.

49. See Stefan Elbe, Anne Roemer-Mahler, and Christopher Long, "Securing Circulating Pharmaceutically: Antiviral Stockpiling and Pandemic Preparedness in the European Union," *Security Dialogue* 45, no. 5 (2014): 440–457.

50. The Vigilant Citizen, "'Contagion' or How Disaster Movies 'Educate,'" paragraph 1.

51. Manohla Dargis, "A Nightmare Pox on Your Civilized World," *The New York Times*, last modified September 8, 2011, paragraph 2, http://www.nytimes.com/2011/09/09/movies/contagion-steven-soderberghs-plague-paranoia-review.html?_r=0.

52. Ibid., paragraph 4.

53. Manohla Dargis has described this character as a "unscrupulous blogger." Dargis, "A Nightmare Pox on Your Civilized World," paragraph 1.

54. Ibid., paragraph 6.

55. Ibid., paragraph 8.

56. David Denby, "Call the Doctor," *The New Yorker*, last modified September 19, 2011, paragraph 1, http://www.newyorker.com/magazine/2011/09/19/call-the-doctor-david-denby.

57. Dr. Anthony Fauci, quoted in Robert Roos, "'Contagion' Portrays Extreme But Not Impossible Scenario," *Center for Infectious Disease Research and Policy*, last modified September 9, 2011, paragraph 3, http://www.cidrap.umn.edu/news-perspective/2011/09/contagion-portrays-extreme-not-impossible-scenario.

58. Bill Hanage, quoted in Tia Ghose, "Contagion: Science Fact?" *The Scientist*, last modified September 16, 2011, paragraph 4, http://www.the-scientist.com/?articles.view/articleNo/31179/title/Contagion—Science-Fact-/.

59. Ghose, "Contagion," paragraph 4.

60. Barbara Reynoldsm, quoted in Ghose, "Contagion: Science Fact?" paragraph 8.

61. Ghose, "Contagion," paragraph 5.

62. Ibid., paragraph 6.

63. Elijah Wolfson, "Ebola and Climate Change: Are Human Beings Responsible for the Severity of the Current Outbreak?" *Newsweek*, last modified August 12, 2014, paragraph 4, http://www.newsweek.com/climate-change-ebola-outbreak-globalization-infectious-disease-264163.

64. Dargis, "A Nightmare Pox," paragraph 1.

65. Ghose, "Contagion," paragraph 7. Earlier in the film a researcher who had looked at the virus's cell structure had remarked, "The wrong pig met up with the wrong bat." Denby, "Call the Doctor," paragraph 2.

66. Nicholas Fontané and Frédéric Keck, "How Biosecurity Reframes Animal Surveillance," *Revue d'anthropologie des connaissances* 9 no. 2 (2015): https://www.cairn.info/revue-anthropologie-des-connaissances-2015-2-page-a.htm.

67. Ibid., paragraph 1.

68. Ghose, "Contagion," paragraph 1.

69. Ibid., paragraphs 13–14.

70. Juliet Musabeyezu, Yusuph Mkangara, and Hamma Amanuel, "The 'Africanization' of Ebola," *Harvard Political Review*, last modified February 25, 2015, http://harvardpolitics.com/world/africanization-ebola/.

71. Ibid., paragraph 1.

72. Ibid., paragraph 4.

73. Ibid., paragraphs 3–5.

74. Rumbi Mushavi, quoted in Musabeyezu, Mkangara, and Amanuel, "The 'Africanization' of Ebola," paragraph 7.

75. See, for example, World Health Organization, "Nigeria Is Not Free of Ebola Virus Disease," World Health Organization International, last modified October 20, 2014, http://www.who.int/mediacentre/news/ebola/20-october-2014/en/index1.html. For purposes of contrast, notice the detailed discussion of many African Ebola "fighters" that appeared in *Time*'s coverage of their 2014 Person of the Year. David von Drehle and Aryn Baker, "The Ebola Fighters," *Time*, December 10, 2014, http://time.com/time-person-of-the-year-ebola-fighters/. The *Time* coverage included visual material that allowed African doctors, nurses, and victims to explain their experiences in detail.

76. Lisa Lynch, "The Neo/bio/colonial Hot Zone, 233–252, 248.

77. Graham Harrison, "The Africanization of Poverty: A Retrospective on 'Making Poverty History,'" *African Affairs* 109, no. 436 (2010): 391–408. doi: 10.1093/afraf/adq025.

78. Steven Weinstein, "The Stigma of Ebola Remains Virulent in New York's African Community," *The New York Observer*, last modified November 11, 2014, paragraphs 5–6, http://observer.com/2014/11/the-taint-of-ebola-remains-virulent-in-new-yorks-african-community/.

79. Ibid., paragraph 1.

80. Carrilho, quoted in Thomas, "This Illustration," paragraph 4.

81. Ibid., paragraph 4.

82. Christopher Hooton, "'The ISIS of Biological Agents?': CNN is Asking the Stupid Ebola Questions," *The Independent*, last modified October 7, 2014, paragraph 4, http://www.independent.co.uk/news/world/americas/the-isis-of-biological-agents-cnn-is-asking-the-stupid-ebola-questions-9779584.html.

83. See, for example, the commentary that was provided by Alexander Garza, an associated dean of public health at the St. Louis University College of Public Health and Social Justice. He argued that Ebola was "no ordinary communicable disease," and that it was "the ISIS of biological agents." Alexander Garza, "Much More Vigorous Government Response to Ebola Is Needed," *The New York Times*, last modified October 3, 2014, paragraph 3, http://www.nytimes.com/roomfordebate/2014/10/02/how-to-stop-the-spread-of-ebola/much-more-vigorous-government-response-to-ebola-is-needed.

84. Stanley McChrystal and Kristina Talbert-Slagle, "How to Treat Threats of Ebola and ISIS,' CNN.com, last modified October 1, 2014, http://www.cnn.com/2014/10/01/opinion/mcchrystal-talbert-slagle-ebola-isis/.

85. Ibid., paragraph 1.

86. Ibid., paragraph 1.

87. Ibid., paragraph 3.

88. Ibid., paragraph 2.

89. Ibid., paragraph 2.

90. Ibid., paragraph 7.

91. Ibid., paragraph 2

92. For readers who might be interested to see how some of this fusion of military and medical rhetorics that were based on threats of infectious diseases have been around since at least 1976, see Andrew Lakoff, "The Generic Biothreat, or, How We Became Unprepared," *Cultural Anthropology* 23, no. 1 (2008): 399–428.

93. McChrystal and Talbert-Slagle," How to Treat Threats," paragraph 5.

94. Ibid., paragraph 7.

95. Ibid., paragraph 13.

96. Natalie D. Baker, Spyridon Samonas, and Kristine Artello, "(Not) Welcome to the U.S.: Hyper-Ebola and the Crisis of Misinformation," ISCRAM 2015 Conference-Kristiansand, May 24–27, 2015, http://iscram2015.uia.no/wp-content/uploads/2015/05/4-10.pdf.

97. Almudena Marí Sáez Ann Kelly and Hannah Brown, "Notes from Case Zero: Anthropology in the Time of Ebola," *Somatosphere: Science, Medicine, and Anthropology,* September 16, 2014, http://somatosphere.net/2014/09/notes-from-case-zero-anthropology-in-the-time-of-ebola.html.

98. Richard Preston, "The Ebola Wars," *The New Yorker,* last modified October 27, 2014, http://www.newyorker.com/magazine/2014/10/27/ebola-wars.

7

✛

Liberia's 2014 Autoimmunization of the West Point Suburb and the Return of the Colonial *Cordon Sanitaire*

In *La Peste* (The Plague), Albert Camus provided readers with an existential novel of how doctors, travelers, citizens, and even criminals in the Algerian city of Oran coped with the realization that they were dealing with an epidemic. The novel is written in a Kafkaesque style that focuses on the absurdity of trying to find secular or sacred rationalizations for why Oran has to suffer from the plague. Even though some realists tried to historicize the novel, Camus preferred to focus on the open-ended nature of his allegorical tales. He argued in one letter to his friend Louis Guilloux that what "counterbalances the absurd is the people struggling against it."[1]

The horrors associated with the recent "West African" Ebola outbreak of 2013–2015 have revived interest in the contemporary relevance of *La Peste*, and in many ways they have also raised questions regarding what type of local, regional, national, and international communities we want to identify with when we face the Sisyphean task of trying to control Ebola epidemics. More specifically, during periods of massive (in)security, what types of communal struggles would we like to see carried out in the name of public safety, health, and welfare? At the same time, in the age of the "Ebola apocalypse," what measures should we avoid taking as we think about the hopes and fears of endangered individuals or populations?

Given the nature of the transcontinental legal, political, medical, and economic arguments about Ebola that I have presented in previous chapters, readers are well aware that much of this theorizing about how to maintain one's humanity during epidemic crises involves more than abstract speculations. Throughout 2014 and 2015, West African leaders and populations had to make some agonizing choices between competing principles as they dealt with both the Ebola virus as well as the spread of fear and panic. While audiences in the global North flocked to movie theaters so that they could vicariously experience what it was like to live through plagues, those in global South did not always have that luxury.

On August 1, 2014, at an emergency meeting called by the Mano River Union, representatives of the three countries hardest hit by the latest Ebola outbreak—Guinea, Sierra Leone, and Liberia—agreed to a drastic emergency plan that would isolate a tri-region where the three countries met. This was a place where some 70 percent of the reported cases of EVD were found. By this time this tri-region, sometimes characterized as the "epicenter" of the outbreak, had witnessed almost 1,900 known cases and more than a thousand deaths from EVD, and representatives who attended the Mano River Union meeting decided to put in place what the Europeans once called a *cordon sanitaire*.[2] This was all taking place while foreign doctors were reporting in their medical journals that the number of cases in the current outbreak had exceeded the number from all previous Ebola outbreaks since 1976.[3] Western medical venues also contained commentaries on some of the indirect effects of the epidemic, including the disruption of standard medical care, interference with malaria containment efforts, and social upheavals.[4]

Ebola phobias in countless global contexts meant that even those nations that had not reported major EVD outbreaks could still use probabilistic or possibilistic arguments to rationalize the preventive actions that they took to make sure that the "West African" Ebola outbreak did not become an "African," or international pandemic. At the same time that the West African nations were trying to control their own borders, nations like Kenya were restricting plane flights in and out of Guinea, Liberia, and Sierra Leone. Talk of all sorts of voluntary or draconian "public health emergencies" were in the air, and cutting off land, sea, and air travel were all parts of these often heated conversations. Humanitarian concerns about mobility rights clashed with perceived collective necessities.

A Foucauldian review of the *dispositifs* that circulated during these periods show that at the center of many of these debates were the conversations about the cordons.

The French phrase *cordon sanitaire* literally means "sanitary barrier," and it refers to the usage of troops, blockades, border closings, or other drastic isolation strategies that are put in place when all else fails. The use of that phrase dates back to at least the early nineteenth century, when some 30,000 French troops were sent to the Pyrenees to stop a fever that was raging in Spain, and the troops were supposed to prevent the fever from crossing into French territory. Almost two centuries later, in the Kailahun and the Kenema districts of Sierra Leone, military blockades were set up where West African soldiers took the temperatures of those who were trying to get in and out of their country.[5]

Bioethicists, legal scholars, health experts, cultural anthropologists, and others who have studied *cordons sanitaires* have often expressed their suspicions about the usage of these tactics, and our colonial archives, tropical disease records, and global health histories are littered with examples of the use and abuse of these tactics. Just a week after WHO declared that the Ebola outbreak in West Africa was an "international public health emergency,"[6] Laurie Garrett explained that she had seen a *cordon sanitaire work* during the 1995 Zaire outbreak. Using immunizing language that pitted the Ebola virus against the West African states, Garrett opined,

> Three impoverished, tiny West African nations are in a collective state of siege, their people surrounded by a microbial enemy, the Ebola virus. In response to months of inaction, followed by ineffective measures, the governments of Sierra Leone, Liberia and Guinea have escalated their counterattack on the virus, imposing *cordons sanitaires* aimed at isolating entire regions . . . in hopes of containing the enemy. It may slow the virus' spread, but it will not be sufficient to stop Ebola or lift the state of siege.[7]

Garrett, perhaps sensing possible international pushback, argued that Congolese officials who used some of these methods to control the 1995 outbreak in "Zaire" had shown this could be "heartless but effective." What she may or may not have known is that her referencing of the "state of siege" could trigger the referencing of all sorts of martial solutions to health problems that had been used in European circles for centuries.

Yet many of those who read or heard about the Mano River Union decisions regarding their *cordon sanitaire* realized that these were desperate times that required unusual and extra-ordinary measures. For example, Liberia had a population of some 4 million people, and by August of 2014 they had fewer than 259 doctors in the entire country. Seven doctors had already contracted Ebola, and two of them died. Moreover, months earlier, dozens of foreign researchers and doctors thought that that they had put out the "West African" outbreak by May of that year, and their exodus thinned the ranks of experienced Ebola "hunters." As Raphael Frankfurter, the executive director of Wellbody, a clinical service for diamond-miners, explained, "The 'locals' seeing this mass exodus of expatriates has contributed to the sense that there's an apocalypse happening and they're in it on their own."[8] Others still held out hope that vaccines, like ZMapp, might help protect at least some of the thousands of health workers or volunteers in Liberia, Sierra Leone, and Guinea, but for now what was known as "supportive therapy" was the primary way of coping with a disease that had somewhere between a 50 percent and 90 percent morality rate.

The usage of cordons was thus considered to be one more potential strategy that could be used by soldiers and police who worked alongside local ministers, health care volunteers, and NGO personnel who were trying to stop the spread of EVD. Dr. Martin S. Cetron, the CDC chief quarantine expert, thought that the Mano River plan "might work," but he quickly qualified these remarks by explaining that it "also has a lot of potential to go poorly if it's not done with an ethical approach." By this, he meant that we no longer lived in "that era anymore" where you just let a disease burn itself out without "considering "the price of controlling it.'"[9]

While many natural scientists, social scientists, and humanists are still debating the efficacy and legality of taking this approach in EVD contexts, the May 2015 announcement that Liberia was "free" of Ebola seemed to provide evidence that vindicated the West Africans' usage of those drastic tactics. Yet by early July of that same year, three new EVD cases in Liberia ended that hollow hope.

The Mano River Union decisions have also revived interdisciplinary interest in studies of the nature, scope, and limits of the use of national or international public health restrictions during EVD outbreaks, and this particular chapter provides a critical cultural analysis of one key feature of some of the cordoning assemblages that would be put in place during the 2013–2015 Ebola outbreak. More specifically, it analyzes what happened just weeks after the Mano River Union meeting, when the Liberian President Ellen Johnson Sirleaf, and the Liberian military, decided to cordon off an entire suburb of Monrovia, the capital. It also juxtaposes those actions with those of foreign governments that started to impose travel restrictions on those who planned to go to West Africa.

As I will argue in more detail below, all of these interrelated nationalistic decisions have much to tell us about the ideological and rhetorical nature of these biosecuritizing measures.

Some of the key nodal points in these biosecurity assemblages are the mass-mediated representations of a Liberian suburb in Monrovia, called "West Point," that was inhabited by somewhere between 50,000 to 70,000 residents. For several weeks residents living in that suburb clashed with police, and they complained to reporters that they were being treated like prisoners, viruses, or slaves. These figurations became a part of what Adia Benton has called the "immune-logic" that categorizes who should, or should not, be controlled during Ebola outbreaks.[10]

Obviously I am not the first rhetorician or critical cultural scholar who has been interested in unpacking dense Ebola *dispositifs*. For example, Professor Bass, in 1998, argued that popular science stories about lethal viruses like Ebola often employ the racist entailments of European colonialism to "present ideologically charged images of the Third World and its relationship to the West as objectively based scientific 'fact.'"[11] Several years later Rebecca Waldon remarked that part of the fear of the "predatorial virus," known as Ebola, comes from the ways that communities use their imaginations to conjure up visions of plagues that will wipe out humanity "should Ebola ever become aerosol."[12] Professor Ayotte, in a more recent work, explained that when publics try to understand public health threats, they do not always adopt the "positivistic epistemological frameworks of public health officials" because they have their own horizons of meaning and some "established context of cultural knowledge about killer viruses."[13] These insightful comments on the importance of studying both elite and vernacular rhetorics in infectious disease contexts seem to provide examples of the "biocriticism" that Lisa Keränen was calling for in her own studies of bioterrorist discourses.[14]

This chapter will add to this growing interest in Ebola rhetorics, and I'll be intervening in the interdisciplinary debates that are taking place as scholars argue about the strengths and weaknesses of particular Ebola prevention, containment, or eradication strategies. Although there are a number of heuristic approaches that might be adopted by those who are interested in the study of cordons, quarantines, or other isolation strategies, I am convinced that an extension of the work of Jacques Derrida on "autoimmunity," Roberto Esposito on "immunitas," and Peter Sloterdijk on "immunology of spheres"[15] provides the necessary theoretical scaffolding for that type of intervention.

With this in mind, the rest of this chapter will be divided into four major sections. I begin by providing an overview of the theoretical relevance of the work of Derrida, Esposito, and Sloterdijk in Ebola contexts, and then I supply readers with a segment that unpacks the ideological features of West African configurations of West Point. The third section then explains how some international communities started to perform their own acts of auto-immunity as they were restricting travel to and from Guinea, Liberia, and Sierra Leone. The final, concluding section then provides a discussion of some of the alternative approaches that need to be considered as elites and publics converse about how to help get populations more involved in humanitarian Ebola containment efforts.

A BRIEF THEORETICAL DISCUSSION OF IMMUNITY, AUTOIMMUNITY, AND THE WORK OF ESPOSITO, DERRIDA, AND SLOTERDIJK

When philosophers and other critics use the term "immunity" in Ebola contexts they are often referring to the nexus that exists between the prophylactic measures that are needed to protect the individual body and the larger prevention or management strategies that might be used by populations dealing with infectious diseases. "Autoimmunity," explains Inga Mutsaers, "is a biological concept that refers to an immune response directed against a body's own cells and tissues."[16] From a critical vantage point, the porous boundaries that exist between literal, material viruses and the figurative, symbolic control of those viruses are inextricably linked, and studies of immunity and autoimmunity help us get at the persuasive aspects of the *dispositifs* that are created when social agents use this type of language in public health contexts.

Roberto Esposito, Jacques Derrida, and Peter Sloterdijk talk about the relevance of immunity or autoimmunity for the study of biopolitics, states of insecurity, and control of twenty-first-century plagues, and they like to philosophize about the constructive, as well as the destructive, ways that societies argue about the health and well-being of individual bodies or populations. Esposito, who comments on the importance of *communitas* and *immunitas*, explains how *communitas* refers to political communities that share risks, enjoy eventful lives, and understand the importance of shouldering egalitarian obligations in a positive sense.[17] When Esposito turns his attention to the notion of *immunitas*, he seems to be dwelling on some of the darker dimensions of human nature that manifest themselves during times of perceived insecurity. For example, he refers to those situations where a select few believe or act as if they are "immune" to the risks that befall others, and this in turn suggests that they are "safe from obligations or dangers that concern everyone else."[18] In sum, what Esposito calls the "immunology paradigm" has both biopolitical and thanatopolitical dimensions.

Jacques Derrida's own ruminations on "autoimmunity" complements and complicates Esposito's work, and he invites us to rethink how we write and talk about medicalization, stigmatization, and the immunization of salient social controversies. As Derrida pointed out before his death, the idea that the state can use discourses of self-protection and self-destruction, or that human beings can carry out policies based on talk of remedies and poisons, has been around a long time. He evidenced this by referencing the ancients' usage of the term *"pharmakon"* that Derrida viewed as an "old name" for "autoimmunitary logic."[19] Perhaps the most famous applied example of what Derrida meant by these terms can be found in his discussion of the appearance of repetitive "autoimmunity" aggression after September 11, 2001.[20]

Both Esposito and Derrida were sensing that the beginning of the twenty-first century was witnessing the advent of a new trend—the obsessive securitization rhetorics that underscored the importance of the immunization of Western populations. In *Bios* Esposito ruminated about how select European states employed an "exasperating immunitary conception of biopolitics that became a form of paroxysmic thanatopolitics, that is, a politics of death."[21] Writing just weeks after 9/11, Derrida opined that one could find logics of autoimmunology at work in the "inevitable perversion of technoscientific advances," where commentaries about "weapons of mass destruction" were linked to concerns about terrorism.[22] The United States after all, had to respond to the figurative infection that came when bin Laden's minions invaded America.

Sloterdijk adds to this mix when he contends that whether we realize it or not, our cultures and societies construct various protective "immunization spheres,"[23] that become *spatial* biosecurity defenses that function like biological, somatic immune systems. Certain immunization practices— that can include anything from our choice of dwellings to the types of cities or world views that we adopt—"act as *immune systems* or *immune responses* against possible threats from the outside world [emphasis in the original]."[24]

Peter Sloterdijk's notion of the "immunology of spheres" underscores the parallels that exist between epidemiological and virological ways of viewing immunity and the responses of larger cultural or political forces in society. Sloterdijk is interested in analyses of both the structures that are used for physical protection, as well as the more ideological features of our rhetorically crafted world. In order to help ground his claims, Sloterdijk points out how the epidemiological ideas of Pasteur and Koch have influenced the material and ideological ways that we think about old and emerging infectious disease threats, and he shows us how our talk of vaccines, health insurance, and other related *epistemes* or assemblages become a part of these immunological spheres.

These types of theoretical analyses have set the stage for critical cultural or legal studies of the phenomenological features of immunological thinking that sadly taps into societies' contemporary feelings of (in)security, where nations are willing to spend billions of dollars on possibilistic bioterrorist threats, while they throw a few million dollars in the direction of those actually fighting Ebola overseas.

The heuristic value of autoimmunity theoretical frames for critical studies stems from their diagnostic features that allow critics to see how some protective measures end up being more destructive than the original threats that they were trying to counter. Some forms of immunization, instead of maintaining healthy bodies and protecting political states, may end up becoming "a major threat to social (political) life itself."[25]

Fears and anxieties that circulate during times of perceived disaster lead to the creation of these immunizing and autoimmunity rhetorics. Derrida explained in one of his key critiques that societies that are worried about the need for immunities constantly create "events" that allow governments to provide publics with assurances about defense necessities or offensive capabilities. Derrida elaborated by noting that sometimes combatting terrorism involved the necessary deployment of "semantic, lexical, and rhetorical" skills. [26]

I now turn my attention to the ideological features of Liberia's attempt autoimmunizing of that nation during the 2013–2015 Ebola outbreak.

LIBERIA IMMUNIZING ITSELF FROM THE CONTAGIONS IN THE WEST POINT "SLUM"

In many neo-liberal tales that are told about the need for "legal" health containment practices, decision makers often try to demonstrate that they made a good-faith effort to use persuasive, "soft" techniques before they have to use more coercive strategies. When a few residents in the West African township of West Point started complaining about Ebola patients being brought to their suburb from other areas, and when Liberian officials heard rumors that some in that township believed that Ebola was a hoax,[27] then this seemed to provide authorities with evidence that the time for "palaver"(talk) had ended.[28] Anecdotal evidence of denialism and other dangerous activities in West Point seemed to warrant necessitous Liberian interventionism.

What were some of the events in West Point that demonstrated to Liberian authorities that they were running out of choices in their battle with Ebola? Many of the occupants of West Point were survivors and refugees of the Civil Wars and "conflict diamond" conflicts that had taken the lives of hundreds of thousands of West Africans, and even before the cordoning off of their suburb they been surveilled by both Tolbert Nyenswah, the Liberian assistant minister of health and social welfare, and President Ellen Johnson Sirleaf. For example, during the middle of August 2014, some kept on eye on several hundred people in West Point who had broken through the gates of a former school that had been converted into an "Ebola center" that housed suspected EVD victims. The Liberian Ministry of Health and Social Welfare, in Liberian Situation Report No. 94 for August 17, claimed that "West Point Community Leadership" had agreed to the reopening of the center as well as the transfer of some suspected Ebola patients to the John F. Kennedy ETU.[29] This created the impression that the majority of law-abiding Liberians living in West Point were peacefully following the dictates of the Liberian government, and those who were not complying constituted threats.

However, more vernacular "on the spot" testimonials and other coverage of these events showed that not everyone accepted the fact that West Point needed to have its own Ebola center. Samuel Tarplah, a Liberian nurse who was running the center, said that the protesters were trying to shut it down because they did not "want an Ebola holding center" in their community. The intruders reportedly stole mattresses, personal protective gear, and even buckets of chlorine.[30] One senior police officer, who spoke to the BBC on condition of anonymity, explained how the theft of these items could contribute to the spread of the virus.[31]

Derek Gregory, in his extension of the work of Derrida, has argued that some "immunitary" logics are clearly ideological when they involve "speech-acts" that are trying to save lives,[32] and West Point became the spatial condensation symbol for all of the cultural threats that endangered Liberians. President Ellen Johnson Sirleaf used a permutation of these immunitary arguments when she rationalized the quarantining of this portion of Monrovia. "We have been unable to control the spread due to continued denials, cultural burying practices, disregard for the advice of health workers and disrespect for the warning of government," she said.[33] For those who may still have had doubts she elaborated by noting that "due to the large population concentration" EVD "has spread widely in Monrovia and environs."[34] Her blend of ecological, epidemiological, and cultural claims made it appear as though West Point obstructionism prevented the Liberian containment of EVD.

Critical cultural scholars pay attention to both grammatical presences and absences, and it should be noted that President Sirleaf did not go into great detail explaining the exact pathogenic reasons why those in the West Point suburb were acting in atypical ways that uniquely threatened Liberian populations outside the "slum." She assumed that illegal West Point behavior looked nothing like legal Liberian behavior. She did not provide any specific examples of varying transmission rates, but she seemed to be implying that there was something phantasmagoric about that particular section of the capital. "May God bless us all and save the state," she said later exclaimed,[35] clearly signaling that she believed that the survival of her country was at stake. This was an example of what Sloterdijk calls the immunity of the "we," where immunization practices are no longer geared toward the preservation of individual life, but rather the communitarian goal of state preservation.

Some Liberians echoed President Ellen Johnson Sirleaf's autoimmunity messages. "There was a level of denial that needed, in our mind, shock therapy," noted one member of her administration, because people in West Point needed to be "awakened" to the facts about EVD deaths so that they realized that this was "no hanky-panky business."[36] Granted, there were studies that showed that many Liberians doubted that Ebola was a problem, and some went so far as to argue that foreign health workers brought EVD, but wasn't this a pervasive issue that involved many other Liberian suburbs or West African rural communities?

As one might imagine, the residents of West Point were divided when they were asked about the raids on the Ebola center in that suburb. Issac

Toe, a hygienist who worked at the center, recalled being terrified at the time of the "invasion," when the "entire West Point community"—"men, women, children, boys, and girls"—broke into the center.[37] Christiana Williams, who lived behind the center, recalled how her neighbors were bewildered by the fact that their neighborhood school had been turned overnight into an Ebola Center. She noted that many locals were terrified of the center, and Williams remembered hearing cries coming from the inside of the center as suspected Ebola victims claimed that they were getting sprayed and were not eating.[38]

It was not only the theft of these abject objects that worried Liberian health workers—former Ebola "inmates" who were quarantined in the West Point holding center had mysteriously vanished from the suburb. Days after the reportage of the quarantining, Liberia's Information Minister, Lewis Brown, told Western media outlets that seventeen of thirty-seven suspected Ebola victims had gone "back to their communities."[39] During a time when Liberian doctors and foreign advisers were talking and writing about how a *single* recalcitrant family, or how the touching of bodies at a major funeral, might prevent the national containment of contagion, the acts of vandalism and flight out of the Ebola center in West Point looked like intentionally transgressive acts. Anxious public officials, who had already been given emergency powers for border cordons, could now deploy the police or the military to protect the public health of the Liberian nation.

One August morning West Point residents woke up to find that Liberian soldiers and police officers, all wearing riot gear, were blocking the roads into their Monrovia suburb. The waterfront was cordoned off by the Liberian Coast Guard, and this prevented residents from setting out in canoes. Barbed wire barricades were set up in streets and alleys as the government announced that it was placing this entire area under strict quarantine.[40] West Point had suddenly turned into a spatialized "Patient Zero," and the Liberian military and police were helping autoimmunize their nation.

Virological, epidemiological, and political rationales were merged together into the public heath *dispositifs* that were used to rationalize the segregation and isolation of West Point. In theory, the quarantine was supposed to last at least twenty-one days, Ebola's maximum incubation period.

International photographers took pictures of the clashes that erupted as hundreds of angry youths in West Point hurled rocks and stormed the barricades. David Anan, a 34-year-old resident of the suburb, asked the heavily armed police and soldiers who were enforcing the quarantine if "you fight Ebola with" arms?[41] Four people were injured when the police or the soldiers fired their weapons, and one teenager, Shakie Kamara, fifteen, died from leg wounds. "This is messed up," said Lieutenant Colonel Abraham Kromah, the Liberian head of operations for the national police, and he talked of how "a group of criminals" had injured one of the police officers.[42]

Some mainstream journalists, who wrote in that positivist style that Professor Ayotte referenced, still tried to provide a not-so-veiled critique of some of these immunizing measures. Norimitsu Oneshi of the *New York Times*, who did an excellent job of contextualizing these affairs, explained to his readers that usually Ebola outbreaks happened in rural areas, but that authorities had to change their focus when EVD spread to major cities like Conakry in Guinea or Monrovia in Liberia. "The risks that Ebola will spread quickly" are multiplied in dense urban environments Oneshi explained, especially in places where health systems had collapsed and where residents "appear increasingly distrustful of the government's approach to the crisis."[43]

The quarantining of West Point was openly defended by Liberian governmental authorities and public health officials as necessitous measures that had to be taken during dire circumstances. Meanwhile, residents did what they could to resist and circumvent these efforts. After just a few days, prices for food staples skyrocketed in the West Point suburb, and some individuals managed to swim in and out of the quarantined zone.[44] More than a few residents bribed their way out of West Point by paying fees to soldiers, and one's personal appearance, circumstances, and even gender were said to be factors in determining how much one paid to travel in and out of West Point. Christian Verre had to pay $6 to get out, while he was charged $4.25 for his girlfriend. While those less fortunate had to stay within the cordon, Verre and his partner managed to move into a shack that was just a few blocks outside of West Point.[45]

When President Ellen Johnson Sirleaf visited West Point during the quarantine period she was surrounded by armed guards who were wearing surgical gloves. This may not have been the official personal protective equipment (PPE) that was supposed to be worn by those who handled Ebola victims, but in this age of *perceptual (in)security* it must have offered some peace of mind for those police who guarded the president. "We suffering! No food, Ma, no eat, we beg you, Ma!" one man yelled at Ms. Sirleaf during her visit,[46] but for days, residents had to fend for themselves.

After ten days the *cordon sanitaire* around West Point was "prematurely" lifted, some eleven days before the required twenty-one-day incubation period. The Liberian government tried to place a positive spin on matters by commenting on how lessons had been learned and how West Point had quieted down, but Abubaker Bah, who managed a drug dispensary, said that most people believed that there wasn't any Ebola in West Point, and that the government left because they didn't find any EVD.[47] Apparently there was more than one form of denialism spreading in that suburb.

While some observers argued that President Sirleaf and the Liberian army had caved in to international pressure, Liberian officials provide the press with other explanations for the lifting of the quarantine. At the same time that crowds cheered and danced in the streets after the end of this particular quarantining, Lewis Brown, Liberia's information minister said that decision was made because it appeared that health authorities could now identify suspected Ebola victims and that the West Point community was "cooperating" with those officials who were fighting the disease.[48] Brown reasoned that this decision did not in any way signal that there was no Ebola in this "shanty town," and he seemed to leave open the possibility that sometime in the future Monrovia might once again have to resort to cordons or quarantines in order to try to protect itself against this enclave.

Interestingly enough, Liberians would soon be complaining that foreigners were turning Liberia into a pariah state. Law abiding Liberians may have wanted to segregate West Point from Monrovia, but foreigners were viewing the Liberian capital through different lenses. The outbreaks in Monrovia, unlike the ones in the Guinean capital of Conakry, or the one in the Sierra Leonean capital of Freetown, where configured by scientists and journalists in the mainstream press as unpredictable, inexplicable, and mysterious. There was something about the body politic in Monrovia, or the people's social or hygienic habits, that seemed to be contributing to the uncontrolled spread of EVD. Dr. Armand Sprecher, an Ebola expert working with Doctors Without Borders, provided a typical commentary on Monrovia when he noted that there was "something in the disease transmission behaviors in Monrovia that has done this. . . . We've never seen this kind of explosion in an urban environment before."[49] Scientific ambiguity and uncertainty thus provided one more rationale for defending needed cordons.

THE "NORTH" IMMUNIZES ITSELF FROM THE EVD THREATS COMING FROM GUINEA, LIBERIA, AND SIERRA LEONE

Ironically, at the very same time that West African nations were trying to set up cordons in order to immunize themselves from places like West Point, other parts of the world were worrying about the EVD that might be coming out of Liberia, Guinea, or Sierra Leone. In spite of the fact that the CDC constantly argued that the Ebola virus could only be spread through direct contact with the blood or fluids of an infected person and not through "airborne transmission," countries like Canada were following the recommendations of their own nation's public health agencies in recommending that Canadians "avoid all non-essential travel" to West Africa.[50]

Mainstream and alternative press coverage of West Point and these flight restrictions allowed journalists, bioethics, public health officials, doctors, and others to debate about the nature and limits of various isolation or restriction schemes. Those in the "North" could experiment and fine-tune their arguments as they argued from a distance about the EVD in the "South." Empowered global communities who rarely dealt with EVD could critique everything from the continued resonance of "apocalyptic" outbreak narratives to the legality of *cordons sanitaires*. William Wallis of the *Financial Times*, for example, opined that the photos of the Liberian Ebola Task Force enforcing the quarantine on the West Point "slum" showed that the older "dystopic" visions that were conjured up in movies such as "*Outbreak* and *Contagion*" were "creeping closer to reality."[51] Wallis contextualized Liberia's cordoning off of its own suburb by noting that Senegal had closed its borders to Liberia, and that that nation had banned air travel and shipping to Guinea, Sierra Leone, and Liberia.

Officials in Senegal could argue that they meant no affront and that they were just being prudent, and they could always claim that they were simply following the lead of nations such as Chad, the Ivory Coast, South Africa, Kenya, and other African states that had already imposed some forms of travel restrictions and trade regulations on those who were coming in and out of the three West African nations.[52] Members of the African Union, who apparently wanted to show that there were pan-African solutions to Ebola problems, announced that any threats to law and order that were posed by the disease would be handled by the deployment of a "military and humanitarian mission comprised of doctors, nurses, and other medical and paramedical personnel."[53]

President Sirleaf's attempt to immunize the rest of Monrovia by quarantining a part of her own city provides an example of what Professor McKerrow once called the "social regulation of space,"[54] and this also seemed to be a part of a much larger wave of draconian assemblages as nation after nation sought to institute symbolic or material immunizing measures. Even Nigeria, a relatively wealthy nation that had seventeen confirmed cases of Ebola (as well as a reputation for successfully preventing outbreaks), found that Cameroon was closing its border with Nigeria. This postcolonial move was itself filled with plenty of ironies, given the fact that during the earlier colonial years Cameroon was once treated as a "laboratory" for European studies of sleeping sickness.[55]

The adoption of critical cultural approaches to all of this talk of travel restrictions, quarantines, cordons, and other isolation strategies underscores the ideological nature of the contested medical knowledges that became hopelessly entangled in some of this decision making. "The word Ebola conjures up more fear than any other word in the medical vocabulary," said Gregory Hartl of WHO, and few of those who were implementing flight restrictions were listening to the warnings of those who talked of panic, food, and fuel problems, and the counterproductive nature of some of these national and international measures.[56] How, after all, were expert logicians, virologists, epidemiologists, foreign health care administrators, or strategic communication experts supposed to get into these areas if travel and trade restrictions were in place? Scientific rationales could be used for these cordons as well as for the lifting of travel restrictions.

Some critics of the West Port quarantines remarked that all of these performances were reminiscent of the "plague villages" that were once used by those in "medieval Europe" who battled the Bubonic Plague. Writers for *National Public Radio*—in an essay that included references to both the quarantining of "Typhoid Mary" and the *cordon sanitaire* of West Point—quoted a representative of Doctors Without Borders who opined that "lockdowns and quarantines do not help control Ebola," because they ended up driving "people underground and jeopardizing the trust between people and health providers."[57] Other opponents of the quarantines and cordons argued that contact tracing, the use of "support" therapies, strategic communication with civic leaders, and airport screenings would do more to help end the spread of EVD in the long run.

In the weeks following the end of the West Point quarantine volunteer health workers went door-to-door asking if residents knew of any sick Ebola suspects. "We are here on health matters," one volunteer explained on a typical visit, and then he proceeded to ask if anyone in that home was suffering from malaria, fever, or typhoid. "We got no sick persons here," one resident replied, and the health workers went on to follow other leads.[58] Although no one seemed to know exactly how many residents in West Point had actually contracted Ebola, and few had access to research on how those statistics compared with the rest of Monrovia or West Africa in general, contact tracers were out in force. In early September of 2014 these tracers believed that they were going to have to check up on 150 people, who were linked to areas of some thirty suspected cases.[59]

CONCLUSION: RESTORING *COMMUNITAS* IN EBOLA CONTEXTS

At this point I want to make explicit what I have been arguing implicitly throughout this chapter—that the use of many of these coercive, immunizing strategies during Ebola outbreaks are both unnecessary and ineffectual. These are exactly the times when you need the cooperation of local populations, when it is contact tracers or other local workers who make the difference when they gain the trust of those who are suspicious of governmental practices. Liberia's quarantining of West Point, that looks as though it was punitive in nature, is an example of what Esposito called *immunitas* and what Derrida characterized as *autoimmunity*. As Inge Mutsaers has recently argued in her critique of a different biosecurity context, sometimes "defensive immunization responses" of countries "bring about considerable collateral damage."[60]

Eventually West Point residents, after the lifting of the quarantine, worked on their own with buckets and buckets of chlorine to try to help clean up their own suburb, and the use of draconian measures only delayed the temporary "end" of the Liberian portion of the West African outbreak.

We can readily understand when nation-states, faced with the loss of thousands of lives, declare emergencies and impose cordons and quarantines that are based on epidemiological or clinical rationales for massive isolation of populations. However, this well-intentioned, if myopic way of viewing an epidemic or pandemic, does not take into account the ideological, the cultural, the psychological, and the social nature of these same biopolitical or thanatopolitical *dispositifs*. As Esposito observed, focusing too much on *immunitas*, and not worrying about the social formation of *communitas*, is a recipe for disaster.

It is therefore incumbent that critical cultural scholars or critical legal researchers join the ranks of the interdisciplinary communities who are trying to pay attention to what Hannah Brown and Ann Kelly call the "material proximities" of "hot spots," those spaces where researchers study the political dimensions of convergences that bring together the "mundane interactions that create the condition of pathological possibility."[61] This is why it is so important that critics try to uncover the reasons why Liberia tried to autoimmunize itself from a part of its body-politic with the cordoning of West Point, and why we need to juxtapose that decision with the actions of other nations that tried to restrict West African air travel.

Much of this had more to do with the spread of fear than the existential threats posed by EVD. Lisa Keränen once argued that "rhetoricians and critical communication scholars can at the very least play a more significant role in explaining" some of the discourses that are "reproducing the very bio(in)insecurity that gives it power and meaning,"[62] and case studies like this complement the work of theorists, as well as practitioners, who worry about excessive immunization. "To completely seal off" and prevent planes from traveling "in or out of the West African countries," noted Dr. Anthony Fauci, Director of the National Institute of Allergy and

Infectious Diseases, "paradoxically make things much worse in the sense that you can't get supplies in, you can't get help in, [and] you can't get the kind of things in there that we need to contain the epidemic."[63]

As I will note in other chapters, local communities and nation-states need not adopt problematic "airborne" transmission Ebola epidemiological theories as they try to rationalize their closing of airports or borders. The adoption of these types of measures often infuriate populations that view them as punitive in nature. A critical review of various *cordons sanitaires* underscores the importance of using imperfect strategies that allow African and other health planners to work with, rather than against, the contagious "other."

There are at least two recent examples of how national communities might be able to avoid some excessive *"immunitas"* while they successfully fight EVD outbreaks. Take, for example, the cases of Nigeria and Senegal, that used two different, but related strategies to gain the warranted assent of their populations as they sought to contain Ebola outbreaks. In Nigeria, massive problems with EVD transmission could have occurred when a Liberian diplomat, Patrick Sawyer, traveled to Lagos, the largest city in Nigeria, which had an overcrowded population of 21 million. Health officials in Nigeria did not panic and few talked about immunizing their country from the infectious diseases that ravaged poorer nations. In the same way that Camus once wrote about how doctors in Oran had the herculean task of dealing with a plague they did not understand, Nigerian public officials dealt with their own virological uncertainties.

Airport staff were unprepared when Sawyer first landed in Nigeria, and during July of 2014 Sawyer managed to pass along Ebola to the officer who escorted him to the hospital, as well as nine of the doctors and nurses who attended him.[64] However, the Nigerians assessed the risks, and as Karen Weintraub explains, public health specialists made sure that there would not be any "apocalyptic outbreak" in Lagos.[65]

Instead of panicking, Nigerians applied preparedness strategies that were used to contain other infectious diseases. They performed airport screenings, and thousands got involved in massive contact tracing of potential Ebola victims and those who may have touched them. Dr. Ameyo Adadevoh became a martyred heroine in many Nigerian circles when she successfully diagnosed Sawyer's Ebola case, and she kept him in the hospital despite his protestations. She later died from Ebola herself, but by sounding the alarm in her nation Nigerians were able to prevent a "doomsday scenario" by tracing the three hundred or so people who had been in direct or indirect contact with the diplomat.[66] The CDC reported that Nigerian health officials and volunteers went to more than 26,000 households of people who were living with, or around the contacts of Ebola patients. Sameul Matkoka, the Ebola operations manager in Nigeria for the International Federal of Red Cross and Red Crescent Societies (IFRC), admitted that at first Nigeria was not really prepared for the Ebola outbreak, but he explained how his nation became Ebola "free" after the "swift response" from the federal government, state governments in Nigeria, and international communities.[67] Twenty Nigerians would become infected, and seven would die, but these would be some of the last reported cases.

The Nigerian elites and publics did not ostracize Ebola victims, and their efforts included "house-to-house leafleting, messages on local radio stations, and enlisting 'Nollywood' stars to delivery health messages."[68] Faisal Shuaib and his co-authors, writing for the CDC's *Morbidity and Mortality Report*, also explained that Nigeria's response had profited from the rapid use of its national public health care infrastructures (NCDC), as well as from some of the lessons that were learned during a major lead poisoning response campaign in 2010 and earlier polio eradication efforts.[69]

Senegal, is a poverty-stricken nation that does not have Nigeria's economic resources, but it was nevertheless able to contain a potential Ebola outbreak. The government there, led by President Macky Sall, provided counseling, and officials handed out needed supplies and food to those who may been in contact with suspected Ebola patients. Public health officials in Senegal also worked to protect the identities of Ebola suspects. As J. Peter Pham, director of the Atlantic Council's Africa Center observed, "they didn't turn them into pariahs," and this was "good policy" and the "right thing to do."[70]

The indexing case in this outbreak narrative began when a young man traveled to Dakar, by road, from Guinea, where WHO officials believe he had direct contact with an Ebola victim. Senegal's response plan involved the identification and monitoring of seventy-four close contacts of the traveler from Guinea, and that nation also put in place stricter surveillance measures at the borders. Teams of epidemiologists from WHO and Médecins sans Frontières helped provide needed staff and testing, and when the traveler recovered he returned to Guinea on September 18, 2014.[71]

Initially Senegal put in place a controversial cordon at the 200-mile long border with Guinea, but after being pressured by the UN and other international officials, Senegal established an "air corridor" that allowed in many humanitarian organizations that needed to ferry in medical supplies and personnel.[72] Officials in Guinea need to be given partial credit for their communitarian actions in this case, because they were the ones who alerted Senegal about the possible arrival of a travel who may have been exposed to Ebola.[73]

Beginning in October of 2014, public health officials in Sierra Leone, Liberia, and Guinea were finally given tens of millions of dollars in foreign aid, and some of this was spent on protective gear and Ebola treatment kits, so that those who refused to visit Ebola treatment centers could at least protect themselves and their loved ones. This was described by some journalists as a "last-ditch, do-it-yourself version of trace, isolate, and treat" strategies that had been used since the 1976 Zaire outbreak.[74]

With the benefit of hindsight, it could be argued that the Liberian army, and the government officials who favored imposition of the *cordons sanitaires*, had forgotten one of the most important lessons of successful auto-immunization efforts—the need to gain the support of the populace. Dr. Jean-Jacques Muyembe, a Congolese physician who was one of the heroes who helped "discover" the "Zaire" Ebola virus in the 1970s, argued that placing the "police and the army in charge of the quarantine was the worst things you could do," because this made those inside West Point feel as though they were being oppressed instead of helped.[75]

Some of the actions in Nigeria and Senegal perhaps provide examples of what Exposito was looking for with his discussions of "*communitas*." "Derrida yearned for a different sort of immune system," argued Warwick Anderson, "one that harbored radical alterity: a commune system,"[76] and while these nations have their own issues, they were at least trying to work with their populations as they battled EVD.

For critical rhetoricians and others who are interested in taking up Lisa's Keränen call for new investigations of biocriticism, the work of Derrida, Esposito, and Sloterdijk presents us with a novel way of configuring a host of immunization and biosecuritization *dispositifs*. Instead of taking at face value the claims of officials that their quarantines, cordons, or other mechanisms have succeeded in stopping the spread of outbreaks like Ebola, a critical perspective invites us to ask more pointed questions. As Inge Mutsaers explained, now the critic has to ask whether certain types of immunization measures risked "destroying not only the alleged enemy outside, but first and foremost the social 'body' it is meant to protect."[77]

In July of 2015, three cases of Ebola were reported in Liberia. Like Camus, those in West Africa will once again have to decide how to rally around each other as they face yet another potential plague.

NOTES

1. Erin Tremblay Ponnou-Delaffon, "In and Out of Place: Geographies of Revolt in Camus's *La Peste*," *Studies in 20th & 21st Century Literature*, 39 no. 1 (2015): 1–13, 10.

2. Donald G. McNeil Jr., "Using a Tactic Unseen in a Century, Countries Cordon Off Ebola-Racked Areas," *The New York Times*, last modified August 12, 2014,

paragraphs 1–5, http://www.nytimes.com/2014/08/13/science/using-a-tactic-unseen-in-a-century-countries-cordon-off-ebola-racked-areas.html?_r=0.

3. Elizabeth Shell, "Ebola Outbreak Now Responsible for More Than Previous Combined," *CCTV America,* last modified September 4, 2014, http://www.cctv-america.com/2014/09/04/ebola-outbreak-now-responsible-for-more-deaths-than-previous-combined.

4. See, for example, Thomas R. Frieden, et al., "Ebola 2014—New Challenges, New Global Response and Responsibilities," *The New England Journal of Medicine* 371 (2014): 1177–1180, doi: 10.1056/NEJMp1409903.

5. McNeil, "Using a Tactic Unseen in a Century," paragraphs 8–9.

6. Kim Willsher, "WHO Declares Ebola Outbreak a Global Health Emergency," *Los Angeles Times,* last modified August 8, 2014, paragraph 1, http://www.latimes.com/world/europe/la-fg-ebola-outbreak-20140808-story.html.

7. Laurie Garrett, "Heartless but Effective: I've Seen 'Cordon Sanitaire' Work against Ebola," *The New Republic,* August 14, 2014, paragraph 1, http://www.newrepublic.com/article/119085/ebola-cordon-sanitaire-when-it-worked-congo-1995.

8. Sheri Fink, "With Aid Doctors Gone, Ebola Fight Grows Harder," *The New York Times,* last modified August 16, 2014, paragraph 5, http://www.ny-times.com/2014/08/17/world/africa/with-aid-doctors-gone-ebola-fight-grows-harder.html.

9. Dr. Martin S. Cetron, quoted in McNeil, "Using a Tactic Unseen in a Century," paragraph 6.

10. Adia Benton, "Race and the Immuno-Logics of Ebola Response in West Africa," Somatosphere.net, September 19, 2014, http://somatosphere.net/2014/09/race-and-the-immuno-logics-of-ebola-response-in-west-africa.html.

11. Jeff D. Bass, "Hearts of Darkness and Hot Zones: The Ideologeme of Imperial Contagion in Recent Accounts of Viral Outbreaks," *The Quarterly Journal of Speech* 84 (1998): 430–447, 430, doi: 10.1080/00335639809384231.

12. Rebecca A. Weldon, "An 'Urban Legend' of Global Proportion: An Analysis of Nonfiction Accounts of the Ebola Virus," *Journal of Communication* 6 (2001): 281–294, 281.

13. Kevin J. Ayotte, "A Vocabulary of Dis-Ease: Argumentation, Hot Zones, and the Intertextuality of Bioterrorism," *Argumentation and Advocacy* 48 (Summer 2011): 1–21, 2–3.

14. Lisa Keränen, "Concocting Viral Apocalypse: Catastrophic Risk and the Production of Bio(in)security," *Western Journal of Communication* 75, no. 5 (2011): 451–472.

15. For an intriguing extension of Peter Sloterdijk's work that applies it to "One-Health" interspecies approaches, see Inge Mutsaers, "One Health Approach as Counter-Measure against 'Autoimmune' Responses in Biosecurity," *Social Science & Medicine* 129 (2015): 123–130.

16. Inge Mutsaers, "One Health Approach as Counter-Measure," 124.

17. Roberto Esposito's most famous works appear in a trilogy that provides the general contours that shape his immunization paradigm. Roberto Esposito, *Communitas: The Origin and Destiny of the Community,* translated by Timothy Campbell (Redwood City, CA: Stanford University Press, 2004); Roberto Esposito,

Bios: Biopolitics and Philosophy, translated by Timothy Campbell (Minneapolis: University of Minnesota Press, 2007); Roberto Esposito, *Immunitas: The Protection and Negation of Life*, translated by Zakiya Hanafi (Cambridge: Polity, 2011). For an excellent overview of how these different books uniquely add to his discussions of immunology, see Rossella Bonito Oliva and Timothy Campbell, "From the Immune Community to the Communitarian Immunity: On the Recent Reflection of Roberto Esposito," *Diacritics* 36, no. 2 (Summer 2006): 70–82.

18. Roberto Esposito, in Robert Esposito and Anna Paparcone, "Interview," *Diacritics* 36, no. 2 (Summer 2006): 49–56, 50.

19. Jacques Derrida, "Autoimmunity: Real and Symbolic Suicides," in *Philosophy in a Time of Terror: Dialogues with Jürgen Habermas and Jacques Derrida*, interviewed by Giovanna Borradori (Chicago: University of Chicago Press, 2003), 85–136, 124.

20. Derrida, "Autoimmunity: Real and Symbolic Suicides," 85–136.

21. Esposito and Paparcone, "Interview," 52.

22. Derrida, "Autoimmunity: Real and Symbolic Suicides," 124.

23. Peter Sloterdijk, *Spharen I Mikrospharologie: Blasen*. (Frankfurt: Suhrkamp Verlag 1998).

24. Inge Mutsaers, "One Health Approach as Counter-Measure," 124.

25. Inge Mutsaers, "One Health Approach as Counter-Measure," 124.

26. Derrida, "Autoimmunity, Real and Symbolic Suicides," 105.

27. BBC News, "Ebola Crisis: Liberia Confirms West Point Patients Missing," BBC.com, last modified August 19, 2014, http://www.bbc.com/news/world-africa-28841040.

28. Liberians were not the only African populations who were willing to discuss the need for federal isolation or quarantine orders. A few Nigerian lawyers who worried about Ebola spilling over from Liberia, also wanted their country to take drastic action. See, for example, Clement Udegbe, "Overcoming the Ebola Palaver," Vanguardngr.com, last modified August 15, 2014, http://www.vanguardngr.com/2014/08/overcoming-ebola-palaver/.

29. Ministry of Health and Social Welfare, *Liberia Ebola Situation Report*, no. 94, August 17, 2014, page 17, http://mohsw.gov.lr/documents/Liberia%20 Ebola%20SitRep%2094%20Aug%2017,%202014.pdf.

30. Samuel Tarplah, quoted in Fink, "With Aid Doctors Gone," paragraph 10.

31. BBC News, "Ebola Crisis: Liberia Confirms," paragraph 15.

32. Derek Gregory, "Theory of the Drone 3: Killing Grounds," Geographical Imaginations, July 29, 2013, paragraphs 16, 27, http://geographicalimaginations.com/2013/07/29/theory-of-the-drone-3-killing-grounds/.

33. Ellen Johnson Sirleaf, quoted in the *LA Times*, "Liberia Imposes Ebola Quarantine and Curfew in a Monrovia Slum," *Los Angeles Times*, last modified August 19, 2014, paragraph 4, http://www.latimes.com/world/africa/la-fg-africa-ebola-liberia-curfew-20140819-story.html.

34. Ibid., paragraph 4.

35. Ibid., paragraph 5.

36. Lewis Brown, quoted in Anne Look, "Liberia Struggles to Isolate Suspected Ebola Cases," Voanews.com, last modified September 5, 2014, paragraph 21,

http://www.voanews.com/content/liberia-struggles-to-find-isolate-suspected-ebola-cases/2440164.html.

37. Issac Toe, quoted in Norimitsu Onishi, "Clashes Erupt as Liberia Sets an Ebola Quarantine," *The New York Times*, last modified August 20, 2014, paragraph 19, http://www.nytimes.com/2014/08/21/world/africa/ebola-outbreak-liberia-quarantine.html?_r=0.

38. Onishi, "Clashes Erupt as Liberia Sets," 20.

39. Lewis Brown, quoted in BBC News, "Ebola Crisis: Liberia Confirms," paragraph 17. Mainstream Western newspapers seemed to have been confused on the exact numbers who left the Ebola center. The *Los Angeles Times*, for example, was reporting that "37 patients who were supposed to be under surveillance left," and that health officials were reporting that they "all later returned." *Los Angeles Times*, "Liberia Imposes Ebola Quarantine," paragraph 6. If this was the case, this undermined some of the rationales for singling out West Point in the first place.

40. Onishi, "Clashes Erupt as Liberia Sets," paragraph 1.

41. Ibid., paragraph 37.

42. Abraham Kromah, quoted in Onishi, "Clashes Erupt as Liberia Sets," paragraph 4.

43. Onishi, "Clashes Erupt as Liberia Sets," paragraph 6–7.

44. Norimitsu Onishi, "As Ebola Grips Liberia's Capital, a Quarantine Sows Social Chaos," *The New York Times*, last modified August 28, 2014, http://www.nytimes.com/2014/08/29/world/africa/in-liberias-capital-an-ebola-outbreak-like-no-other.html.

45. Ibid., paragraphs 2–3.

46. Ibid., paragraph 6.

47. Abubakar Bah, quoted in Norimitsu Onishi, "Quarantine for Ebola Lifted in Liberia Slum," *The New York Times*, last modified August 29, 2014, paragraph 8, http://www.nytimes.com/2014/08/30/world/africa/quarantine-for-ebola-lifted-in-liberia-slum.html.

48. Gabriella Joxwiak, "Liberia Lifts Ebola Slum Siege," *The Sunday Times*, last modified August 31, 2014, http://www.thesundaytimes.co.uk/sto/news/world_news/Africa/article1453042.ece.

49. Armand Sprecher, quoted in Onishi, "As Ebola Grips Liberia's Capital," paragraph 22.

50. *Toronto Star*, "A Guide for Canadians Worried about Ebola Outbreak," Thestar.com, last modified August 5, 2014, http://www.thestar.com/news/world/2014/08/05/a_guide_for_canadians_worried_about_ebola_outbreak.html.

51. William Wallis, "*Cordon Sanitaire* Tightens around West African States to Beat Ebola," *Financial Times*, last modified August 22, 2014, paragraph 1, http://www.ft.com/cms/s/0/d7419538-2a0e-11e4-8139-00144feabdc0.html#axzz3vw1Up4pA.

52. Ibid., paragraphs 2–3.

53. Ibid., paragraph 19.

54. Raymie E. McKerrow, "Space and Time in the Postmodern Polity," *Western Journal of Communication* 63, no. 3 (1999) 271–290, 278.

55. Daniel R. Headrick, "Sleeping Sickness Epidemics and Colonial Responses in East and Central Africa, 1900–1940," *PLOS Neglected Tropical Diseases* 8, no. 4 (April 2014): 1–8.

56. Ibid., paragraph 10.

57. NPR, "Awful Moments in Quarantine History: Remember Typhoid Mary?" NPR.com last modified October 30, 2014, paragraph 30, http://www.npr.org/sections/goatsandsoda/2014/10/30/360120406/awful-moments-in-quarantine-history-remember-typhoid-mary.

58. Look, "Liberia Struggles to Isolate," paragraphs 1–5.

59. Ibid., paragraph 22.

60. Mutsaers, "One-Health Approach," 124.

61. Hannah Brown and Ann H. Kelly, "Material Proximities and Hotspots: Toward an Anthropology of Viral Hemorrhagic Fevers," *Medical Anthropological Quarterly* 28, no. 2 (2014): 280–303, 281–282.

62. Keränen, "Concocting Viral Apocalypse," 468.

63. Anthony Fauci, quoted in Julia Belluz and Steven Hoffman, "Why Travel Bans Will Only Make the Ebola Epidemic Worse," Vox.com, last modified October 17, 2014, paragraph 15, http://www.vox.com/2014/10/13/6964633/travel-ban-airport-screening-ebola-outbreak-virus.

64. Karen Weintraub, "From Senegal and Nigeria, 4 Lessons On How to Stop Ebola," *National Geographic*, October 25, 2014, paragraph 3, http://news.nationalgeographic.com/content/news/en_US/news/2014/10/141024-ebola-nigeria-outbreak-lessons-virus-health.html.

65. Ibid., paragraph 4.

66. Camullus Eboh and Angela Ukomadu, "Nigeria Declared Ebola-free, Holds Lessons for Others," Reuters, last modified October 20, 2014, http://in.reuters.com/article/2014/10/20/health-ebola-nigeria-idINKCN0I90UN20141020.

67. Eboh and Ukomadu, "Nigeria Declared Ebola-free," paragraphs 11–12.

68. Weintraub, "From Senegal and Nigeria," paragraph 55.

69. Faisal Shuaib et al., "Ebola Virus Disease Outbreak-Nigeria, July-September 2014," *Morbidity and Mortality Weekly Report* 63, no. 39 (October 3, 2014): 867–872, 869.

70. J. Peter Pham, quoted in Alexandra Zavis, "Ebola-Free: How Did Nigeria And Senegal Do It?" *Los Angeles Times*, October 22, 2014, paragraph 24, http://www.latimes.com/world/africa/la-fg-nigeria-senegal-ebola-20141022-story.html. Zavis, "Ebola-Free, How Did Nigeria and Senegal," paragraph 24.

71. World Health Organization, "Who Congratulates Senegal on Ending Ebola Transmission," *World Health Organization, International,* last modified October 17, 2014, http://www.who.int/mediacentre/news/statements/2014/senegal-ends-ebola/en/.

72. Zavis, "Ebola-Free: How Did Nigeria and Senegal," paragraph 8.

73. Ibid., paragraph 14.

74. Weintraub, "From Senegal and Nigeria," paragraph 29.

75. Dr. Jean-Jacques Muybembe, quoted in Onishi, "As Ebola Grips Liberia's Capital," paragraph 10.

76. Warwick Anderson, "Tolerance," Somatosphere, October 27, 2014, paragraph 6, http://somatosphere.net/2014/10/tolerance.html.

77. Inge Mutsaers, "One Health Approach as Counter-Measure," 125.

8

✛

Belated Military Humanitarianism and American "Ebola Exceptionalism" during the West African Ebola Outbreak

After the August 2014 WHO declaration that Ebola had become a global health emergency many nations around the world, embarrassed by their belated interventionism, scrambled to make up for lost time. Dr. Joanne Liu, the president of Médicines sans Frontières, remarked during the early fall of 2014 that it's "like wartime," and pleaded for more active humanitarian interventionism.[1] While NGOs like Doctors Without Borders continued to circulate Cassandra-like clarion calls for humanitarian relief, less shrill voices demanded that the World Bank, the IMF, the United Nations, and many other organizations try to show that they could set aside their political or economic differences in the name of more transcendent, humanitarian goals. "If the outbreak is not stopped now, we could be looking at hundreds of thousands of people infected" opined U.S. President Barack Obama, and he went on to assert that "it's a profound threat to global security . . . if people panic."[2] In this age of insecurity, he did not hesitate to blend together military and medical humanitarian rhetorics.

Some of the aid that flowed into Liberia, Sierra Leone, and Guinea came from those who were usually talking about non-military aid or civilian humanitarianism, and it did not escape the notice of some that this aid was coming from communities who consistently defended the vaunted principles of impartiality and non-neutrality. However, the global anxieties about a spreading pandemic, that could kill regardless of one's morals, mobilized both realists and idealists,[3] and all of this contributed to the formation of some unusual alliances in the battle against Ebola. As I mentioned in chapter 1, this led to the reluctant advocacy of military solutions to apparently massive logical problems.

For several generations, going back at least to colonial times, countless conversations had taken place regarding the exact nature and scope of the military solutions that were proffered during humanitarian crises. This was especially true on the African continent, where those who celebrated decolonization during the early 1960s were not always sure of what to make of the French, Belgian, Portuguese, British, or American soldiers who got caught up in the civil wars and resource conflicts of the period.

As noted in previous chapters, some of the medical humanitarian principles that were espoused by organizations like Médicines sans Frontières had to do with the cross-border reporting of any violations of human rights protections, which meant they were sometimes the "watchdogs on the state."[4] In the past some of MSF's political entanglements with governmental military or state policies, that interfered with the freedom of movement of medical humanitarians, had occasionally forced the withdrawal of doctors from places like Ethiopia[5] and North Korea. Those who read "along the grain" of the dominant humanitarian *epistemes*[6] were suspicious of the military authorities who had historically claimed to be working in the name of medical humanitarianism.[7]

The American elites and members of the public who defended U.S. military and medical interventionism in Africa entered into this prefigured world, and they tried to argue that global audiences need not fear America's various "overseas contingency operations." For those who believed in the nobility of these causes, U.S. interventionism in Africa, for counterterrorist or public health purposes, was just a natural extension of the ways that Americans had always helped those who were interested in democratic governance or freedom from want. As the nation's commander-in-chief would explain, Americans realized that whenever "a disaster or a disease strikes, the world looks to us." President Obama was sure that the world would see that it was "American values" that made U.S. efforts "exceptional."[8] The dominant narratives, at least in Anglo-American communities, continually emphasized the point that there was nothing incompatible between multilateral notions of medical humanitarianism and American notions of unilateral or bilateral military humanitarianism.

Oftentimes "dual purposes" motivated those who wanted to ensure the survival of those in the "third world" at the same time that they fought against "Jihadist" terrorism, and any potential contradictions in principles could be papered over by those who were sure that anti-Americanism should not stand in the way of military humanitarianism. Many neo-liberals, who supported all types of needed foreign interventionism during times of emergency, apparently sensed that they were hearing counternarratives that went against the grain. Dane Erickson and Alice Friend complained in November of 2014,

> After almost fifteen years of unprecedented political stabilization and economic development in Africa, the ravages of Ebola and a spike in military coups in places like Burkina Faso and Mali are ominous signs of a continent backsliding under the weight of corruption and political conflict. Pundits and reporters in the United States are framing these events with concerns about the "militarization" of U.S. Africa policy. but the modest level of American security assistance in Africa is not to blame for recent developments in West Africa. If we learn anything from recent civil-military conflicts, it should be that Africa needs more U.S. security assistance, not less.[9]

At the same time, Erickson and Friend argued that very little of the nearly $7 billion that was being designated by the State Department to go to sub-Sahara Africa was really related to securitization that might hurt civilian-military relationships. They calculated that maybe 6 percent of these allocations were going to security, and they were adamant that the U.S. Africa Command had no interest in talking over economic, development, or humanitarian investments in the region. As far as Erickson and Friend were concerned, critics of the Americans needed to remember that "many African militaries are corrupt and weak, with poor human rights records and histories of threatening democratic rule, and that it was Boko Haram al-Shabaab And Al Qaeda that were the real military threats and corrupting powers in the region."[10]

In this particular chapter, I will be discussing how various American, British, and other communities reacted to all of these defenses of what scholars are now calling the "militarization" or securitization of Ebola.[11] I will use a case study of the American public relations campaigns that reviews the controversies that swirled around "Operation United Assistance" (OUA), and I will use those reviews as entrée points for critiquing the operative military logics that went into effect during the "Ebola surge."[12]

Were some critics right when they saw this surge as just a public relations ploy that extended the reach of the U.S. Africa Command (AFRICOM), or was this a sincere and novel form of military humanitarianism, that followed in the wake of WHO calls for a "military-like" response to Ebola?[13] From a critical legal vantage point, did the members of mainstream Anglo-American journalistic circles conceal as much as they revealed about the impacts of this interventionism?

It may be decades before we can see some of the Pentagon memos that may have circulated in Washington, D.C., circles during this latest Ebola outbreak, but we have been left with fragmentary texts that indicated that

by September of 2014 many disheartened members of NGOs were join-
ing those who felt a sense of urgency. As I noted in the first two chapters
of this book, I personally believe that they underestimated the cultural
changes that were taking place at the community levels as West African
citizens took matters in hand, but this was clearly not the way that many
military leaders configured the Ebola outbreak.

To be fair to these military leaders, we need to recall that for several
weeks leaders of West African countries had been sending out global
calls for more aid so that former colonial powers in the United Kingdom
and France would send more personnel and equipment to Sierra Leone
and Guinea, and those who supported President Obama's efforts could
not help highlighting just how American money had been earmarked for
Ebola relief. "The amount for which we requested was about $100 million
a month ago and now it is $1 billion so our asking has gone up 10 times in
a month," explained Dr. David Nabarro of the United Nations. He elaborated by explaining that the advanced stage of the Ebola outbreak meant
that the "level of surge we need" is "massive" and "unprecedented."[14]

Even those who usually balked at the idea of working with military
personnel realized that compromises might need to be made in the name
of global medical necessities. Dr. Joanne Liu explained in a special briefing to the United Nations how the epidemic had outstripped the capacity
of her organization to provide needed aid:

> Today, in Monrovia, sick people are banging on the doors of MSF Ebola care
> centers, because they do not want to infect their families and they are desper-
> ate for a safe place in which to be isolated. Tragically, our teams must turn
> them away. We simply do not have enough capacity for them. Highly infec-
> tious people are forced to return home, only to infect others and continue the
> spread of this deadly virus. All for a lack of international response.[15]

As noted elsewhere, many doctors working for her organization espoused
their continued allegiance to the humanitarian principles of *témoignage*,
neutrality, impartiality, but some felt that this was an exceptional time of
emergency. While pundits were mulling over the potential consequences
of supporting military interventionism, experts were estimating that
somewhere between 20,000 and 1.5 million people might be infected by
the next month if drastic actions were not taken.[16]

This larger figure, for many Anglo-Americans, could be derived from
realistic appraisals of statistical information and a medical calculus that
seemed to indisputably point toward necessitous interventionism. Helping West African Ebola fighters was deemed a moral as well as a medical
imperative. In the same way that Americans used international law principles of "defense" as they went after Al Qaeda or Taliban terrorists, they

now talked of how they had to intervene overseas so that they could fight Ebola before it "jumped" continents and came their way.

The Americans deployed Ebola *dispositifs* that melded together fragments from the archives of both military humanitarian histories and medical humanitarian genealogies as they justified what they viewed as their "leadership" role in Operation United Assistance. In theory, the Obama part of the surge would serve as the "backbone" that would give other countries the "confidence to send in supplies and money to help."[17] The U.S. commander-in-chief, and those in his chain of command, were fond of saying that that the U.S. leadership efforts had a "multiplier" effect on the aid from other countries that flowed into Liberia, Guinea, and Sierra Leone. This, of course, often assumed that *civilian initiatives* couldn't have been led by the United Nations, WHO, the European Union, African Union, Chinese or Cuban officials. True believers were convinced that there was something special about American military leadership that might turn the tide in the battle against Ebola.

It is often said that beggars can't be choosers, and that any form of aid, even military humanitarian aid, provides life-saving measures in times of great medical distress. However, in this chapter what I would like to argue is that before readers reach any definitive conclusions regarding the short-term and long-term costs or rewards of any particular military humanitarian intervention they need to factor in the empirical evidence of the impact of that intervention, the motivations for that activity, and the unintended consequences of that military interventionism. As Alberto Toscano has explained in another context, "among intellectuals of a more oppositional cast, the idea that reference to human rights has served as a threadbare cloak for both *realpolitik* and depoliticization is uncontroversial."[18] Moreover, it may be possible that if the Ebola was already under control, then allowing in the military only contributes to the formation of more moral hazards.

When mainstream newspapers wrote about the advent of Operation United Assistance they sometimes showed readers pictures of Liberian Red Cross health care workers wearing protective suits as they carried bodies of victims of EVD in places like Monrovia, but these were not going to be the co-workers who would be standing beside American military personnel in these same places and in these same battles. Anglo-American mainstream outlets might show television viewers or newspaper readers images of newly minted Ebola centers or hospital facilities, but what they often ignored were the relatively marginal roles that foreign interventionists played in the overall schemes that were needed to contain this latest Ebola outbreak.

This, obviously, was not going to be the way that American and U.K. military forces were going to contextualize their own social agency.

THE ADVENT OF OPERATION UNITED ASSISTANCE AND THE DEFENSES OF U.S. MILITARY HUMANITARIANISM

Even before President Ellen Johnson Sirleaf and President Obama were talking about the importance of massive infusions of American aid during the fall of 2014, there were countless NGO personnel, politicians, journalists, and others who were using military metaphors to contextualize the spread of Ebola virus disease in West Africa. Sarah Crowe of UNICEF, for example, self-identified as a fighter on the "frontline" in Liberia's "biological war," talked as if Ebola was the personification of some terrorist threat:

> When I was in Liberia in 2006 it was to work on reintegration of child soldiers. . . . Ebola has turned survivors into human booby traps, unexploded ordnance—touch and you die. Ebola psychosis is paralyzing. . . . In the car with colleagues, they talk nostalgically about the long civil war here—a time when the enemy was seen, the rockets were heard, the bullets could be dodged.[19]

The invisibility of the Ebola enemy only underscored the importance of having allies who could render visible EVD threats.

For most of September and October of 2014, America's mainstream newspapers provided their readers with a steady stream of information that often came from the representatives of USAID or the Department of Defense. This all could be used to outline the American preparedness plans for what would be called Operation United Assistance. Between three thousand and four thousand U.S. military personnel would be sent to West Africa so that they could provide medical, security, and logical support.

However, it was not always clear exactly how many of these U.S. travelers would be the doctors and nurses who would actually help those who tracked, isolated, and diagnosed EVD on the "frontlines." The use of these quantitative figures made it appear as if each and every one of these volunteers was aiding this particular "surge" and military humanitarian effort.

Talking about the numbers of personnel or the amount of the money that was being spent during the Obama Ebola "surge" was not the only way that military leaders could put on display the significance of Operation United Assistance. Generals and subalterns who were interviewed could also talk about the need to quickly build hospitals that contained at least twenty-five beds. Building something known as the "modular hospital," or what in military parlance was called an expeditionary medical support system (EMED), was a popular topic of discussion, and readers were told of how it was going to be constructed near an airport outside of Monrovia.[20] J. Freedom du Lac, a reporter for the *Washington Post*, provided a typical summary of American efforts when he wrote this byline during the second week of October: "The U.S. Military's New Enemy, Ebola: Operation United Assistance Is Now Underway."[21] More than a month later the military personnel who traveled overseas were now being called the "U.S. Ebola fighters."[22]

Some four thousand individuals volunteered to be a part of the U.S. civilian portion of Operation United Assistance, and they realized that someone had to staff the seventeen ETUs that were going to be built. USAID reported that while it was unclear just how many civilians would make it through the entire vetting process, some of those who stepped up to be vetted had experience working with the International Medical Corps, Save the Children, the International Organization, and the International Rescue Committee.[23] If you take into account their willingness to serve, this indeed looked like "united assistance."

By the time that Americans started to actually send troops overseas almost six thousand West Africans had already died from EVD, but this did not dampen the spirit of many Anglo-Americans who talked about this latest "mission." Although there were some commentators who openly questioned how ordinary U.S. soldiers were going to help those who needed doctors, nurses, and other public health care workers, there plenty of supporters who were convinced that this was the next Haiti, and that Americans had to shoulder their extraordinary global responsibilities.

At places like Fort Campbell, Kentucky, pictures were taken of soldiers being trained at the U.S. Army Medical Research Institute of Infectious Diseases, and all of this helped allay the fears of some who worried that the members of the 101 Airborne Division (Air Assault) were being sent in to fight an enemy that was different from Al Qaeda, the Taliban, or ISIS. This, however, did not prevent the reporting of descriptive information that showed that the Pentagon was planning on sending engineers to set up treatment centers in Liberia, each with a 100-bed capacity.[24]

It is telling that the U.S. military, and those who defended American military intervention, seemed to assiduously avoid discussing whether any of these American military personnel were going to be looking for the next "Patient Zero," or whether they would be working in the forest regions of the tri-state area that was considered to be the epicenter of this Ebola outbreak. Yes, observers could see pictures of them talking to West Africans, building Ebola treatment centers, but where were the photos of medical doctors *actually treating any suspected or confirmed EVD patients*? Would the members of Operation United Assistance work alongside West African health care workers, and would they be the wearing the same exact personal protective gear that would be worn by MSF or local African workers?

While a few sources indicated that some military medical doctors might be helping do that type of work, most of the essays that appeared in mainstream newspapers between September and October of 2014 did not provide any detailed discussions of how these American personnel were actually putting themselves at risk. These particular American versions of Ebola rescue narratives were crafted by those who listed the number of beds that would be prepared, the treatment units that would be built, and the amount of supplies that would be shipped by U.S. cargo planes.

During this same period the nation's commander in chief announced that the U.S. military was going to "lead" the fight against Ebola in West Africa, and he promised that some $750 million was going to be dedicated to the effort. One newspaper tried to contextualize the American initiative as one that a reluctant nation shouldered because few others were overseeing "what has been a chaotic and widely criticized response to the worse Ebola outbreak in history."[25] Readers of the *Washington Post* were assured that an American general would be sent over from U.S. Africa Command, and that he would lead Operation United Assistance. The general would head a regional command that would be based in Liberia, and this command would then be used to coordinate U.S. and international relief efforts while a separate regional staging base was set up to help accelerate logistics with the transportation of needed equipment, supplies, or personnel. Talk of the goals of AFRICOM in general, and Operation United Assistance in particular, were often linked together as examples of beneficent, and benign, military humanitarian efforts.

It was telling that few, if any, of these mainstream Anglo-American newspapers contained any stories about how West Africans or NGO personnel had explicitly asked that the United States *lead* humanitarian efforts during the fall of 2014. Surely any help was appreciated, but questions could be raised about how American funds were getting spent by West African recipients. An obvious question, given the fact that the Liberians had been fighting Ebola for many months, is why U.S. troops, engineers, and doctors were not being placed at the disposal of the Liberian military or civilian authorities. Weren't these Liberian authorities representatives of democracies, and weren't international relations scholars always discussing the importance of state "sovereignty"? Even though there was evidence that President Sirleaf had asked for aid, it was not always clear that her views represented those of most Liberians or others who battled EVD on a daily basis.

Many journalists who worked for mainstream Anglo-American television stations or newspapers tried to be supportive in their contextualization of Operation United Assistance. They circulated materials that were supplied by the White House, USAID, or the Department of Defense, and only occasionally did investigative reporters question the decisions that were made to militarize Ebola containment efforts. A fairly bland, and typical commentary regarding U.S. national interests was supplied by Lena Sun and Juliet Eilperin when they remarked in September that Obama's decision to enlist the U.S. military reflected the concern of U.S. officials that "unless greater force is brought to bear, the epidemic could wreak havoc on the continent."[26] Perhaps the privatization of health care, and the fragmented nature of civilian containment efforts, had underscored the importance of finding military solutions to Ebola problems.

The pictures that were used to adorn some of these mainstream stories about Operation United Assistance made it clear that the U.S. military would be staying under Obama's command, and that American generals and others would be the ones making the decisions about how, when, and where they needed to carry out their missions. There were photo opportunities that put on display the cooperative nature of these efforts as U.S. engineers were photographed talking to Liberian airport workers, and some news articles contained commentaries on how West Africans were grateful recipients who appreciated these efforts.

In earlier chapters I have described the constitutive rhetorical creation of many of the antecedent "man versus microbe" rhetorics, and the recirculation of these figurations helped pave the way for the *naturalization* of U.S. military humanitarian efforts. The fight against Ebola was depicted as a typical military engagement, and one photograph that accompanied the J. Freedom du Lac essay showed a group of U.S. Air Force airmen preparing a barbed wire fence in Monrovia. Audiences could enthymematically infer that in the same way that troops in Iraq or Afghanistan had to put up barbed wire to keep out Taliban insurgents, Americans fighting Ebola had to set barriers in portions of Monrovia.

To its credit, *Voice of America* at least admitted that not everyone was enamored with this American intervention, and some hinted that all of this might be serving as nice public relations for anxious audiences back in the United States. After all, those back home were still reading about the struggles in America of Nina Pham, Thomas Eric Duncan, or Kent Brantly. Benno Muchler, who reported on how the United States was the largest foreign contributor to Ebola efforts in West Africa, explained that this was the biggest military operation for America since the withdrawal of forces from Somalia in 1993. He went on, however, to admit that local "residents had mixed feelings about the military involvement as the first uniformed soldiers arrived here at the end of September."[27] What went unsaid was the fact that those who expressed any reservations had little say in any of this decision making.

Like many other foreigners who had been involved in both the first and the second interventions to fight Ebola in 2014, the Americans often configured the spread of EVD as a problem that could be attributed to local ignorance and misunderstanding. This way of conceptualizing the problem could then be tethered to commentaries that presumed that the military offered the solution to those local problems.

Oftentimes this supposed lack of West African understanding could also become the entrée point for commentaries on the irrationality of other misperceptions. Major General Darryl Williams, who led the U.S. "humanitarian military operation" in Liberia, said that he believed that most Liberians liked Americans, but that he understood that any military venture might be unpopular. He said that his troops were prepared to cope with these feelings. Muchler, after quoting Williams, then explains that "a lack of information about the virus led to the quick spread of Ebola in Liberia, Sierra Leone, and Guinea" when this outbreak first began in December of 2013.[28] Muchler then linked these two statements together and said that U.S. forces seemed to know that they were in an "information war," where earlier suspicions and lack of education had led to the killing in Guinea of some health care workers.

This type of commentary served several rhetorical functions. First of all, it could be used to summarily dismiss the notion that American military personnel did not belong in West Africa. Second, it allowed military leaders to pose as knowledgeable parties who knew about Ebola virology or pathogenesis. Third, by commenting on how this was an "information" war, this created the impression that the beneficent American military was using some of the same "hearts and minds" strategizing that had worked in Iraq or Afghanistan. Moreover, the commentary on attacks on MSF and other health care workers made it appear as though any problems that the U.S. military encountered were the normal and typical problems that confronted all foreigners who were working in this region.

The implication was clear—more than a few Americans believed that they were on a righteous mission to help the Liberians fight Ebola, and only a minority of West African resented their interventionism. Given the popularity of the American military in the United States, as well as the resonance of many U.S. military humanitarian discourses, it is understandable that many academics not only accepted, but applauded the Obama Ebola "surge." For example, political scientist Maryam Zarnegar Deloffre published an essay that contained a panoptic view of the room where President Obama was speaking about the international response to Ebola epidemic during the 69th session of the UN General Assembly in New York. Writing just a few weeks after the UN Security Council (UNSC) held an unprecedented emergency meeting on the topic of a public health crisis, Deloffre wrote about how Obama's deployment plans included the training of some five hundred health care workers per week.[29]

Employing very formalistic rhetorics that touched on the topic of "human security" Deloffre contextualized Obama's surge as an example of how human security now meant more than just single sovereign nation-states protecting their people, borders, economic stability, or political interests. The phrase "human security," according to Deloffre, now meant that the world paid attention to the collective needs and the multi-lateral efforts of the collectives who worried about health pandemics, global poverty and climate related disasters that impacted the lives of many.[30]

Perhaps anticipating that suspicious parties might wonder about the unilateral nature of America's efforts, Deloffre invited her readers to think about the novel features of this particular military intervention. She tried to argue that neither Operation United Assistance, nor the UN Mission for Ebola Emergency Response (UNMEER),[31] were like other previous militarized humanitarian missions. She was convinced that the emphasis that was being placed on concretizing the abstract notion of "human security" represented some type of watershed moment, a chance for a paradigm shift, where non-government organizations and the military "work together in a partnership."[32]

Some defenders of America's military humanitarianism were puzzled by all of the criticism that was directed at President Obama or the Pentagon when they talked of the security needs of both West Africa and the United States. Dan Murphy, for example, said that the U.S. military excelled at the type of work that was needed to fight Ebola, and yet he was convinced that if you paid attention to cable news you would find "both calls for the Obama administration to ramp up its military effort to 'destroy' the so-called Islamic State in Iraq and Syria" as well as "warnings that the president's deployment of up to 4,000 troops to help contain Ebola" was a "disaster waiting to happen."[33] Clearly some conservatives thought that we were fighting the wrong foe, but Murphy explained that the pundits in the press were getting this all backward—Iraq and Syria were complex messes, where the military had to deal with "competing ethnicities, ideologies, religious sects, and divergent interests among so-called allies." Murphy thought that the lessons learned from some past incursions shows that the United States had trouble trying to kill "ideologies in foreign societies" but it could excel when other countries needed American expertise, discipline, and the ability to mobilize resources in the service of an "achievable goal."[34] These types of Ebola outbreak narratives contextualized EVD containment as an opportunity that needed to be seized by Americans during a period when they could provide humanitarian relief without having to battle the "isms" that so often got in the way. This, from a critical vantage point, hid Murphy's own "isms."

Previous medical histories and colonial archives were used by Murphy to illustrate how Operation United Assistance was just one small part of a lengthy, linear legacy of military involvement in the international containment of diseases. Murphy could point out that George Washington and his troops faced the threat of smallpox epidemics, and U.S. medical teams helped build the Panama canal by controlling the spread of malaria. Later on, Murphy explained, the U.S. military medical research had helped with the development of vaccines for strains of hepatitis and typhoid, and other military medical researchers and doctors helped improve the treatment of diseases.

In the next section I survey some of the commentary that came from those who were willing to read "against the grain" as they critiqued the Obama Ebola surge.

MODERATE AND HARSH CRITIQUES OF MILITARY HUMANITARIANISM AND PUBLIC ATTACKS ON AFRICOM' S INVOLVEMENT IN WEST AFRICAN AFFAIRS

While many mainstream journalists pointed out that Liberia's president Ellen Johnson Sirleaf had asked that President Obama and other leaders of more prosperous nations increase their aid efforts, there were no shortage of critics who worried that the "militarization" of humanitarian aid did little to actually help the people of Liberia, Guinea, or Sierra Leone. "America's response to Ebola," wrote law professor Karen Greenberg, "looks disturbing similar to the War on Terror."[35] She contextualized the Obama surge as an act that reprised the Petraeus surge in Iraq in 2007, and she tied this medical adventurism to Obama's interest in increasing security at the Mexico-U.S. border, drone attacks overseas, and other defenses of the homeland. Greenberg was bothered by the "ease" with which U.S. elites and publics were accepting the words of "non-medical authorities" who were using the now familiar discourse on the global war on terrorism to produce a "default template for Ebola" that was allowing the country to uncritically march "down the road" to war against a disease.[36]

Some academics reminded readers that this was not the first time that those in the "North" found reasons to rescue those in the "South." Alex de Waal, writing in the *Boston Review*, complained that Operation United Assistance might look altruistic and benign, but he pointed out some of the long-term implications of using military rhetorics and policies that reframed the attempts at stopping the spread of EVD:

> This is worryingly authoritarian, bad for the public and strategically counter-productive. Despite its impressive logistics, the army makes only a marginal contribution to international disaster relief—and often makes things worse. Nor do soldiers "fight" pathogens—and the language of warfare risks turning infected people and their caretakers into objects of fear and stigma.[37]

While Obama and other defenders of Operation United Assistance often tried to underscore how the U.S. military was coordinating with USAID and was working alongside others overseas in the fight against Ebola, de Waal mentioned several points that were often glossed over by journalists writing in the mainstream presses. For example, he pointed out that military commanders were going to be the ones giving the orders during Operation United Assistance, and that some humanitarian workers actually refused to be seen with soldiers.[38]

Critics like Alex de Waal were willing to grant the importance of having military aid in the form of *logistical support*, but he realized that their military aid came with a price—securitized goals and motives would clash with medical humanitarian efforts, and the U.S. military, and not the Liberian civilian authorities, were going to the ones leading this "surge." Matte Peppe, writing in March of 2015, questioned how Rear Admiral John Kirby could call the Department of Defense Ebola mission a success when "the troops did not treat a single patient, much less save a single life."[39] This may have been a slight exaggeration, but it nevertheless conveyed the argument that some were trying to take too much credit for the work of others.

Some critics tried to emphasize the point that there were alternative civilian humanitarian options that were overlooked by those who rushed to rationalize military solutions. Kim Yi Dionne, Laura Seay, and Erin McDaniel, for example, understood that Liberian President Ellen Johnson Sirleaf had asked for some military-like assistance, but they worried about the adverse impact of this particular response.[40] Charles Ellison, writing just a few weeks after some of the first U.S. troops were landing in Liberia, asked, Why send "the military and not medicine" to Ebola-stricken parts of Africa?[41] During a discussion that included Ellison, Peter James Hudson, and Jemima Pierce the three of them talked of how the American response could be contrasted with the efforts of the Cubans, who were sending over some three hundred doctors who joined the 461 who were already in West Africa. This raised the prospect that the U.S. response to Ebola was actually a very small part of some broader securitizing strategizing on the part of the Obama administration, that began as far back as some of President George W. Bush's initiatives in 2008. Hudson opined that part of the motivations for Obama's latest surge came from security preparations for the "threat" of China's presence in any future scramble for scarce African resources, and he pointed out that by that time the United States had a military presence in just about every African nation.[42] Was it possible that post–Cold War logics were become entangled in contemporary rhetorics about twenty-first-century medical humanitarian campaigns?

In sum, some of the academics who watched the progress of Obama's military humanitarian surge argued that sending in the military so that they could handle what some regarded as a purely medical emergency made it difficult for some of these aid workers to follow the traditional medical humanitarian principles of neutrality and impartiality.

Readers can guess that those who supported Operation United Assistance, especially after December of 2014, ignored most of these complaints.

HAGIOGRAPHIC REMEMBRANCES OF OPERATION UNITED ASSISTANCE AND TAKING CREDIT FOR "ENDING" THE LIBERIAN EBOLA OUTBREAK

Although there would be skeptics who talked of the belated nature of what they viewed as a largely irrelevant American Ebola "surge," most writers for popular press magazines, mainstream newspapers, and academic outlets, when they did use temporal types of frameworks, invited their readers to believe that the U.S. troops arrived right on time, and that their mobilization efforts were a total and unqualified success.

In some cases observers went even further and claimed that things *could have been much worse* if the Americans hadn't mounted Operation United Assistance. David Francis, a contributor to *Foreign Policy*, wrote an essay in February of 2015 that admitted that Ebola's toll had been horrific, but he was sure that it could have been worse. President Obama isn't declaring "that Africa's Ebola crisis is over," Francis opined, but "he's making clear that he believes that the spread of the virus, which public health workers once feared could infect hundreds of thousands, has been largely stopped in its tracks."[43] Naturally, the Americans were given credit for this stoppage.

Many of these American celebrations of the efficacy of Operation United Assistance magnified the nature of the perceived threats before the surge, and then they allowed the American military, and USAID, to take the bulk of the credit for helping contain this latest outbreak. Accounts like those that were written by David Francis mentioned in passing the contributions of the Chinese or personnel from the EU but the bulk of their commentaries made little mention of the sacrifices of thousands of contact tracers, local missionaries, tribal leaders, West African health officials, and many others who were on the scene long before the Americans stepped foot in Liberia. Instead, essays like the Francis essay mentioned Obama's social agency, and how he was at a "celebratory news conference" praising the U.S. troops and doctors who had traveled to Africa to fight the disease.[44]

In some cases the medical reports that documented the "lessons learned" from Operation United Assistance used their own politicized chronologies of past military identification of "infectious disease threats" as they outlined how the U.S. military research and development had worked at dealing with malaria, diarrhea-bacteria, dengue fever, Rift Valley Fever, and other infectious diseases.[45] Writing in *Military Medicine* in June of 2015, Colonel Clinton Murray and his co-authors could use the notion of "infectious disease threats" to focus on what could have happened, rather than what did happen, during OUA:

> Those deployed in support of OUA are at substantial risk of developing infectious complications in addition to potential exposure to Ebola. The most likely threats would be diarrheal diseases and respiratory infection, which place a high priority on hygiene measures. Vector-borne diseases are also of concern, placing a premium on PPM [public private mix]. Malaria presents the greatest risk given the high attack rate and potential for severe diseases necessitating command emphasis on PPM and malaria chemoprophylaxis adherence with clinicians required to provide early and accurate diagnosis and therapy for malaria.[46]

In the same way that U.S. military medical chroniclers once wrote about the challenges that confronted American military forces during the building of the Panama Canal or the policing of the Philippines, twenty-first-century military medical reports contained narratives of new "infectious disease threats."

Intentionally or unintentionally, these types of militarized medical stories, with their strategic adaption of the generic Ebola "rescue" plot lines, provided permutations of outbreak narratives that made it appear as though American soldiers placed themselves at risk while others reported on how their interventionism *was the key* factor in turning the tide against Ebola.

Many of these American rescue narratives used before-and-after narratives that contrasted the dystopia of places like Monrovia before the Obama "surge" with the utopian afterimages of the cleanliness and the orderliness that came in the wake of foreign military interventionism. In laudatory, selective chronologies neoliberal writers could write about how there once had been bodies lying in the streets, gangs threatening to burn hospitals, and conditions that led one ambassador to warn about an "apocalyptic urban outbreak." Stability appeared on the horizons in these biopolitical tales as U.S. authors waxed eloquently on the healing that would come after West Africans learned of the $6.2 billion that the Obama administration had committed to spending on combating disease in West Africa and in the United States.[47]

Many of the critics of OUA ridiculed this mission by pointing out that many facilities that were built were emptied, but defenders of the operation like David Francis tried to argue that this was proof that the earlier dire predictions were wrong, and that massive deaths were not inevitable. In his contextualization of American medical interventionism, it was the media that had gone overboard in overhyping the potential dangers in the first place.

A related strategy that was used by defenders of OUA involved focusing on a specific list of military goals that were assigned to those who carried out the Obama Ebola surge, and then those who took this approach could argue that the United States decided to leave after accomplishing those goals. For example, one publication explained that when Major General Gary Volesky arrived and assumed command had been handed a "to-do list by the U.S. Agency for the International Development (USAID) and the Liberian government" that included the need to (1) build seventeen temporary treatment facilities across the country; (2) train a mixture of local Liberian and international health care workers to staff them; and (3) use some of the Pentagon's "high end medical equipment to test patients' blood for the deadly virus."[48] Brian Castner then explained that when Volesky and his forces checked off nearly all of those items by January of 2015, they could either go home, stay and wait and see if the outbreak worsened, or they could move on to Sierra Leone or Guinea and use a similar list.[49]

Conspicuously absent in this type of review was any commentary on the specific contributions or day-to-day work of the medical doctors, or the numbers of Ebola patients that they actually treated. Instead, readers were told about how Major General Gary Volesky once flew around in his Black Hawk helicopter from Monrovia to small places like Bopulu in northern Liberia in order to oversee the progress that had been made in the construction of one of the Army's Ebola treatment facilities.

By this time the Pentagon had decided to build fifteen instead of seventeen facilities, and each of them only needed to hold fifty beds instead of a hundred, and all of this was chalked up to the fact that what had once been an "out of control crisis" had now become a "more focused strategy of stamping out flare-ups."[50] The Bopulu initiative was configured as a part of the "vital part of the ring of outposts" that were being built around northern Liberia that were going to "guard Monrovia and the cities along the coast against migrants from Sierra Leone and Guinea who may carrying the virus with them."[51]

This type of revised framing of OUA deflected attention away from what the Americans *were not doing* so that readers could congratulate the military for their securitization of the perimeter at the same time that they provided logical support and medical supplies. This was one more way of magnifying the contributions of the United States for those who could forget that some of the earlier outbreaks in West Africa took place in regions where there had been porous borders, lax cordons, quarantines, and isolationist practices. Now the troops who participated in Operation United Assistance could argue that they, and their USAID colleagues, had provided civilian/ military cooperation that made possible the efforts of the Ebola fighters who were actually providing medical care to EVD patients.

In many ways, Major General Volesky's very presence served as a reminder of the symbolic and material links between the 2007 Iraq "surge" of President Bush and General Petraeus and the Obama "surge" in 2014. Volesky, who told reporters that "we are fighting an enemy" and that enemy is Ebola, had served four tours of duty in Iraq (dating back to the 1991 Persian Gulf War) and in 2004 he had been awarded a Silver Star as a young battalion commander who lead a rescue mission in Sadr City.[52]

Writers like Castner could write with pride about how soldiers like Major General Volesky had made sure that they finished training some 1,200 health workers before they headed home. NGOs like Partners in Health and International Medical Corp were going to take over the Ebola treatment centers built by the Army, and the World Food Program stepped in and arranged for the transportation of supplies for blood testing. As Castner explained to his readers, by January of 2015 it looked like it was time to come home. "For Volesky and his soldiers," this writer averred, the "next item may well involve" declaring "victory."[53]

The decisions regarding when this victory over Ebola took place, and who were the victors, was an easy one to make for military humanitarians.

CONCLUSION

Months before the White House, USAID, and the Department of Defense were heralding the role that American exceptionalism had played in "ending" the spread of Ebola in Liberia, there were many commentators who were convinced that the militarization of EVD finally provided health care workers with the optimal strategizing that was needed. Circulating an example of what Stephen Collier and Andrew Lakoff call "vital systems security" rhetoric,[54] Tom Koch argued that pundits who studied American medical military histories would find that the containment of Ebola vulnerabilities was indeed a "war":

> To combat the expanding bacterium or an advancing, viral incursion has always required military style thinking. To survive, a microbe requires potential hosts who can be effected just as invading armies require supplies if they are to advance. To tame a microbial incursion requires containment procedures that will deny it new hosts, new supplies.[55]

A critical cultural analysis of this type of rhetoric would point out the constitutive nature of this discourse, that worked in recursive ways. It could magnify and personify the existential dangers of Ebola so that fighting EVD looked like symmetrical warfare. At the same time, it could help those who fought Ebola feel as though they were in combat, fighting a war, and this implied that they needed to be congratulated for their services to their country.

Make no mistake, I understand the *perceptual sense of urgency* that motivated those who sought military solutions to Ebola problems in September of 2014. During that period perhaps few members of the American public realized that local West African community initiatives were gradually working, and that cultural and attitudinal changes were contributing to the efficacy of African containment efforts. What obviously bothers me are the problematic Western media representations that made it appear as though military forces from the United States or the United Kingdom played a major role, or the leading role, in these containment efforts.

Sadly, at the same time that Western pundits complained about the supposed waste and corruption of West African authorities who did not always keep track of all of the money that was flowing in during these turbulent times, little effort was expended tracking the flow of the billions of dollars of Obama "surge" money. Instead of turning over a large portion of those dollars to West Africans so that they that could rebuild their health care infrastructures—that would have interfered with the structural readjustment—strings were attached to the foreign aid.

At the same time, some of that Obama surge money was actually being earmarked for *expensive U.S. Ebola* preparedness programs. This helped calm American anxieties but it did little to help impoverished communities in Guinea, Liberia, or Sierra Leone who needed to build up their own health care infrastructures.

What the Obama "surge" did do was help revitalize interest in clinical and epidemiological studies of Ebola, and this has also contributed to the production of the vaccines that I discuss in my concluding chapter.

The way that OUA was implemented allowed the U.S. military to put on display their muscular prowess, as well as their willingness to take credit for "ending" the 2013–2015 West African Ebola outbreak. The fact that every one of the troops who came home was quarantined for twenty-one days—in ways that went against some CDC advice—also underscored the point that some military leaders were going to follow the "precautionary principle" and the advice of their own military doctors who knew all about the possibilities of "airborne" contagion.

At the same time, the Department of Defense and those who supported this type of interventionism emphasized the "medical" aspects of this adventurism while papering over some of the worries associated with military mission creep. Robert Greene Sands would summarize some of the critics' positions when he noted in March of 2015,

> The EVD outbreak has continued the discussion of the militarization of humanitarian and disaster relief that has been prominent in the press since the 2010 relief efforts in Haiti. Over 10,000 were sent to Haiti, along with aviation

and naval support. Four years later there was much consternation in the media over the involvement of the U.S. military and especially U.S. Africa Command (AFRICOM). . . . DoD and AFRICOM had not engaged in a large-scale outbreak prior to EVD and the ability to meet the challenge questioned . . . . "[t]he militarization" of aid in global contexts can promote partiality . . . [and this could end up] violating two basic premises of aid response—neutrality and impartiality.[56]

Sands responded to these critiques by arguing that those who carried out OUA seemed to be trying to follow the anthropological advice that was supplied by Clifford Geertz, whose study of culture was key to secure local cooperation. Sands went on to note that the "security" footprint of the U.S. military contingent was light, and that the situation was so "dire" that NGOs like Doctors Without Borders had "urged the participation of AFRICOM and other national militaries."[57] Note the conspicuous absence of any detailed discussion of local or regional input regarding decision making from populations who may not have felt that they wanted, or needed, this particular type of AFRICOM interventionism.

All of this leads me to conclude that the OUA served primarily as an image event for the U.S. military, which showed once again that they were a "global force for good." They could remain casualty averse by making sure that they did not have their troops venture into Ebola epicenters, and at the same time they could build impressive-looking Ebola centers or hospital structures that looked very telegenic.

All of this allowed the U.S. military to show the world the beneficence of their own brand of military humanitarianism, that might be a variant of what Michelle Meyer, in another context, called "U.S. Ebola exceptionalism." The label of exceptionalism was earned by those did not wear the same PPE (personal protective equipment), who did not have to visit the same Ebola facilities, did not have to follow the same protocols, or did not have the same freedom of mobility. Meyer explained that in some Ebola contexts similarly situated personnel, who are exposed to similar EVD risks, have to experience "disparate treatment under every actual and proposed policy."[58]

These disparities were obfuscated when different treatment of nationals were rarely mentioned in the euphoria that came with the "ending" of the Liberia portion of the EVD outbreak.

NOTES

1. *Sky News*, "Ebola Epidemic Is Like War Time, Says MSF," *Sky News*, last modified, August 14, 2014, http://news.sky.com/story/1319044/ebola-epidemic-is-like-war-time-says-msf.

2. Barack Obama, quoted in Dan Lamothe, "Meet the New U.S. Military Force That Obama Is Deploying to Fight Ebola," *The Washington Post*, last modified

September 16, 2014, paragraph 3, https://www.washingtonpost.com/news/checkpoint/wp/2014/09/16/meet-the-new-u-s-military-force-that-obama-is-deploying-to-fight-ebola/.

3. By idealists, I meant those who follow certain principles regarding provision of aid that explicitly indicates why military humanitarianism needs to be avoided in most cases. Oxfam, for example, has argued specifically, in its *Policy Compendium Note*, that foreign military forces, including UN peacekeeping operations, should not provide relief or development assistance, other than in exceptional cases. Oxfam, "OI Policy Compendium Note on the Provision of Aid by Foreign Military Forces," April 2012, https://www.oxfam.org/sites/www.oxfam.org/files/file_attachments/story/hpn-provision-aid-military-forces-010412-en.pdf.

4. D. Robert DeChaine, "Humanitarian Space and the Social Imaginary: Médecins Sans Frontières/Doctors Without Borders and the Rhetoric of Global Community," *Journal of Communication Inquiry* 26, no. 4 (October, 2002): 354–369, 355.

5. See, for example, Eyal Weizman, *The Least of All Possible Evils: Humanitarian Violence from Arendt to Gaza* (London: Verso, 2012).

6. In order to explain the complexity of the dominant *epistemes* that can be found in dense archives that have been bequeathed to us by previous generations, Anne Stoler once talked of how metaphors of wood, flowing rivers, pulsing bodies, and a palimpsest could all be used to explain some of the rhetorical features of the archives that could be read "along" the grain. Anne Laura Stoler, *Along the Archival Grain: Epistemic Anxieties and Colonial Common Sense* (Princeton: Princeton University Press, 2009), 51.

7. Note here Professor Ayotte's discussion of how some researchers panic and use threat inflation that in turn contributes to the public's acceptance of militarized solutions to diplomatic or health problems. See Kevin J. Ayotte, "A Vocabulary of Dis-ease: Argumentation, Hot Zones, and the Intertextuality of Bioterrorism," *Argumentation and Advocacy* 48 (Summer 2011): 1–21, 18.

8. President Barack Obama, "Remarks by the President on America's Leadership in the Ebola Fight," Whitehouse.gov, last modified February 11, 2015, paragraphs 3–25, https://www.whitehouse.gov/the-press-office/2015/02/11/remarks-president-americas-leadership-ebola-fight.

9. Dane Erickson and Alice Friend, "The Myth of the Militarization of America's Africa Policy," *The National Interest*, November 17, 2014, paragraph 1, http://nationalinterest.org/feature/the-myth-the-militarization-americas-africa-policy-11691?page=show.

10. Erickson and Friend, "The Myth of the Militarization," paragraphs 3–10.

11. For earlier examples of journalistic or academic worries about how African aid was becoming increasingly militarized, even before Operation United Assistance, see Stephanie McCrummen, "Report: U.S. Aid Is Increasingly Military," *Washington Post*, July 18, 2008, http://www.washingtonpost.com/wp-dyn/content/article/2008/07/17/ar2008071702550.html.

12. Maggie Fox, "Ebola Surge: Obama to Announce Military-Led Fight," NBC News, last modified September 16, 2014, http://www.nbcnews.com/storyline/ebola-virus-outbreak/ebola-surge-obama-announce-military-led-fight-n204106. Obama hinted that he was mulling over something like the surge during an interview that he gave to an NBC journalist during the first week of September. *Meet*

the Press, "President Barack Obama's Full Interview with NBC's Chuck Todd," NBC News, last modified September 7, 2014, http://www.nbcnews.com/meet-the-press/president-barack-obamas-full-interview-nbcs-chuck-todd-n197616.

13. CCTV News, "Interview: WHO Calls for Military-Like Response to Ebola Crisis," *cctv.com*, last modified September 5, 2014, http://english.cntv.cn/2014/09/05/VIDE1409861639281124.shtml.

14. David Nabarro, quoted in Fox, "Ebola Surge," paragraph 4.

15. Joanne Liu, quoted in Fox, "Ebola Surge," paragraph 8.

16. As noted in other chapters the discrepancy in the potential numbers of EVD victims had to do with differing opinions regarding whether or not the populations in West Africa would become cooperative with government officials, NGO workers, and foreign interventionists during the "surge." For example, the worse-case scenarios tried to factor in local resistance, no major changes in cultural traditions allowing the touching of the dead during funerals, the eating of bushmeat, and so on. For a discussion of the more conservative figure of 20,000 potential victims by November of 2014, see WHO Ebola Response Team, "Ebola Virus Disease in West Africa—The First 9 Months of the Epidemic and Forward Projects," *The New England Journal of Medicine* 371 (October 16, 2014): 1481–1495.

17. Fox, "Ebola Surge," paragraph 11.

18. Alberto Toscano, "The Tactics and Ethics of Humanitarianism," *Humanity* 5, no. 1 (Spring 2014): 123–147, 123.

19. Sarah Crowe, quoted in BBC News, "Ebola Virus: 'Biological War' in Liberia," BBC.com, last modified September 11, 2014, paragraphs 3, 9–10, 16, http://www.bbc.com/news/world-africa-29147797. For other critiques of some of this military language, see Gudrun Sif Fridriksdottir, "The 'War' on Ebola," Mats Utas, last modified October 27, 2014, https://matsutas.wordpress.com/2014/10/27/the-war-on-ebola-by-gudrun-sif-fridriksdottir/; Derek Gregory, "Fighting Ebola," *Geographical Imaginations*, last modified November 15, 2014, http://geographicalimaginations.com/2014/11/15/fighting-ebola/.

20. J. Freedom du Lac, "The U.S. Military's New Enemy: Ebola. Operation United Assistance is Now Underway," *The Washington Post*, October 13, 2014, paragraph 7, http://www.washingtonpost.com/news/to-your-health/wp/2014/09/30/the-u-s-military-forces-fighting-the-war-on-ebola/.

21. See, for example, Du Lac, "The U.S. Military's New Enemy."

22. Joel Achenbach and Lena H. Sun, "U.S. Ebola Fighters Head to Africa, But Will the Military and Civilian Effort Be Enough?" *Washington Post*, last modified October 25, 2014, http://www.washingtonpost.com/national/health-science/us-ebola-fighters-head-to-africa-but-will-the-military-and-civilian-effort-be-enough/2014/10/25/1ceba6a8-5b99-11e4-8264-deed989ae9a2_story.html. This is how Achenbach and Sun described this motley crew of Ebola fighters:

> This Ebola corps is a collection of doctors, nurses, scientists, soldiers, aviators, technicians, mechanics and engineers. Many are volunteers with nonprofit organizations or the government, including uniformed doctors and nurses from the little-known U.S. Public Health Service. Most are military personnel, snapping a salute when are assigned to their mission—"Operation United Assistance." It does not qualify for combat pay, only hardship-duty incentive pay, which is about $5 a day-before taxes. (paragraph 2)

23. Achenbach and Sun, "U.S. Ebola Fighters Head to Africa," paragraph 11.

24. Sun and Eilperin, "U.S. Military Will Lead," paragraph 2.

25. Lena H. Sun and Juliet Eilperin, "U.S. Military Will Lead $750 Million Fight against Ebola in West Africa, *Washington Post*, last modified September 16, 2014, Paragraph 1.

26. Sun and Eilperin, "U.S. Military Will Lead," paragraph 4.

27. Benno Muchler, "U.S. Troops Take First Steps to Help Liberia Combat Ebola," *Voice of America News*, last modified September 29, 2014, paragraph 8, http://www.voanews.com/content/us-troops-help-liberia-combat-ebola-/2465887.html.

28. Muchler, "U.S. Troops Take First Steps," paragraphs 11–13.

29. Maryam Zarnegar Deloffre, "Will AFRICOM's Ebola Response Be Watershed Moment for International Action on Human Security?" *Washington Post,* last modified September 29, 2014, paragraph 1, http://www.washingtonpost.com/blogs/monkey-cage/wp/2014/09/29/will-africoms-ebola-response-be-watershed-moment-for-international-action-on-human-security/.

30. Deloffre, "Will AFRICOM's Ebola Response," paragraph 3.

31. *UN News Centre*, "UN Announces Mission to Combat Ebola, Declares Outbreak 'Threat to Peace and Security,'" Un.org, last modified September 18, 2014, http://www.un.org/apps/news/story.asp?NewsID=48746#.Va6WDflVhBd.

32. Deloffre, "Will AFRICOM's Ebola Response," paragraph 2.

33. Dan Murphy, "Ebola: The Kind of Enemy the U.S. Military Excels at Fighting," *Christian Science Monitor*, last modified October 8, 2014, paragraph 1, http://www.csmonitor.com/World/Security-Watch/Backchannels/2014/1008/Ebola-The-kind-of-enemy-the-US-military-excels-at-fighting.

34. Murphy, "Ebola: The Kind of Enemy," paragraphs 2, 6.

35. Karen Greenberg, "America's Response to Ebola Looks Disturbingly Similar to the War on Terror," *Mother Jones*, last modified November 12, 2014, http://www.motherjones.com/politics/2014/11/4-lessons-war-terror-apply-ebola-fight.

36. Greenberg, "America's Response to Ebola," paragraphs 3–6.

37. Alex De Waal, "Militarizing Global Health," *Boston Review*, November 11, 2014, paragraph 2, http://bostonreview.net/world/alex-de-waal-militarizing-global-health-ebola.

38. De Waal, "Militarizing Global Health," paragraph 16.

39. Matt Peppe, "Two Different Approaches, Two Different Results," *Dissident Voice*, last modified March 3, 2015, http://dissidentvoice.org/2015/03/two-different-approaches-two-different-results-in-fighting-ebola/. I believe that military doctors and other military personnel associated with Operation United Assistance actually treated and helped a few dozen EVD victims.

40. Kim Yi Dionne, Laura Seay and Erin McDaniel," AFRICOM's Ebola Response and the Militarization of Humanitarian Aid," *Washington Post*, last modified September 25, 2014, http://www.washingtonpost.com/blogs/monkey-cage/wp/2014/09/25/africoms-ebola-response-and-the-militarization-of-humanitarian-aid/.

41. Charles D. Ellison, "Why Send the Military and Not Medicine to Ebola-Stricken Africa?" *The Root*, last modified October 7, 2014, http://www.theroot.

com/blogs/the_take/2014/10/why_the_military_and_not_medicine_to_ebola_stricken_africa.html.

42. Peter James Hudson, quoted in Ellison, "Why Send the Military," paragraph f5.

43. David Francis, "Ebola's Toll Was Horrific: It Could Have Been Much Worse," *Foreign Policy*, February 11, 2015, paragraph 1, http://foreignpolicy.com/2015/02/11/epidemic-ebola-pentagon-obama-outbreak-africa/.

44. Francis, "Ebola's Toll Was Horrific," paragraph 2.

45. Clinton K. Murray et al., "Operation United Assistance: Infectious Disease Threats to Deployed Military Personnel," *Military Medicine* 180, no., 6 (June, 2015): 626–650, 645.

46. Murray et al., "Operation United Assistance," 645.

47. Francis, "Ebola's Toll Was Horrific," paragraphs 4–5.

48. Brian Castner, "We Are Fighting an Enemy, and the Enemy Is Ebola," *Foreign Policy*, last modified January 14, 2015, paragraph 1, http://foreignpolicy.com/2015/01/14/us-army-general-volesky-fighting-ebola-outbreak-in-liberia/.

49. Ibid., paragraph 1.

50. Ibid., paragraph 2.

51. Ibid., paragraph 2.

52. Ibid., paragraph 6.

53. Ibid., paragraph 16.

54. Stephen J. Collier and Andrew Lakoff, "Vital Systems Security: Reflexive Biopolitics and the Government of Emergency," *Theory, Culture, & Society* 32, no. 2 (2015): 19–51.

55. Tom Koch, "Ebola, Epidemics, Pandemics and the Mapping of their Containment," Remedianetwork.net, September 22, 2014, paragraph 12, http://remedianetwork.net/2014/09/22/ebola-epidemics-pandemics-and-the-mapping-of-their-containment/.

56. Robert Greene Sands, "Local Knowledge, Geertz and the Militarization of Response," *Robert Green Sands*, March 16, 2015, paragraph 6, http://www.rgsands.com/blog/2015/3/16/local-knowledge-geertz-and-the-militarization-of-response. For more on worries about aid neutrality, see Dionne and McDaniel, "AFRICOM's Ebola Response."

57. Sands, "Local Knowledge," paragraph 6.

58. Michelle Meyer, "Will the Real Evidence-Based Ebola Policy Please Stand Up," *The Faculty Lounge*, last modified November 6, 2014, paragraph 108, http://www.thefacultylounge.org/2014/11/will-the-real-evidence-based-ebola-policy-please-stand-up-seven-take-aways-from-maine-dhhs-v-hickox.html. For a more pointed critique that expressly associated Operation United Assistance with American exceptionalism, see Matt Peppe, "Two Different Approaches."

9

The Legal and Cultural Legacies of the 2013–2015 West African Outbreak

As I write this conclusion many transcontinental audiences are celebrating the fact that by the end of 2015, the West African Ebola outbreak seemed to have been contained. Military communities in the United Kingdom and the United States had handed out medals and promoted those who fought Ebola overseas, and public health experts talked about needed reforms and the shifting responsibilities as WHO defenders spoke of major reforms. Nurses' organizations, bioethicists, and others remembered the trials and tribulations of Craig Spencer, Kaci Hickox, and Nina Pham as they wrote about the need to protect health care workers as well as Ebola victims. More than a few hoped that we would never again experience the types of pandemics that some called "slate wipers."[1]

I am also writing at a time when fewer and fewer "new" Ebola cases are reported in Liberia, Sierra Leone, and Guinea. In Sierra Leone, for the first time in over a year, communities are allowed to congregate at dances and other public gatherings. After Sierra Leonean president Ernest Bai Koroma lifted the ban on public gatherings, people could once again go to restaurants, beach bars, outdoor cinemas, travel to night clubs, and play beach football.[2]

Ebola "hunters" and other public health workers were worn down, psychologically and physically, by their battles with the microbes. Journalists wrote about EVD "fatigue" and the need to go on with our lives, but the ever-cautious sentinels at Doctors Without Borders reminded us about the dangers of over exuberance. Joanne Liu, for example, writing in *Nature* in August of 2015, understood that national leaders and health agencies wanted to talk about "lessons learned," but she urged readers to remember that they had to "finish the fight against Ebola":

> Numbers of cases refusing to diminish, new communities being infected, bodies buried in secret. Sound familiar? It should. But these are not just scenes from last year's Ebola epidemic. They are playing out today in West Africa . . . . I have witnessed how a lack of political will undermined the response in the early days of the epidemic. Now, fatigue and a waning focus are threatening the push to end it.[3]

In the same way that the outbreak allegedly began with denialism, stigmatization, cultural misunderstandings, conspiracies, mutual suspicions, and worries about the announcing of an "epidemic" might impact mining companies and touring, the outbreak was ending in ways that still worried those on the "frontlines" of the Ebola battles. Although Joanne Liu did not cite the work of Achille Mbembe as she discussed all of the burial of "infected bodies," humanists who are familiar with scholarly theories on necropolitics and thanatopolitics can easily appreciate some of the difficulties associated with moving away from some of this politics of death. The decisionism that went into the declarations of the beginning and the ending of these emergency states of exception impacted the lives of many global audiences.[4]

In this concluding chapter, I want to take up the question of how critical cultural scholars can evaluate the many claims of "lessons learned" that have circulated since the second wave of foreign interventionism that began in August of 2014. Has the "situational awareness," or the "frontline" experiences of those who worked in Conakry or Kenema changed the ways that researchers and scientists conceptualize Ebola pathogenesis, transmission, DNA or contact tracing? Did the latest outbreak alter global health care organizational politics so that we know who is supposed to take the "lead" in future Ebola epidemics? What jurisprudential norms have changed in the aftermath of the 2013–2015 outbreak, and how has this impacted the legal or rhetorical cultures of elites and publics who still write or talk about EVD?

I'll begin by providing a subsection that comments on how legal scholars and others are advocating that we defend the notion of "global health security" for all.

INSTANTIATING "GLOBAL HEALTH SECURITY" IN FUTURE EBOLA CONTEXTS

As David Heymann and his co-authors have observed, when doctors and decision makers converse about "global health security," they are usually referencing the "non-traditional issues" such as the vulnerability of national populations that comes from unintentionally caused small chains of transmission that might turn into epidemics. Heymann, however, wanted to advance the position that there was a "less appreciated" way of conceptualizing that same ideograph.[5] Why not focus on "individual health security"?

Heymann's defense of the possible instantiation of the notion of some individual right to have "global health security" will be controversial because it touches on a taboo subject that is often glossed over in the hagiographic tales that are told about heroic protagonists in Western outbreak narratives. Heymann elaborates on what he means by "individual" global health security:

> This is security that comes from access to safe and effective health services, products, and technologies. Ebola-infected health workers from developed countries have been repatriated from West Africa for care in their own countries where there is health security for individuals—hospitals that provide safe and effective access to life-saving medicines and services. Meanwhile, Ebola-infected West Africans have had to accept that health care is not always safe, not always effective, and not always accessible—that their own health security is yet again at risk. As the Ebola epidemic has unfolded, the part that has been played by substandard infection control and inadequate access to effective health products and services has clearly demonstrated a wider scope of health security—the intertwining of collective and individual health security.[6]

Militarists, counterterrorist planners, WHO officials, and others were used to talking about the collectivist and the nationalist features of this "global health security," but it looked as though Heymann was trying to add even more connotative meanings to these grammars.

Heymann used a selective review of the history behind "collective health security" to set up his defense of "individual health security." He began with a study of how quarantining, since at least the fourteenth century, had meant that collective efforts had to be made at preventing the bubonic plague from crossing European borders. Then later on, international treaties and conventions were organized to protect collectives from three other additional infectious diseases—cholera, smallpox, and yellow fever. In Heymann's temporal periodization, 1969 was a key year because that was when the "International Health Regulations" were set up to help provide a collaborative global framework for those four infectious diseases. In the name of collective securitization various countries were supposed to report on the presence of plague, cholera, smallpox, or yellow fever, and the "International Health Regulations" included guidelines for predetermined actions at the border.[7]

Heymann's chronology is used to explain how, over time, the International Health Regulations (IHR) were later broadened in scope to include more principles, more "evidence-based actions at borders," and more surveillance of diseases like severe acute respiratory syndrome (SARS) in 2003, but he notes that the regulations were not met by all countries. Moreover, the reformed IHR guidelines were aimed at mitigating and preventing "collective health risk," and they were not put in place to "provide access to goods and health services." This, he contends is a major flaw that overlooks the importance of providing individuals and smaller groups with health security, and he used the 2007 dispute between the Indonesian government and the larger international health community as a transition point for his outright defense of "individual health security."[8]

In 2007 the Indonesian government started to worry that the results of the Avian flu strain tests that were being conducting in that country were contributing to information flows that only helped nations in the global North. In a move that shocked many Western medical authorities the Indonesian government decided to stop sharing information about the influenza strains that came from the tests that were conducted in that country. Heymann uses this example to argue that this shows that attention needs to be paid to matters of "individual" access and need, and he contends that this even led to the "doctrine of equal benefits from equal sharing." Although Heymann admits that the principles regarding individual access that came out of this incident for pandemic influenza preparedness were not "binding," he uses these types of politicized negotiations to underscore that point that we have reached a stage in twenty-first-century planning where we protect individual access to vaccines and other materials so that those in the "developing" world might also benefit from this infectious disease research.[9]

Piero Olliaro, Peter Horby, and Els Torreele, in an essay in *The Lancet* published in May of 2015, tried to go beyond Heymann's suggestion by proffering the notion that this was the time for individual "health security and rights."[10] Their argument was that the latest Ebola outbreak showed how few individuals had any affordable access to effective diagnostics, medicines, or vaccines. They painted a picture of a dystopic world, where some nations used failed models of R&D, marginalized the study of antimicrobial resistance or neglected tropical diseases, and only prepared some for the fights against "superbugs" that were "haunting even the best equipped hospitals."[11] Instead of accepting the traditional neoliberal "market failure" explanations for this lack of more universal access Olliaro, Horby, and Torreele argued that these simplistic explanations masked the real underlying causes of these disparities—"our current medical research and development system, which relies largely on pharmaceutical companies that respond to profit prospects rather than health needs." "Without a health rights frame," and without the necessary leadership, they reasoned, "our current model prioritises the development of blockbuster products that can be marketed to generate maximum risks, sales, even if marginal or superfluous from a medical perspective."[12]

Only time will tell if these are aspirational types of commentaries or the beginnings of the pragmatic instantiation of the notion of some "individual" right to health care, but there is little question that for several years many Africans were bothered by the rumors that only a few privileged individuals got MZapp, other vaccines, or that one's skin color or one's ethnicity determined who would be evacuated out West Africa. Was it any coincidence that while expatriates fled West African doctors, nurses, and contact tracers were left to fight Ebola with often rudimentary equipment?

Neoliberals don't like to hear about topics like "need," entitlements, or access "rights" to public health care, and so I anticipate that for many years "global health security" will become a contested ideograph that is used by Westerners to convey their collective anxieties about traveling EVD. Over the years we will hear more about how every suspected Ebola victim needs to receive similar treatment, and this will be moving in the direction of Heymann's notion of "individual" global health security, but this will run up against the reality that strings are still attached to much of the foreign aid that is flowing into Liberia, Sierra Leone, and Guinea.

For many observers the latest Ebola outbreak provided a watershed movement that needed to catalyze the efforts of cosmopolitans. One blog that was produced by the London School of Hygiene and Tropical Medicine, which was used to comment on Heymann and the essays written by Piero Olliaro, Peter Horby, Els Torreele and others, asked whether the Ebola outbreak could "rejuvenate global health security."[13] The blogger who wrote this essay made the point that since about a quarter of the medicines in low-income countries were believed to be substandard or counterfeit, then the lack of individual access, and the soaring costs of infectious disease medicines, was creating a situation where the sale of fake medicines was undermining the capabilities of governments to deal with both infectious and non-communicable diseases.

Part of the problem that prevented elite and public communities from giving their warrant assent to the notion that all global denizens in the world, regardless of economic, political, or ethnic status, deserved to have "global health security" had to do with the mini-disputation that took place by those who got sidetracked by arguing about other topics. Donal Brown, who was in charge of the British efforts to tackle EVD, explained that part of the reason for the belated interventionism in West Africa had to do with ongoing disputes about whether this was a "health" problem that needed to be led by WHO, or a "humanitarian" matter that required UN leadership.[14] Brown wondered whether talking about a right of individual global health security might help break the impasse that he saw between these communities. In theory, both WHO and the United Nations could be put in charge of ensuring the protection of that *individuated* health security right—regardless of whether it was based on health or humanitarian concerns.

Assume for the moment that organizations like the World Bank, the United Nations, Doctors Without Borders, WHO, and so on, took seriously the idea that every global citizen deserved to have "global health security." How would that impact the ways that we actually protected individuals in concrete, emotive and volatile situations?

Recall, for example, how in earlier chapters, I noted how collectivist worries in places like Liberia led to the quarantining of West Point. As long as Ebola appeared in remote jungle villages, observers didn't need to worry about the use of harsh measures like cordons, mandatory isolation, and so forth, but all of this changed with reports of rising EVD transmission rates in urban areas. "The Ebola outbreak in West Africa is so out of control," Donald G. McNeil Jr., once warned. He went on to explain that this time "governments there have revived a disease-fighting tactic not used in a century: the *'condon sanitaire'* in which a line is drawn around the infected areas and no one is allowed out."[15]

Isolation techniques that had been used during colonial and imperial times were resurrected for presentist needs, and although international pressure was brought to bear on the Liberians to remove the cordons, one wonders about the motivation. I saw few critics discussing individual security rights during that heated disputation. Were these outside powers worried about the individual rights of the residents of the suburb of Monrovia, or were they actually worried that these quarantines were counterproductive and ineffective *communal measures* that raised the risks of EVD spreading to the "North"?

As readers might imagine, instantiating and preserving some "right" to individuated global health security also raised questions of legal liability and the reintroduction of probabilistic thinking, especially in Western legal and media circles. Imagine a situation where lawyers, armed with the knowledge that came from cases like Nina Pham's, now started to sue hospitals for not providing respirators to individual nurses as their lawyers talked about the possibility of "airborne" transmission. Massive numbers of new legal tort claims would create jurisprudential nightmares for American jurists.

In the abstract, talk of "individual" global "health security" seems noble and aspirational, but we need to keep in mind the proliferation of cases that would come when many would claim that the passage of "new" CDC protocol seemed to be geared to protecting "individual" public health care workers who treated Ebola patients. The popularity of the "aerial theories" of transmission,[16] combined with the popularity of talk of individual needs and access, would open up a Pandora's box of lawsuits. "The greatest new epidemic threats are unknown pathogens that spread easily" through "the air," argued *Nature* magazine's Declan Butler in August of 2015, and this in turn meant that they were having to prepare for situations where "humans have little or no immunity."[17]

In the next section I take up questions that have to do with the "cultural lessons" that we may have learned from the 2013–2015 outbreak.

IRONIES, PARADOXES, AND UNANTICIPATED CULTURAL LESSONS

When Donal Brown talked to reporters in the United Kingdom about the challenges that Sierra Leone faced during the latest Ebola outbreak, he indicated that the "UK and the international community can bring all the weapons" they want—labs, and the treatment centers—but they were "foreigners," and only "person-to-person engagement" was going to help with the understanding that was needed to deal with the "subtleties" of West African cultures.[18] While he applauded the fact that his nation was putting together teams of epidemiologists and infection control specialists who would become part of mobile "disease detectives" that would be ready to travel overseas, he underscored the point that the challenges of EVD could not be met by relying on twenty-first-century technological prowess.[19]

Although Donal Brown focused on both problems with belated interventionism as well as the need for African cultural change, he wrote from a stance that assumed that it would be West Africans who would have to take the lead in facilitating African behavioral change. While this avoided some of the usual objectification that treated African communities as passive objects that see through the prisms of Westerner gazers, his commentary made no mention of the fact that perhaps African doctors and nurses might need to reciprocate and help alter UK cultural landscapes.

As I reviewed the Ebola *dispositifs* that appeared in various legal, economic, political, military, media, and other rhetorical venues over the last several years, I couldn't help noticing the appearance of a host of ironies and paradoxes. While contact tracers, West African governmental health workers, and NGO personnel working in the "South" dealt with talk of how Ebola was actually a hoax to secure foreign aid or other forms of denialism, those in the "North" *faced the exact opposite problem.* Western leaders and medical experts dealt with Ebola obsessions, hyperinflation of risks, and other forms of what some have called "Ebolaphobia." West Africans who lived with hundreds of Ebola victims turned away, hid their loved ones, complained about ambulances, interference with burial rites, and so on, while communities in the global North, thousands of miles away, invented counterfactual narratives filled with stories of leaky bodies and porous borders.

Sadly, during a period of time when Westerners could have been learning from Nigerians and others about how to cope with EVD and Ebolaphobia, empowered politicians and others in the global North were using the occasion to write about a host of other border "crises." Take, for example, the discourse that was produced by Phil Gingrey, a doctor who served in the U.S. House of Representatives. In July of 2014, while hundreds were dying in West Africa, he sent this missive to Thomas Frieden of the CDC:

> As you know, the United States is currently experiencing a crisis at our southern border. The influx of families and unaccompanied children at the border poses many risks, including grave public health threats. As a physician for over thirty years, I am aware of the dangers infectious disease pose. . . . [R]eports of illegal migrants carrying deadly diseases such as swine flu, dengue fever, Ebola virus and tuberculosis are particularly concerning. Many of the children who are coming across the border also lack basic vaccinations such as those to prevent chicken pox of measles. This makes those Americans who are not vaccinated—and especially children and the elderly—particularly susceptible.[20]

Gingrey then recommended that the CDC take immediate action and do something to "assess the public risk" that came from the "influx" of unaccompanied children who might be transported by commercial airlines or other forms of transportation into the United States. He also wanted to make sure that border patrol guards were provided with adequate protection, that children be medically screened, and that the appropriate "decontamination efforts" be carried out to "mitigate what could become a public health crisis."[21]

Was Gingrey representing the views of a small group of Americans, or were others willing to raise similar cultural anxieties? Rice professor Bob Stein, during an interview with National Public Radio, expressed his opinion that "our borders are being besieged with people who may have diseases like Ebola."[22] Audiences who were already used to talk of militarizing the Mexico-U.S. borders had little difficulty imagining the needs for securitizing the border in the name of public health necessities.

Remember, all of this was happening during times when the mainstream presses carried outbreak narratives that featured the work of Kent Brantly, Craig Spencer, Amber Vinson, and Nina Pham. Commentary on the patrolling of the U.S.-Mexico border complicated what was already being said about the travelers from Africa. Dr. Gregg Mitman, for example, recalled that it was in late July 2014, after two American health workers in Liberia had become infected, that global headlines first started labeling this an "epidemic," and this in turn triggered all of the talk of quarantines. Mitman elaborated by noting: "Fear of Ebola's escaping the African continent" finally "brought international attention."[23]

As I argued in previous chapters, the Kaci Hickox incident became a metonymic marker for larger Anglo-American debates about the nature and scope of public health protection in similar situations. Like Mary Mallon ("Typhoid Mary") before her, Hickox become a cipher for those who wanted to talk about alleged threat exaggeration, state power, legal coercion, and how to deal with asymptomatic "carriers" of infectious disease.

So if we are going to talk about the need for cultural change, before Anglo-American communities turn their gaze toward Africa and complain about West African traditions, burial practices, and denialism, they need to complement those critiques with analysis of Western cultures that overhype Ebola risks.

An example of the continued resonance of apocalyptic outbreak narratives—in spite of all of the efforts of the CDC and others to talk about only close human-to-human Ebola transmission—appeared in the pages of the prestigious science magazine *Nature*, where Declan Butler contributed an essay in August of 2015 that was titled "The Next Time." This was an essay that was aesthetically adorned with an iconic image of rows of beds in some massive hanger during the period of time when Americans battled the 1918 "Spanish" influenza that killed tens of millions. The essay argued that while the world was ill-prepared for the next pandemic, perhaps the West African Ebola outbreak might become the needed driver for change. While some portions of the essay try to critique the conventional fears associated with the spread of Ebola, this very message was undercut by other parts of the very same essay that used hypothetical scenarios to keep us on our guard. Note, for example, how Declan Butler writes about what might have happened if EVD had spread to many regions of Nigeria during the West African outbreak:

> If there was one point last year when public-health experts held their breath, it was when a Liberian man infected with Ebola virus flew to Lagos, Nigeria, in July. Ebola was already raging uncontrolled through impoverished countries in West Africa, killing half of those it infected. Now a vomiting man had carried it straight to the heart of Africa's largest megacity—with 21 million inhabitants, many of whom live in slums. Experts were horrified at the prospect that the virus might rip through the city—and then, because Lagos is an international travel hub, spread farther afield. "The last thing anyone in the world wants to hear is the two words, 'Ebola' and 'Lagos' in

the same sentence," said Jeffrey Hawkins, the US consul general in Nigeria, at the time. In the end, this apocalyptic scenario did not play out.[24]

To his credit Butler goes on to explain that this was because Nigeria was a focal point of global efforts to eradicate polio and Nigerians knew something about controlling infectious diseases. Nigerians had what Butler called a "decent infrastructure of virology labs and epidemiologists" who had the "capacity to run large public-awareness campaigns."[25] This was supposed to explain why the "vomiting man" who traveled from West Africa to Nigeria did not trigger a pandemic.

Yet the tone and the content of some of Butler's passages creates a rhetorical situation where he becomes a potential purveyor of the possibilistic apocalyptic outbreak narratives. The prestige of *Nature* magazine should not dissuade us from seeing that scientists, as well as science journalists, can also craft apocalyptic narratives, even in cases when fragments in their own texts provide indications that they are aware of the dangers of Ebola sensationalism.

The hyperbolic permutations of Ebola *dispositifs*—and the fragmentary claims, images, arguments, *topoi*, and other shards that are the constitutive parts of those rhetorics—can appear and reappear in many different public, technical, military, medical, social, and entertainment venues.

The reported "end" of the West African outbreak will not end the epidemiological and psycho-social issues that will confront those who will have to deal with future outbreaks, and this in turn means that critical legal scholars and critical cultural scholars need to constantly be pointing out the continued resonance of some of these Ebola *dispositifs*. Note, for example, how Richard Preston once used necropolitical, or thanatopolitical critiques in his 1994 *Hot Zone* to warn the world about the dangers that came from the convergence of environmental degradation, cells looking for hosts, and primordial habitats. Preston used the tale of "Charles Monet" to detail what happened when a Frenchman contracted the Marburg virus as he traveled by plane to Nairobi, Kenya, in search of medical help:

> The airsickness bag fills up to the brim with . . . speckled liquid of two colors, black and red, a stew of tarry granules mixed with flesh red arterial blood. It is hemorrhage, and it smells like a slaughterhouse. The black vomit is loaded with virus. It is highly infective, lethally hot. . . . The bag is bulging and softening, threatening to leak; and he hands it to a flight attendant.[26]

Readers later learn that Monet entered a hospital waiting room, "jammed with bleary-eyed people, Africans and Europeans sitting shoulder to shoulder,"[27] when the "human virus bomb explodes." Monet dies, and then the Marburg virus is given sentient features as it is "trying to find a new host."[28] We can now understand why Preston, a few pages earlier, had argued that all "of the earth's cities are connected by a web of airline routes," that were a "network," and that "Charles Monet and the life form inside him had entered the net."[29]

Decades before Declan Butler was writing about the hypothetical dangers of what might have been in Lagos, with its population of some 21 million, Preston's *Hot Zone* was already taking advantage of earlier *cultural* prefigurations and antecedent rhetorics as Preston used Charles Monet as a signifier for what happens when we don't have in place legal or ethical restraints in a crowded world.

The myths of the traveling disease carriers continue to resonate with many Anglo-American audiences. As Margaret Humphreys once noted in her study of Western sciences, in all of this historical talk of panic, and in all of these formulaic contagion narratives, it is "travelers" who create "panics" when we collectively worry that the "edge of safety cannot be defined."[30] Bill Albertini has similar noted that in these "depictions of free-floating contagion in public space we find the true horror of the doomsday virus narrative: bodies."[31]

One of the many cultural lessons that we can take away from the latest outbreak is that we have no monolithic "science" that is going to be circulated by all scientists as they try to dispel cultural mythologies. Helen Epstein represented some of the most popular positions on Ebola transmission when she wrote that "Ebola is not transmitted through the air like flu or through food and water like cholera and typhoid."[32] However, as I noted in earlier chapters, there are myriad reasons why other scientists, lawyers, politicians, book authors, movie producers, and others want to talk and write about aerosol transmission. The same Donal Brown, who supervised the British Ebola humanitarian efforts, told *The Guardian*'s journalists that he had seen the "consequences in animal populations of airborne diseases" and he couldn't fathom what would have happened if Ebola was transmitted in that way.[33]

From a post-structural vantage point, even Brown's acknowledgment that the people of Sierra Leone, Liberia, and Guinea were not dealing with an airborne threat only served to underscore the dangers that just might come if scientists ever discovered that Ebola *mutated* to the point where it did become airborne. The very raising of those types of possibilistic scenarios—as Andrew Lakoff and others have reminded us—leads not only to threat inflation, but to the spending of billions of pounds and dollars on anticipated biosecurity threats. At the same time, the continued attraction of aerosol versions of outbreak tales impacts the ways that we think about everything from West African burial customs[34] to transcontinental airport traffic.

In the future, if we really care about lessons learned, cultural critics and critical legal scholars will need to join the ranks of other global citizens who continue to worry that various types of sensationalism—regardless of motivation—lead to the "Africanization" of EVD, the stigmatization of Ebola victims, moral panic, pandemic obsessions, and threat inflation in the "North."

Those who keep a watchful eye on geopolitical conditions in West Africa and other locales will need to supplement those critiques of the "North" with analyses of rhetorical situations in the "South" that take into account local perceptions, needs, religions, and social practices. Instead of adopting essentialist epidemiological frames of EVD transmission that automatically blame the spread of disease on the scientific illiteracy of those in Liberia, Sierra Leone, and Guinea, we need to factor in the possibility that those who survive EVD gain a tacit form of knowledge that cannot be found in the pages of *The Lancet* or the *New England Journal of Medicine*. Instead of just congratulating those twenty-first-century progressives who put up billboards that "educate" West Africans so that they can adopt Western cultural habits, we need to acknowledge the fact that those in the "North" and the "South" can educate each other.

Granted, we can understand the concerns of NGOs and politicians who want to put on display the efficacy of large-scale initiatives that may appeal to publics and potential donors, but oftentimes radical change takes place at the micro-levels where the efforts of tens of thousands of individuals are rendered invisible by the spotlights that are placed on inanimate objects. Claudia Evers, who was the emergency Ebola coordinator in Guinea for Médecins Sans Frontières, would tell Reuters' reporters in February of 2015 that there had been a shortage of adequate public health messages during the early stages of the interventions, and that Doctors Without Borders had spent too little time communicating with the West African populations. "Instead of asking for more beds," argued Evers, "we should have asked for more sensitization activities."[35] My chapter on contact tracers and other volunteers was included in this book to make sure that readers take into account the trials and tribulations of those who actually are on the "frontlines" of the "battles" against EVD.

Evers was commenting on one of the major problems that impeded Ebola containment efforts during the West African outbreak, but he was also providing warnings regarding the characterization and treatment of local populations who did not share the customs, the traditions, the religion, the scientific beliefs, or the values of those who came to "rescue" them. As Misha Hussain reminded readers in February of 2015, the "Zaire" Ebola was a type of hemorrhagic fever that sometimes killed two-thirds of the people it infected, and that mistrust of government and health workers had contributed to the miscommunication that took place when communities decided to hide their infected family members instead of cooperating with Ebola task forces.[36] A study of the post-August WHO announcement about the global threats posed by the spread of EVD showed that this "mistrust" became a common theme in many explanatory, anticipatory, and accusatory Western frameworks.

One of the lessons here is that African public and elite *disagreements* over Doctors Without Borders initiatives or WHO edicts from Geneva can be reconfigured by Westerners as matters of communicative *"misunderstanding."* Sakoba Keita, the head of the national Ebola response in Guinea, explained that before anyone was going to get to "zero Ebola" they needed to remember that they had to get to "zero resistance."[37]

For that to happen, several rhetorical cultures needed changing, compassion needed to replace stigmatization, and global communities needed to understand both their vulnerabilities as well as those of the "other."

EPIDEMIOLOGICAL, VIROLOGICAL, AND GENETIC LESSONS THAT COULD BE TAUGHT BY THOSE SEEKING COMPREHENSIVE WAYS OF COPING WITH "BLACK SWAN" EVENTS

There is no doubt that many scientists and science writers, in spite of all of the horrors associated with EVD, were hopeful that this unprecedented Ebola outbreak would also unify members of the national and international health communities so that they could be in a better position to contain future infectious disease outbreaks. Michael Osterholm, Kristine Moore, and Lawrence Gostin, when they looked toward the future of public health in the "age of Ebola," thought this was the opportune time to take on challenges that they said were posed by infectious diseases like AIDS and Ebola. They argued that researchers could profit from Nassim Nichols Taleb's notion of a "Black Swan" event, when human actors had to confront "high-profile, difficult-to-predict, and rare events" in public health settings.[38]

In several ways Taleb's theorizing about unpredictable, potentially catastrophic events seemed to ring true for those who were trying to make sense of the chaos that often swirled around Ebola containment efforts.[39] In 2007, Taleb would explain to readers of his book that

> [w]hat we call here a Black Swan (and capitalize it) is an event with the following three attributes. First, it is an outlier, as it lies outside the realm of regular expectations, because nothing in the past can convincingly point to its possibility. Second, it carries an extreme "impact." Third, in spite of its outlier status, human nature makes us concoct explanations for its occurrence after the fact, making it explainable and predictable.[40]

Osterholm, Moore, and Gostin thought that the latest Ebola outbreak had all of the attributes of a Black Swan event, with the possible exception that this was one time when the global health community was going to have to spend years trying to figure out some of the pathogenic dimensions of this dreaded disease.

Part of the reason that Osterholm, Moore, and Gostin found heuristic value in the conceptual apparatus of the Black Swan theories is that they seemed to provide explanatory frameworks for the ways that some global health organizations had actually responded to the failures of the first stage of the outbreak during the spring of 2014. These authors reminded their readers that at one time WHO—which had accurately reported the appearance of more than 20,000 cases by December of 2014—had to watch as their prognostications were juxtaposed with those of the CDC, that had modelers who once predicted that there would be some 1.4 million cases in Liberia and Sierra Leone in the absence of successful interventionism.[41]

Osterholm, Moore, and Gostin extended Taleb's work on Black Swan events to argue that the global health communities had learned the dangers that were posed by newly "infected, but not ill or only mildly ill, persons" who could "leave the affected countries by foot, automobiles, trains and even plans to move across this continent." This worried them, because with the millions who lived in places like Dakar, Senegal or Abidjan, Ivory Coast the "crowded squalid conditions of poverty in the large slums of major urban centers" meant that circumstances were "ripe for an even larger Ebola epidemic throughout continental Africa."[42] The potential for this type of Black Swan event, they were convinced, meant that we had "learned" from the various stages of this latest outbreak that urban EVD threats were different from rural ones, and that some quarantine efforts had backfired. This, in turn, taught us that infectious disease threats impacted international and regional security, economic stability, and the "overarching public health governance."[43]

In some cases, cultural anthropologists—who often watched as their colleagues lost jobs during previous years when economic declines brought WHO cuts in public health preparedness—thought that the lessons that needed to be learned here had to do with *misplaced* scientific priorities, disciplinary marginalizations, and epistemic miscalculations. The American Anthropological Association's executive director, Edward Liebow provided an example of the contested nature of some of these Ebola scientific rhetorics when he asserted that epidemiologists were "making oversimplified assumptions about transmission," while culturally sensitive anthropologists were supposedly in a better position to "breathe life into the numbers," and "make much more realistic assessments of near-term and longer-term predictions."[44]

In other cases, scientists talked of how DNA studies and genomic research would take the place of subjective contact tracing, and the billions of dollars that were being set aside for future Ebola studies by President

Obama and other empowered communities raised the hopes of those who were glad to see that this "neglected" disease was now becoming a global priority. From an epidemiological standpoint, Ebola virus disease was no longer that exotic disease that was studied by Peter Piot back in 1976, nor was it only a devastating illness that could endanger the lives of hundreds over the course of dozens of years. The reportage of massive morbidity and mortality rates in Liberia, Sierra Leone, and Guinea meant that EVD would receive plenty of attention in the "North."

"EBOLA, ÇA SUFFIT!" ("EBOLA, THAT'S ENOUGH!"): EGALITARIAN GLOBAL HEALTH PREPAREDNESS AND TALK OF VACCINES

During the last days of July 2015 global audiences around the world woke up to some startling news—a Canadian vaccine, that had been sitting on shelves, and that had been bought by Merck, might be the "magic bullet" that was so desperately needed by those who tried to contain the spread of EVD. Could the appearance of this vaccine help with the egalitarian access of individuated health care that would serve the needs of those that may want a "right" to "global health" security?

Talk of the new "rVSV-ZEBOV vaccine" was circulating at the same time that West Africans were reporting on the sporadic appearance of a few more "new" cases in their countries, and science journalists and mainstream reporters wrote euphorically about the efforts of Ana Maria Henao-Restrepo. She and her co-authors announced that their "Guinea Ring" vaccination trials showed 100 percent effectiveness of an rVSV-vector vaccine that might protect future communities ravaged by Ebola. The methodological approach that was used in this study drew from earlier models for recruitment and estimation that were used during the 1970's smallpox eradication campaigns. The uniqueness of this "ring vaccination" trial focused on a "cluster of individuals at high risk for infection," who were connected socially and geographically to the confirmed "index case" of that two-year old who allegedly started this all back in December of 2013.[45]

Excited journalists, scientists, health officials, and administrators wrote about how the work of Ana Maria Henao-Restrepo and her colleagues showed that this latest Merck vaccine could be a "game changer" that would provide just the right help at a crucial time in Ebola containment efforts. In spite of their promising results, Ana Maria Henao-Restrepo and her colleagues urged caution, and indicated that the third phase of their randomized testing of the vaccine—strategically called the *Ebola ça Suffit* ("Ebola, that's enough")—was just getting underway.[46]

By now countless West Africans had suffered from the social stigmas, the psychological traumas, the social fragmentation and the economic destruction that came with coping with EVD realities and Ebola representations, and these researchers, in their strategic naming of their last vaccination trials, clearly sensed the mood of those they were trying to help. The pronouncements about the efficacy of the rVSV-ZEBOV vaccine were coming during a period when so many were tired of hearing about Ebola.

This Ebola fatigue did not hinder the efforts of excited science writers who realized that for years we had witnessed heated debates about the need to accelerate the clinical trials and pharmaceutical developments of drugs like this. Zosia Kmietowicz, writing in the *British Medical Journal*, for example, quoted representatives from the World Health Organization who said that the results of the Ebola vaccine trial—that had involved thousands of Africans—were "extremely promising."[47] Sarah Boseley, a journalist employed by the *Guardian* in the United Kingdom, explained that infectious disease experts were saying that the rapid development and testing of this vaccine might bring the current epidemic to an end as well as help with the control of future outbreaks.[48] Journalists tempered some of this enthusiasm by underscoring the point that the vaccine, while it had been developed and then licensed to Merck & Co., had yet to go through the legal regulatory process that usually preceded vaccine distribution.[49]

Some participants in the legal, cultural, and bioethical debates that took place after the announcement of the efficacy of the new Merck Ebola vaccine argued that this was no time for endangered populations to have to deal with the traditional legal hurdles that were placed in the path of those who needed immediate help. Was this one of those times when the very regulatory and legal procedures, that had been put in place to ensure public safety, were standing in the way of scientific progress or global public health? Why, some argued, after having lost almost 12,000 lives to EVD, were people quibbling about the need to wait until the vaccine had passed through the procedural steps that were laid out for the usual field testing and clinical trials that were performed before the usual dissemination to the population? "It looks about as safe as a flu vaccine," intoned a virologist by the name of Ben Neuman, and he thought that there was no "reasons on humanitarian grounds why it should not be used immediately."[50]

What raised the hopes of many who read these reports were the analyses that underscored the rigorous nature, and the novelty, of the vaccine testing that was used by Guinean public health officials and their supporters who helped Ana Maria Henao-Restrepo. The vaccination studies also rendered visible the leg work of contact tracers and others who had come in contact with "patient zero" and other potential Ebola suspects, and the investigators who carried out the clinical trials determined that none of those who were vaccinated became infected. What made all of this even more interesting was the fact that some of this data had been collected while Ebola "hunters" and others were fighting the disease in Ebola centers, hospitals, and other places.

Elites around the world heralded the arrival of the Merck vaccine. Margaret Chan, the director general of WHO was quoted as saying the credit for the vaccination study needed to go to the Guinean government, the "people living in the communities, and our partners in this project." She went on to explain that the discovery of "an effective vaccine" will provide another "very important tool for both current and future Ebola outbreaks."[51] One of Guinea's leading doctors argued that the Merck vaccine was "Guineas's gift to West Africa and the world."[52]

From a critical vantage point this all seemed to be a type of biopolitics that put on display the benefits that came when "science" rather than "politics" guided humanitarianism. Those who believed in the objectivity of science, and the progress of global health, could gesture in ways that highlighted the benefits that came when local, regional, and national communities worked together to fight infectious diseases. Wasn't this a neoliberal success story that showed how the privatization of vaccines helped, and didn't hinder, egalitarian access to needed treatments?

For several days near the end of July and the beginning of August 2015, mainstream and alternative press outlets contained countless scientific, public, and legal commentaries on the potential of this Merck vaccine. The scientific reportage on the rVSV-ZEBOV vaccine actually began in March 2015, and with the passage of time readers learned that the clinical trials were conducted in one of the few areas in Guinea that were still reporting new cases of EVD.

Many international health organizations had personnel who supported the funding of these particular vaccine trials. To provide readers with some evidence of the amount of money, and the psychic energy, that was invested in this study, as well as the symbolic importance of the public dissemination of these results, consider the fact that this study of the rVSV-ZEBOV vaccine was funded by WHO, with support from the Wellcome Trust (UK), Médecins Sans Frontières, the Norwegian Ministry of Foreign Affairs through the Research Council of Norway, and the Canadian Government through the Public Health Agency of Canada, Canadian Institutes of Health Research, International Development Research Centre, and Department of Foreign Affairs, Trade and Development.

Regardless of whether, in the long run, this vaccine turns out to provide the short-term or long-term protection that is needed, all of the buzz surrounding the various phases of this study spoke volumes about the global hopes and communal desires of many who now demanded that other vaccine trials be carried out in order to help prevent or "end" future outbreaks. The lesson here was many vocal observers were demanding that government officials reorder their priorities so they could circumvent the usual profit motives that stood in the way of producing these types of vaccines for "neglected" diseases. Scientific and public pressure could now be brought to bear in ways that facilitated the clinical trials of Ebola vaccines. Perhaps this was the political will that so many had been looking for.

FUTURE MOBILE RAPID RESPONSES AND THE PROSPECT OF MAJOR INFRASTRUCTURAL HEALTH CARE CHANGES IN WEST AFRICAN CONTEXTS

One of the major lessons that needs to be taken from the latest Ebola outbreak is that those in the "North" can no longer assiduously avoid the task of helping to rebuild West African health care infrastructures while they celebrate the efficacy of their rapid mobile responses during emergencies. The vast majority of infectious-disease research and surveillance that is being carried on in the world is housed, spatially and economically, in the "developed" sites of the "North," while most of the emerging diseases and "re-emerging" diseases are in the "developing" locales in the "South." "We need to be where the diseases are, and where they are likely to emerge," argued David Morens of the U.S. National Institute of Allergy and Infectious Diseases in Bethesda, Maryland, and not be "sitting in labs in U.S. science buildings."[53]

No doubt, as Christian Bréchot explains, major public organizations will be tasked with the responsibility of training the scientists who will need to be in crisis mode in order to confront the next outbreak.[54] However, as noted above, we need reciprocal flows of epidemiological information, so that those who survived Ebola can teach those who can only speculate about how to handle dire situations in rural and urban contexts. Communities in Nigeria and Senegal need to join those in Mali, Guinea, Liberia, Sierra Leone, Spain, and the United States. as they plan for pandemics that should no longer be characterized as an "African" problem that is "aided" by foreigners. The "North" needs to take lessons from the "South" on how to work daily on behavioral change as they put together public health campaigns. Instead of berating supposedly illiterate communities they need to try and gain the cooperation of recalcitrant Ebola victims, families, and neighbors, and Ebola phobias need to be replaced with community-based outreach programs that are sensitive to the needs of survivors, their families, and those who helped them get through this latest crisis.

I hazard to guess that in the coming years global audiences on all the continents will be bombarded with a surfeit of books and articles on the heroic efforts and the successes of the interveners, but few of these will spotlight the selective nature of these Ebola *dispositifs*. As Clár Ní Chonghaile astutely observes, many in the United States, the United Kingdom, and other places will want to reminisce about the amount of monetary aid that they dispensed, but they may be forgetting other visions of what could have been:

> There are other, less quantifiable losses: the number of people who died because they were afraid to go to hospitals for non-Ebola related illnesses; the number of children who will die from preventable illnesses exacerbated by poverty caused when Ebola closed local markets; the number of farmers who have been unable to plant their crops, and now do not have any money to send their children to school. There are also psychological scars. Some people now see hospitals as cursed places. Some children do not want to go back to school because their classrooms were used as Ebola treatment units.[55]

These are not matters that can be handled by those who focus only on rapid response, swoop down with their planes, put up some tents, build some treatment centers or hospitals, and then get back on those planes and return to their foreign bases.

THE NEED TO DEFEND MEDICAL HUMANITARIANISM AND THE NEED TO PROBLEMATIZE THE NOTION OF "MILITARY HUMANITARIANISM"

The growing resonance of martial rhetorics that trumpet the beneficence and efficacy of "security" oriented rapid military responses during crises like Haiti and West Africa will continue to bedevil those who need the logical support, but not the paternalism, that comes from U.S. and other foreign interventionism.[56] As Stefan Elbe noted several years ago the "securitizing" of infectious diseases often brings unique forms of "haggling over viruses," where we have disputation between populations from the global North and South who have very different ways of viewing ownership of contested knowledge about vaccines, anti-viral medicals, leadership during internal health crises and the role that diplomacy plays during potential pandemics.[57] "Biosecurity" is an alluring ideograph, but that does not mean that it cannot be unpacked and critiqued.[58]

It is imperative that critical legal scholars and critical cultural scholars constantly attend to the ways that military humanitarian adventurism does more than just build some tents, hospitals, "air bridges," and so forth, during health care epidemics. As noted in earlier chapters, projects like Operation United Assistance also promote the idea that the U.S. military is a global force for "good," and that a major American footprint in Africa, evidenced by the growth of AFRICOM, can help provide the securitized bases that are needed in this "pivot" area to fight not only diseases but terrorists. Is it any wonder that CNN, in spite of all of the levity and sarcasm that they suffered at the hands of competitive networks or alternative press outlets, can have personnel, with straight faces, compare Ebola with ISIS? This is *because of the populist acceptance* of the dense layers of rhetorical figurations about U.S. medical military involvement in disease control—in places like Panama, Cuba, or the Philippines—that have become a part of the public memories co-produced by generations of Americans who believed in American military exceptionalism.

No doubt the belated arrival of WHO, Obama's military "surge," and so on, may have helped West Africans psychologically and materially as they battled EVD, but as I noted in previous chapters we need to be circumspect in the ways that we marginalize the efforts of the contact tracers, the African public health care workers, and others who were in the "hot zones" risking their lives. There is a great deal of difference between claiming that you were at the "frontlines" of the metaphoric battles that were fought against Ebola, and actually coming into contact with suspected or confirmed Ebola patients.

Some of those who reflected back on dire 2014 forecasts—that had warned of a possible scenario where global communities would have to cope with ten thousand cases[59]—congratulated all of the donors, soldiers, and volunteers who had intervened to make sure that matters did not get completely out of hand. Yet Clár Ní Chonghaile openly wondered whether recent medical and military humanitarian efforts that did not involve any "sustainable, long-lasting donor commitments to health systems" would leave much of a "positive legacy" from the millions of dollars that had been spent.[60] Tom Dannatt, the founder of the United Kingdom's charity *Street Child*, claimed that well-intentioned interventionists were focusing on the wrong dimensions of the Ebola problems:

> The flat-footedness of the entire [aid] structure has been dramatically exposed by almost every stage of this crisis. As to the investment made in the past six months, it doesn't have any longevity beyond Ebola. The ETCs (Ebola treatment centres) and holding centres and all the rest are viewed with ambiguity by locals because they are almost all temporary structures. . . . When this outbreak is over, they will be folded down, burnt down or knocked down. I don't understand why we invested so much in a hardware-based response when it seemed quite obvious that the key things were behavioural, and attitudinal and educational. . . . That has basically been proven because, by the time all these clinics became operational, they weren't needed.[61]

Tom Dannatt, of course, was assuming that the EVD victims themselves were both the primary beneficiaries, as well as the targets, of all of the Ebola interventionism that took place during what MSF calls that second stage of Ebola interventionism, which began in August of 2014 and started to wind down by February of 2015.

My focus on the role that *realpolitik* interests, disparate power, and media access plays in Ebola contexts leads me to conclude that there were other considerations involved when foreign interventionists paid a visit to West Africa during that second stage. One of the reasons that many may have wanted to build those type of structures that Dannatt was talking about may have to do with *their telegenic nature*, where philanthropic donors, Congressional or Parliamentary leaders, scientists, and members of the public *could see* how their money was being spent. If the billions of dollars that had been spent on researchers, lab preparedness, logistics, PPE, troop salaries, and so forth, had been spent in the ways that Tom Dannatt was suggesting, then this might have helped West Africans but it did not render visible the heroism and the sacrifices of the rescuers. How, after all, does one put on display the spending for behavioral or attitudinal change that was needed at the local, micro levels? How will it help the Ebola "exceptionalists" when you spend money on contact tracers' salaries instead of paying for expensive Ebola research, pharmaceuticals, and the like?

Visibility, strategic communication, and the promotion of Western-oriented, neoliberal health targets and assessment tools simply plays well at home, even in cases where there is a disconnect between what West African communities need and what Westerns *think they need*. What Western audiences wanted to see were some of the ETCs that Dannatt was complaining about. In other words, Dannatt was touching on some of *the psycho-social features* of EVD outbreaks when he provided his normative critique of how donated funds should be spent.

The vast majority of Western authors and researchers who look back on the "lessons learned" from the 2013–2015 outbreak do mention, in passing, the need for drastic changes in public health infrastructural systems in Guinea, Liberia, and Sierra Leone, but these are usually presented in ways that gloss over this topic as they congratulate the donors and the interveners who supposedly risked their lives in the name of transcendent principles like the "responsibility to protect." The Western mediascapes that put on display rows of neat tents and hospital beds resonated with those who could say that they had made a difference, but in the future, critical scholars will need to spend years evidencing how talk of the efficacy of rapid response teams will be used *to avoid* spending in other ways that might interfere with the austerity measures, and the strings that have been attached, to the aid that comes from financial institutions like the World Bank and the IMF.

In the future, critical cultural scholars and critical legal researchers will also need to deconstruct the notion that it was the militarization of Ebola that turned the tide in the "war" against Ebola. They will need to find ways of deterritorializing and demystifying the arguments that they will hear in the future about how the American military had applied the containment lessons that they had learned from the pandemic of avian influenza during the 1990s, the anthrax attacks in 2001 in the United States, and the outbreak of SARS in 2003. These critics will need to confront military permutations of the outbreak narratives that will contrast the older, probabilistic civilian isolationist practices with the "new" ways of talking about resilience, possibilistic reasoning, and the biosecurity preparedness.

Not surprising, those who conversed about these topics in Pentagon, Congressional, or private corporate hallways were oftentimes some of the very social agents who were asked to come up with the twenty-first-century plans for containing these same "bioterrorist" or other threats. Reportage on Ebola outbreaks, and other health care "emergencies," led to the convergence of public health rhetorics and securitization discourses that called for stronger national public health capabilities.[62]

CONCLUSION

Hope springs eternal and more than a few cosmopolitan citizens around the world will pray that the belated interventionism and other medical, political, and legal conundrums that manifested themselves during the latest West African outbreak can teach all nation-states and their populations some key lessons. There are signs of progress when we hear about the possible funding of a massive Ebola emergency fund or when we hear there are plans afoot for the revision of the World Health Organization's 2005 "International Health Regulations."[63]

However, if I am right then these types of formalistic changes will accomplish very little if we don't change the rhetorical cultures of those in the "North" who implement these plans. If we continue to use neo-Malthusian rhetorics that highlight the importance of "emergency" assistance, then we will continue to be reactive instead of proactive in Ebola contexts. I am talking about recrafting the pandemic *dispositifs* that once treated "Guinea haemorrhagic fever" as something that morphed into the "West African outbreak" and that only worried major global powers when it became what Margaret Chan of WHO called a "crisis for international peace."[64]

Talk of mobility, preparedness, and rapid response may resonate with those who enjoy knowing that their nation helped with bilateral or international "rescue" but this often masks the more isolationist, austerity-driven, triage-oriented ways of handling global pandemics that avoids grappling with the structural violence that is often at the heart of the containment measures that are used in endemic and epidemic situations.[65]

The chapters in this book have illustrated some of the reasons why we can no longer view Ebola fighting as some epidemiological or clinical battle that will be won or lost by those who can modify the behavior of West Africans. It is the multi-faceted, sedimented, and protean nature of the various Ebola rhetorics that I have studied that makes it so difficult for well-intentioned interventionists to make any long-term difference in epidemic contexts.

If this is indeed the "age of Ebola," or the time of the "Ebola apocalypse," then the future contests that have to be fought against both EVD and the anxieties this disease generates will need to take into account mutual vulnerabilities of those living in the global South and the global North.

NOTES

1. For a brilliant critique of some of the myriad cellular and geographic dimensions of Preston's work that appears in *The Hot Zone*, see Bill Albertini, "The Geographies of Contagion," *Rhizomes: Cultural Studies in Emerging Knowledge* 19 (Summer 2009): n.p., http://www.rhizomes.net/issue19/albertini.html.

2. Michael Wilson, "Sierra Leone's First Party in 12 Months," Global Citizen, last modified August 11, 2015, https://www.globalcitizen.org/en/content/sierra-leones-first-party-in-12-months/.

3. Joanne Liu, "Finish the Fight," *Nature* 524 (August 6, 2015): 27–29, 27.

4. One of the intriguing topics that future researchers need to take up is the role that corruption and politics played during all of this decisionism. Fodei Batty hints at some of this in Fodei Batty, "Ebola Epidemic's Legacy of Fear and Corruption," *Hartford Courant*, last modified August 11, 2015, http://www.courant.com/opinion/op-ed/hc-op-batty-ebola-scam-in-west-africa-20150811-story.html.

5. David L. Heymann, et al., "Global Health Security: The Wider Lessons from the West African Ebola Virus Disease Epidemic," *The Lancet* 385 (May 9, 2015): 1884–1887, 1884.

6. Ibid., 1884.

7. Ibid., 1884.

8. Ibid., 1884–1885.

9. Ibid., 1885.

10. Piero L. Olliaro, Peter Horby, and Else Teorreele, "Health Security and Rights in Times of Emerging Health Threats," *The Lancet* 385 (May 9, 2015): 1892–1893.

11. Ibid., 1892.

12. Ibid., 1892.

13. London School of Hygiene and Tropical Medicine, "Can the Ebola Outbreak Rejuvenate Global Health Security," London School of Hygiene and Tropical

Medicine, last modified May 8, 2015, http://www.lshtm.ac.uk/newsevents/news/2015/ebola_outbreak_rejuvenate_health_security.html.

14. Donal Brown, quoted in Sam Jones, "U.K. Expert Warns of Disaster If Lessons Are Not Learned from Ebola Outbreak," *The Guardian*, last modified June 17, 2015, paragraph 4, http://www.theguardian.com/global-development/2015/jun/17/uk-expert-warns-of-disaster-if-lessons-are-not-learned-from-ebola-outbreak.

15. Donald G. McNeil Jr., "Using a Tactic Unseen in a Century, Countries Cordon Off Ebola-Racked Areas," *The New York Times*, last modified August 12, 2014, paragraph 1, http://www.nytimes.com/2014/08/13/science/using-a-tactic-unseen-in-a-century-countries-cordon-off-ebola-racked-areas.html.

16. These included hunger strikes as well as strikes by nurses. British Broadcasting Corporation "Ebola Crisis: Guinea Hunger Strike at Village Occupation." BBC News, last modified November 11, 2014, http://www.bbc.com/news/health-30004362.

17. Declan Butler, "The Next Time," *Nature* 524 (August 6, 2015): 22–25.

18. Donal Brown, quoted in Sam Jones, "U.K. Expert Warns of Disaster," paragraphs 10–12.

19. Ibid., paragraph 9.

20. Phil Gingrey, "Letter to Thomas R. Frieden," *Think Progress*, last modified July 7, 2014, http://thinkprogress.org/wp-content/uploads/2014/07/gingrey_letter_to_cdc_on_public_health_crisis.pdf.

21. Ibid., 4–6.

22. Wade Goodwin, "In U.S., Ebola Turns from A Public Health Issue to a Political One," NPR, last modified October 9, 2014, http://www.npr.org/2014/10/09/354890869/in-u-s-ebola-turns-from-a-public-health-issue-to-a-political-one.

23. Gregg Mitman, "Ebola in a Stew of Fear," *New England Journal of Medicine* 371, no. 9 (November 6, 2014): 1763–1765, 1764. DOI: 10.1056/NEJMp1411244.

24. Butler, "The Next Time," 23.

25. Ibid., 23.

26. Richard Preston, *The Hot Zone* (New York: Random House, 1994), 13.

27. Ibid., 16.

28. Ibid., 16–17.

29. Ibid., 11–12.

30. Margaret Humphreys, "No Safe Place: Disease and Panic in American History," *American Literary History* 14, no. 4 (2002): 845–857, 847. For other relevant studies of the perceptual dangers often associated with travel and contagion, see Laura Otis, *Membranes: Metaphors of Invasion in Nineteenth-Century Literature, Science, and Politics* (Baltimore, MD: Johns Hopkins University Press, 1999); Howard Markel, *When Germs Travel: Six Major Epidemics That Have Invaded America Since 1900 and the Fears They Have Unleashed* (New York: Pantheon Books, 2004).

31. Albertini, "The Geographies of Contagion," paragraph 23.

32. Helen Epstein, "Ebola in Liberia: An Epidemic of Rumors," *The New York Review of Books,* last modified December 18, 2014, paragraph 6, http://www.nybooks.com/articles/archives/2014/dec/18/ebola-liberia-epidemic-rumors/.

33. Donal Brown, quoted in in Sam Jones, "U.K. Expert Warns of Disaster," paragraph 7.

34. During both the first and second interventions, when foreign advisors and NGOs traveled overseas to combat EVD, many scientists, public health officials, infectious disease experts and journalists presented us with their views on why local fears, superstitions, religious traditions, and other cultural or social factors prevented the accurate recording of the "real" transmission of Ebola, but a critical study of this period also reveals that many social actors had a hand in interfering with these efforts.

35. Claude Evers, quoted in Misah Hussain, "MSF Says Lack of Public Health Messages on Ebola, 'Big Mistake,'" Reuters, last modified February 4, 2015, paragraph 5, http://www.reuters.com/article/2015/02/04/us-health-ebola-msf-idUSKBN0L81QF20150204.

36. Hussain, "MSF Says Lack of Public Health Messages."

37. Sakoba Keita, quoted in Hussain, "MSF Says Lack of Public Health Messages," paragraph 11.

38. Michael T. Osterholm, Kristine A. Moore, and Lawrence O. Gostin, "Public Health in the Age of Ebola," *The Journal of the American Medical Association* 175, no. 1 (January, 2015): 7–8, doi:10.1001/jamainternmed.2014.6235.

39. For an excellent journalist essay that reviews some of the governmental, societal, and cultural chaos that swirled around this latest Ebola outbreak, see Kevin Sack, Sheri Fink, Pam Belluck, and Adam Nossiter, "How Ebola Roared Back," *The New York Times*, last modified December 28, 2014, http://www.nytimes.com/2014/12/30/health/how-ebola-roared-back.html?_r=0.

40. Nassim Nicholas Taleb, *The Black Swan: The Impact of the Highly Improbable* (New York, Random House, 2010), xxi, xxii.

41. Martin I. Meltzer, Charisma Y. Atkins, Scott Santibanez, et al., "Estimating The Future Number of Cases in the Ebola Epidemic—Liberia and Sierra Leone, 2014–2015," *Morbidity and Mortality Weekly Report* 63, no. 3 (2014): 1–14.

42. Osterholm, Moore, and Gostin, "Public Health in the Age of Ebola," 7–8.

43. Ibid., 7–8.

44. Edward Liebow, quoted in Kari Lydersen, "Ebola Teams Need Better Cultural Understanding, Anthropologists Say," *Discover*, December 9, 2014, paragraph 13, http://blogs.discovermagazine.com/crux/2014/12/09/ebola-cultural-anthropologists/#.VXHoY89VhBd.

45. Ann-Maria Henao-Restrepo et al., "Efficacy and Effectiveness of an rVSV-vector Vaccine Expressing Ebola Surface Glycoprotein: Interim Results from the Guinea Ring Vaccination Cluster-Randomised Trial," *The Lancet* 386, no. 9996 (August 29/September 4 2015): 857–866.

46. Ibid., 2.

47. Zosia Kmietowicz, "Ebola Vaccine Trial Results Are 'Extremely Promising,' Says WHO," *British Medical Journal* 351 (July 31, 2015): h4192, doi: http://dx.doi.org/10.1136/bmj.h4192.

48. Sarah Boseley, "Ebola Vaccine Trial Proves 100% Successful in Guinea," *The Guardian*, last modified July 31, 2015, http://www.theguardian.com/world/2015/jul/31/ebola-vaccine-trial-proves-100-successful-in-guinea. We all need to temper some of this enthusiasm and remember that even the reportage of successful trials is often followed by years of wrangling over licensing, development, and marketing. See, for example, the commentary on this that appears in Bruce Y. Lee et al., "Is

the World Ready for an Ebola Vaccine," *The Lancet* 385, no. 9964 (January 17, 2015): 203–204, DOI: http://dx.doi.org/10.1016/S0140-6736(14)62398-9.

49. Maria Cheng, "Ebola Vaccine Seems Effective, Could Stop Current Outbreak and Prevent Future Disasters," *Minneapolis Star Tribune*, last modified August 1, 2015, paragraph 6, http://bigstory.ap.org/article/2a57470b0b714f8da98c3 4add847ba15/experimental-ebola-vaccine-could-stop-virus-west-africa.

50. Ben Neuman, quoted in Cheng, "Ebola Vaccine Seems Effective," paragraph 14.

51. Margaret Chan, quoted in Kmietowicz, "Ebola Vaccine Trial Results," 1.

52. WHO, "World On the Verge of an Effective Vaccine," WHO, last modified July 31, 2015, http://www.who.int/mediacentre/news/releases/2015/effective-ebola-vaccine/en/.

53. David Morens, quoted in Butler, "The Next Time," 23.

54. Christian Bréchot, "Train Africa's Scientists in Crisis Response," *Nature* 524 (August 6, 2015): 7.

55. Chonghaile, "Ebola Spending," paragraphs 12–13.

56. For an example of a contextualization that is very different from my own, that uses historical research to argue that military involvement helps with public health responses and outcomes, see Christopher Watterson and Adam Kamradt-Scott, "Fighting Flu: Securitization and the Military Role in Combating Influenza," *Armed Forces & Society* (2015); 1–15, DOI: 10.1177/0095327X14567364.

57. Stefan Elbe, "Haggling Over Viruses: The Downside Risks of Securitizing Infectious Diseases," *Health Policy and Planning*, 25, no. 6 (2010): 476–485.

58. As several critical scholars have pointed out, by focusing on bioterrorism and biosecurity threats elites have spent billions elsewhere that could have been spent on African public health care infrastructures.

59. Sarah Bosely, "WHO Warns 10,000 New Cases of Ebola a Week Is Possible," *The Guardian*, last modified October 14, 2014, http://www.theguardian.com/world/2014/oct/14/who-new-ebola-cases-world-health-organisation.

60. Clár Ní Chonghaile, "Ebola Spending: Will Lack of a Positive Legacy Turn Dollars to Delour?" *The Guardian*, last modified February 13, 2015, paragraphs 2–4, http://www.theguardian.com/global-development/2015/feb/13/ebola-spending-positive-healthcare-legacy-west-africa.

61. Tom Dannatt, quoted in Chonghaile, "Ebola Spending," paragraphs 6–9.

62. Gian Luci Burci, "Ebola, The Security Council and the Securitization of Public Health," *Questions of International Law*, December 23, 2014, paragraph 12, http://www.qil-qdi.org/ebola-security-council-securitization-public-health/.

63. World Health Organization, *International Health Organization* (Geneva: World Health Organization, 2005).

64. Margaret Chan, quoted in Nick Cumming-Bruce, "WHO Chief Calls Ebola Outbreak a "Crisis for International Peace," *The New York Times*, last modified October 13, 2014, http://www.nytimes.com/2014/10/14/world/africa/ebola-virus-outbreak.html?_r=0.

65. For a detailed discussion of the role that structural violence has played in infectious disease contexts both before and during the 2013–2015 West African outbreak, see Annie Wilkinson and Melissa Leach, "Briefing: Ebola-Myths, Realities and Structural Violence," *African Affairs* 114, no. 454 (2014): 136–148.

Bibliography

BOOKS

Agamben, Gorgio. *"What Is an Apparatus?" and Other Essays*. London: Stanford University Press, 2009.

Appadurai, Arjun. *Modernity at Large: Cultural Dimensions of Globalization*. Minneapolis, MN: University of Minnesota Press, 1996.

Arendt, Hannah. *The Origins of Totalitarianism*. (1951). New York: Harcourt, Inc., 1973.

Arnold, David. *Imperial Medicine and Indigenous Societies*. New York: Manchester University Press, 1988.

Barnett, Michael, and Thomas G. Weiss. *Humanitarianism Contested: Where Angels Fear to Tread*. New York: Routledge: 2011.

Benton, Adia. *HIV Exceptionalism: Development through Disease in Sierra Leone*. Minneapolis: University of Minnesota Press, 2015.

Boas, Morten. *The Politics of Conflict Economies: Miners, Merchants, and Warriors in the African Borderlands*. New York: Routledge, 2015.

Condit, Celeste M., and John L. Lucaites. *Crafting Equality: America's Anglo-African Word*. Chicago: University of Chicago Press, 1993.

Cooney, Daniel, Vincent Wong, and Yaneer Bar-Yam. *Beyond Contract Tracing: Community-Based Early Detection for Ebola Response*. Cambridge: New England Complex Systems Institute, 2015.

De Walle, Nicolas Van. *African Economies and the Politics of Permanent Crisis, 1979–1999*. New York: Cambridge University Press, 2001.

Esposito, Roberto. *Bios: Biopolitics and Philosophy*. Translated by Timothy Campbell. Minneapolis: University of Minnesota Press, 2007.

Esposito, Roberto. *Communitas: The Origin and Destiny of the Community*. Translated by Timothy Campbell. Redwood City, CA: Stanford University Press, 2004.

Esposito, Roberto. *Immunitas: The Protection and Negation of Life*. Translated by Zakiya Hanafi. Cambridge: Polity, 2011.

Farmer, Paul. *AIDS and Accusation: Haiti and Geography of Blame*. Berkeley: University of California Press, 2006.

Farmer, Paul. *Infections and Inequalities: The Modern Plagues* Berkeley: University of California Press, 2001.

Foucault, Michel. *The History of Sexuality, Vol. 1: The Will to Knowledge*. Translated by Robert Hurley. London: Penguin, 1998.

Foucault, Michel. *"Society Must Be Defended": Lectures at the Collège De France, 1975–1976*. Translated by David Macey. New York: Picador, 2003.

Gross, Jean-Germain. *Healthcare Policy in Africa: Institutions and Politics from Colonialism to the Present*. Lanham, MD: Rowman & Littlefield, 2015.

Harvey, David. *A Brief History of Neoliberalism*. Oxford: Oxford Univ. Press, 2005.

Markel, Howard. *When Germs Travel: Six Major Epidemics That Have Invaded America Since 1900 and the Fears They Have Unleashed*. New York: Pantheon Books, 2004.

Moeller, Susan D. *Compassion Fatigue: How the Media Sell Disease, Famine, War and Death*. New York: Routledge, 1999.

Otis, Laura. *Membranes: Metaphors of Invasion in Nineteenth-Century Literature, Science, and Politics*. Baltimore, MD: Johns Hopkins University Press, 1999.

Preston, Richard. *The Hot Zone*. New York: Random House, 1994.

Rankin, F. Harrison. *The White Man's Grave: A Visit to Sierra Leone, in 1834*. London: Richard Bently, 1836.

Redfield, Peter. *Life in Crisis: The Ethical Journal of Doctors Without Borders*. Berkeley: University of California Press, 2013.

Rowden, Richard. *The Deadly Ideas of Neoliberalism: How the IMF has Undermined Public Health and the Fight against AIDS*. London: Zed Books, 2009.

Schwöbel, Christine. *Critical Approaches to International Criminal Law*. New York: Routledge, 2014.

Sloterdijk, Peter. *Bubbles: Spheres Volume I: Microspherology*. Translated by Wileland Hoban. Cambridge, MA: MIT Press, 2011.

Stoler, Anne Laura. *Along the Archival Grain: Epistemic Anxieties and Colonial Common Sense*. Princeton: Princeton University Press, 2009.

Taleb, Nassim Nicholas. *The Black Swan: The Impact of the Highly Improbable*. New York, Random House, 2010.

Wallis, Braithwaite Wallis. *The Advance of Our West Africa Empire*. (1903). New York: Negro Universities, 1969.

Eyal Weizman. *The Least of All Possible Evils: Humanitarian Violence from Arendt to Gaza*. London: Verso, 2012.

World Health Organization. *International Health Organization*. Geneva: World Health Organization, 2005.

BOOK CHAPTERS

Ayotte, Kevin J., Daniel Rex Bernard, and H. Dan O'Hair. "Knowing Terror: On the Epistemology and Rhetoric of Risk." In *Handbook of Risk and Crisis Com-*

munication, edited by Robert L. Heath and H. Dan O'Hair, 607–628. New York: Routledge, 2009.

Derrida, Jacques. "Autoimmunity: Real and Symbolic Suicides." In *Philosophy in a Time of Terror: Dialogues with Jürgen Habermas and Jacques Derrida*, interviewed by Giovanna Borradori, 85–136. Chicago: University of Chicago Press, 2003.

Foucault, Michel. "Nietzsche, Genealogy, History." In *The Foucault Reader*, edited Paul Rabinow, 76–100. Harmondsworth: Penguin, 1984.

Foucault, Michel. The Confession of the Flesh. In *Power/Knowledge: Selected Interviews and Other Writings, 1972–1977*, edited by Colin Gordon, translated by Colin Gordon, Leo Marshall, John Mepham, and Kate Soper, 194–228. New York: Pantheon Books, 1980.

Foucault, Michel. "Truth and Power." In *Power/Knowledge: Selected Interviews and Other Writings, 1971–1977*, edited by Colin Gordon, translated by Colin Gordon, Leo Marshall, John Mepham, and Kate Soper, 109–133. New York: Pantheon Books, 1980.

Kegters, Llewellyn J., Linda H. Brink, and Ernest T. Takafuji. "Are We Prepared for a Viral Outbreak Emergency?" In *Emerging Diseases*, edited by Stephen S. Morse, 269–282. New York: Oxford University Press, 1993.

JOURNAL ARTICLES AND LAW REVIEWS

Bill Albertini, Bill. "Contagion and the Necessary Accident." *Discourse* 30, no. 3 (Fall, 2008): 443–467.

Appadurai, Arjun. "Disjuncture and Difference in the Global Cultural Economy." *Public Culture* 2, no. 2 (1990): 1–24. doi: 10.1215/08992363-2-2-1.

Ayotte, Kevin. J. "A Vocabulary of Disease: Argumentation, Hot Zones, and the Intertextuality of Bioterrorism." *Argumentation and Advocacy* 48, no. 1 (Summer, 2011): 1–21.

Bah, Elhadj Ilbrahima. "Clinical Presentation of Patients with Ebola Virus Disease in Conakry, Guinea." *The New England Journal of Medicine* 372 (2015): 40–47.

Baize, Sylvain, et al. "Emergence of Zaire Ebola Virus Disease in Guinea." *New England Journal of Medicine* 371, no. 15 (2014):1418–1425. doi.org/10.1056/NEJ Moa1404505.

Bass, Jeff. D. "Hearts of Darkness and Hot Zones: The Ideogeme of Imperial Contagion in Recent Accounts of Viral Outbreaks." *The Quarterly Journal of Speech* 84 (1998): 430–447. doi: 10.1080/00335639809384231.

Bergstresser, Sara M. "Health Communication, Public Mistrust, And the Politics of 'Rationality.'" *The American Journal of Bioethics* 14, no. 4 (2015): 57–59. doi: 10.1080/15265161.2015.1009570.

Berry, John M. "Pandemics: Avoiding the Mistakes of 1918." *Nature* 459 (May 21, 2009): 324–325. doi: 10.1038/459324a.

Boozary, Andrew S., Paul E. Farmer, and Ashish K. Jha. "The Ebola Outbreak: Fragile Health Systems and Quality as a Cure." *The Journal of the American Medical Association* 312, no. 18 (November 12, 2014): 1859–1860.

Bréchot, Christian. "Train Africa's Scientists in Crisis Response." *Nature* 524 (August 6, 2015): 7.

Brown, Hannah, and Ann H. Kelly, "Material Proximities and Hotspots: Toward an Anthropology of Viral Hemorrhagic Fevers." *Medical Anthropological Quarterly* 28, no. 2 (2014): 280–303.

Burkle, Frederick M., Jr., and Dan Hanfling. "Political Leadership in the Time of Crises: *Primum non Nocere*." *PLOS Currents* 7 (May 29, 2015): doi: 10.1371/currents.dis.fd8aaf6707cd5dd252e33c771d08b949.

Bussolin, Jeffrey. "What Is a *Dispositif?*" *Foucault Studies* 10 (2010): 85–107.

Butler, Declan. "The Next Time," *Nature* 524 (August 6, 2015): 22–25.

Campbell, Timothy. "'Bios,' Immunity, Life: The Thought of Roberto Esposito." *Diacritics* 36, no. 2 (Summer, 2006): 2–22.

Chan, Kit Yee, and Daniel D. Reidpath, "'Typhoid Mary' and 'HIV Jane': Responsibility, Agency and Disease Prevention." *Reproductive Health Matters* 11, no. 22 (November 2003): 40–50. doi:10.1016/S0968–8080(03)02291-2.

Chandler, Clare, et al. "Ebola: Limitations of Correcting Misinformation." *The Lancet* 384 (April 4, 2015): 1275–1276.

Chiappelli, Francesco, et al. "Ebola: Translational Science Consideration." *Journal of Translational Medicine* 13, no. 11 (2015): 1–29.

Chua, Arlene C., et al., "The Case for Improved Diagnostic Tools to Control Ebola Virus Disease in West Africa and How to Get There." *PLOS Neglected Tropical Diseases* (June 11, 2015): 1–6.

Cisneros, David. "Contaminated Communities: The Metaphor of 'Immigrant as Pollutant' in Media Representations of Immigration." *Rhetoric & Public Affairs* 11, no. 4 (2008): 569–602.

Cloud, Dana L. "The Null Persona: Race and the Rhetoric of Silence in the Uprising of '34." *Rhetoric & Public Affairs* 2, no. 2 (Summer, 1999): 177–209.

Collier, Stephen J., and Andrew Lakoff. "Vital Systems Security: Reflective Biopolitics and the Government of Emergency." *Theory, Culture, & Society* 32, no. 2 (2015): 19–51.

Condit, Celeste M., John Lynch, and Emily Winderman. "Recent Rhetorical Studies in Public Understanding of Science: Multiple Purposes and Strengths." *Public Understanding of Science* 21, no. 4 (2012): 386–400. doi: 10.1177/0963662512437330.

Conteh-Morgan, Earl. "Globalization, State Failure, and Collective Violence: The Case of Sierra Leone." *International Journal of Peace Studies* 11, no. 2 (Autumn/Winter, 2006): 87–103.

DeChaine, D. Robert. "Humanitarian Space and the Social Imaginary: Médecins Sans Frontières/Doctors Without Borders and the Rhetoric of Global Community." *Journal of Communication Inquiry* 26, no. 4 (October, 2012): 354–369.

Delicath, John W., and Kevin Michael DeLuca. "Image Events, the Public Sphere, and Argumentative Practice: The Case of Radical Environmental Groups." *Argumentation* 17 (2003): 315–333.

Doyle, Michael W. "A Few Words on Mill, Walzer, and Noninterventionism." *Ethics & International Affairs* 23, no. 4 (December, 2009): 349–369.

Drazen, Jeffrey M., et al. "Ebola and Quarantine." *The New England Journal of Medicine* 371 (November 20, 2014): 2029–2030.

Dudziak, Mary L. "Oliver Wendell Holmes, Jr., as a Eugenic Reformer: Rhetoric in the Writing of Constitutional Law." *Iowa Law Review* 71, no. 3 (March, 1986): 833–868.

Elbe, Stefan. "Haggling over Viruses: The Downside Risks of Securitizing Infectious Diseases." *Health Policy and Planning*, 25, no. 6 (2010): 476–485.

Elbe, Stefan, Anne Roemer-Mahler, and Christopher Long. "Securing Circulating Pharmaceutically: Antiviral Stockpiling and Pandemic Preparedness in the European Union." *Security Dialogue* 45, no. 5 (2014): 440–457.

Erni, John Nguyet. "A Legal Realist View of Citizen Actions in Hong Kong's Umbrella Movement." *Chinese Journal of Communication* 8, no. 4 (2015): 412–419.

Esposito, Roberto, and Anna Paparcone. "Interview." *Diacritics* 36, no. 2 (Summer 2006): 49–56.

Etuk, E. E. "Ebola: A West African Perspective." *Journal of the Royal College of Physicians, Edinburgh* 45 (2015): 19–22.

Fins, Joseph J. "Ideology and Microbiology: Ebola, Science, and Deliberative Democracy." *The American Journal of Bioethics* 15, no. 4 (2015): 1–3. doi: 10.1080/15265161.2015.1023119.

Fontané, Nicholas, and Frédéric Keck. "How Biosecurity Reframes Animal Surveillance." *Revue d'anthropologie des connaissances* 9 no. 2 (2015): https://www.cairn.info/revue-anthropologie-des-connaissances-2015-2-page-a.htm.

Frankel, Stephen, and John Western. "Pretext or Prophylaxis? Racial Segregation and Malarial Mosquitos in a British Tropical Colony: Sierra Leone." *Annals of the Association of American Geographers* 78, no. 2 (June, 1988): 211–228.

Frieden, Thomas R., et al. "Ebola 2014—New Challenges, New Global Response and Responsibilities." *The New England Journal of Medicine* 371 (2014): 1177–1180. doi 10.1056/NEJMp1409903.

Gatter, Robert. "Ebola, Quarantine, and Flawed CDC Policy." *University of Miami Business Law Review* (2015): 375–397.

Gonsalves, Gregg, and Peter Staley. "Panic, Paranoia, and Public Health—The AIDS Epidemic's Lessons for Ebola." *The New England Journal of Medicine* 371 (December 18, 2014): 2348–2349.

Gupta, Sanjeev. "Response to 'The International Monetary Fund and the Ebola Outbreak.'" *The Lancet* 3, no. 2 (January 5, 2015): e78.

Hasian, Marouf, Jr. "Critical Legal Rhetorics: The Theory and Practice of Law in a Postmodern World." *Southern Communication Journal* 60, no. 1 (1994): 44–56.

Hayden, Erika Check. "MSF Takes Bigger Global-Health Role." *Nature* 522 (June 4, 2015): 18–19.

Headrick, Daniel R. "Sleeping Sickness Epidemics and Colonial Responses in East and Central Africa, 1900–1940." *PLOS Neglected Tropical Diseases* 8, no. 4 (April 2014): 1–8.

Heath, J. Benton. "Global Emergency Power in the Age of Ebola." *Harvard International Law Journal* 57, no. 1 (July 6, 2015): http://papers.ssrn.com/sol3/papers.cfm?abstract_id=2587720.

Henao-Restrepo, Ann-Maria, et al. "Efficacy and Effectiveness of an rVSV-vector Vaccine Expressing Ebola Surface Glycoprotein: Interim Results from the Guinea Ring Vaccination Cluster-Randomised Trial." *The Lancet* 386, no. 9996 (August 29/September 4 2015): 857–866.

Heymann, David L., et al. "Global Health Security: The Wider Lessons from the West African Ebola Virus Disease Epidemic." *The Lancet* 385 (May 9, 2015): 1884–1887.

Hickox, Kaci. "Caught between Civil Liberties and Public Safety Fears: Personal Reflections from a Healthcare Provider Treating Ebola." *Journal of Health & Biomedical Law* 11 (2015): 9–23.

Huber, Lindsay Pérez, and Daniel G. Solorzano. "Visualizing Everyday Racism: Critical Race Theory, Visual Micro-aggressions, and the Historical Imagery of Mexican Banditry." *Qualitative Inquiry* 21, no. 3 (2015): 223–238, doi: 10.1177/1077800414562899.

Humphreys, Margaret. "No Safe Place: Disease and Panic in American History," *American Literary History* 14, no. 4 (2002): 845–857.

Inniss, Lolita Buckner. "A Critical Legal Rhetoric Approach to *In Re African-American Slave Descendants Litigation*." *St. John's Journal of Legal Commentary* 24 (2009): 649–696.

Joffe, Hélène, and Georgina Haarhoff. "Representations of Far-Flung Illnesses: The Case of Ebola in Britain." *Social Science and Medicine* 54, no. 6 (2002): 988–969. doi: 10.1016/S0277-9536(01)00068-5.

Jones, Jared. "Ebola, Emerging: The Limitations of Culturalist Discourses in Epidemiology." *Journal of Global Health* 1, no. 1 (Spring, 2011): 1–6.

Kekulé, Alexander S. "Learning from Ebola Virus: How to Prevent Future Epidemics." *Viruses* 7 (2015): 3789–3797.

Kentikelenis, Alexander, Lawrence King, Martin McKee, and David Stuckler. "The International Monetary Fund and the Ebola Crisis." *The Lancet* 3 (February 2015): e69–e70.

Keränen, Lisa. "Concocting Viral Apocalypse: Catastrophic Risk and the Production of Bio(in)security." *Western Journal of Communication* 75, no. 5 (2011): 451–472.

Keränen, Lisa. "Review Essay: Addressing the Epidemic of Epidemics: Germs, Security, and a Call for Biocriticism." *The Quarterly Journal of Speech* 97, no. 2 (2011): 224–244. doi: 10.1080/00335630.2011.565785.

Kmietowicz, Zosia. "Ebola Vaccine Trial Results are 'Extremely Promising,' Says WHO." *British Medical Journal* 351 (July 31, 2015): h4192, doi: http://dx.doi.org/10.1136/bmj.h4192.

Kupferschmidt, Kai. "On the Trail of Contagion." *Science* 347 I6218 (January 9, 2015): 120–121.

Lakoff, Andrew. "The Generic Biothreat, or, How We Became Unprepared." *Cultural Anthropology* 23, no. 1 (2008): 399–428.

Leach, Melissa. "Time to Put Ebola in Context." *Bulletin of the World Health Organization*, 88, no. 7 (July 1, 2010): 481–560. doi: 10.2471/BLT.10.030710.

Leavitt, Judith Walzer. "Typhoid Mary Strikes Back: Bacteriological Theory and Practice in Early Twentieth- Century Public Health." *ISIS* 83, no. 4 (December, 1992): 608–629.

Lee, Bruce Y., et al. "Is the World Ready for an Ebola Vaccine." *The Lancet* 385, no. 9964 (January 17, 2015): 203–204. doi: http://dx.doi.org/10.1016/S0140-6736 (14)62398-9.

Lemke, Thomas. "Foucault, Governmentality, and Critique." *Rethinking Marxism* 14, no. 3 (2002): 49–64.

Liu, Joanne. "Finish the Fight," *Nature* 524 (August 6, 2015): 27–29.

Livingstone, David N. "Race, Space and Moral Climatology: Notes Toward a Genealogy." *Journal of Historical Geography* 28, no. 2 (2002): 159–180.

Lombardo, Paul A. "Facing Carrie Buck." *The Hastings Center Report* 33, no. 2 (March/April, 2003): 14–17. doi: 10.2307/3528148.

Lynch, Lisa. "The Neo/bio/colonial Hot Zone: African Viruses, American Fairytales." *International Journal of Cultural Studies* 1, no 2 (1998): 233–252.

Matonock, Almea, et al. "Ebola Virus Diseases among Health Care Workers Not Working in Ebola Treatment Units-Liberia, June-August, 2014." *Morbidity and Mortality Weekly* 634, no. 46 (November 21, 2014): 1077–1081.

McCarthy, Michael. "CDC Rejects Mandatory Quarantine for Travelers Arriving from Ebola Stricken Nations." *British Medical Journal* 349 (2014): g6499.

McCarthy, Michael. "Maine Judge Refuses to Quarantine Nurse Who Cared for Ebola Patients." *British Medical Journal* 349 (November 3, 2014): g6606.

McCarthy, Michael. "Nurse Says She Will Fight Ebola Quarantine." *British Medical Journal* (2014): 349: g6555.

McDorman, Todd F. "Challenging Constitutional Authority: African American Responses to *Scott v. Sandford*." *The Quarterly Journal of Speech* 83, no. 2 (1997): 192–209, doi: 10.1080/00335639709384180.

McGee, Michael C. "The 'Ideograph': A Link between Rhetoric and Ideology." *The Quarterly Journal of Speech*, 66, no. 1 (1980): 1–16, doi: 10.1080/00335638009383499.

McKerrow, Raymie E. "Space and Time in the Postmodern Polity." *Western Journal of Communication* 63, no. 2 (1999): 271–290.

Meltzer, Martin, et al. "Estimating the Future Number of Cases in the Ebola Epidemic—Liberia and Sierra Leone, 2014–2015." *Morbidity and Mortality Weekly Reports, Supplements*, 63, no. 3 (September 26, 2914): 1–14.

Mitman, Gregg. "Ebola in a Stew of Fear." *New England Journal of Medicine* 371, no. 9 (November 6, 2014): 1763–1765. doi: 10.1056/NEJMp1411244.

Murdocca, Carmela. "When Ebola Came to Canada: Race and the Making of the Respectable Body," *Atlantis* 27, no. 2 (Spring/Summer 2003): 24–31.

Murphy, William P. "Military Patrimonialism and Child Soldier Clientalism in the Liberia and Sierra Leonean Civil Wars." *African Studies Review* 46, no. 2 (2003): 61–87.

Murray, Clinton K., et al., "Operation United Assistance: Infectious Disease Threats to Deployed Military Personnel." *Military Medicine* 180, no., 6 (June, 2015): 626–650.

Murray, Stuart J. "Myth as Critique: Review of Michel Foucault's "Society Must be Defended." *Qui Parle* 13, no. 2 (Spring/Summer, 2003): 203–221.

Murray, Stuart J. "Thanatopolitics: On the Use of Death for Mobilizing Political Life." *Polygraph* 18 (2006): 191–215.

Mutsaers, Inge. "One Health Approach as Counter-Measure against 'Autoimmune' Responses in Biosecurity." *Social Science & Medicine* 129 (2015): 123–130.

Nunnenkamp, Peter, and Hannes Öhler. "Throwing Foreign Aid at HIV/AIDS in Developing Countries: Missing the Target?" *World Development* 39, no. 10 (2011): 1704–1723.

Oberdabernig, Doris A. "Revisiting the Effects of IMF Programs On Poverty and Inequality." *World Development* 46 (June, 2013): 113–142.

Obilade, Titilola T. "The Political Economy of the Ebola Virus Disease (EVD); Taking Individual and Community Ownership in the Prevention and Control of EVD." *Healthcare* 3 (2015): 36–49.

Olliaro, Piero L., Peter Horby, and Else Teorreele. "Health Security and Rights in Times of Emerging Health Threats." *The Lancet* 385 (May 9, 2015): 1892–1893.

Ono, Kent A., and John M. Sloop. "The Critique of Vernacular Discourse." *Communication Monographs* 62 (March, 1995): 19–46.

Osterholm, Michael T., Kristine A. Moore, and Lawrence O. Gostin. "Public Health in the Age of Ebola." *The Journal of the American Medical Association* 175, no. 1 (January, 2015): 7–8. doi:10.1001/jamainternmed.2014.6235.

Petherick, Anna. "Ebola in West Africa: Learning the Lessons." The *Lancet* 385, no. 9968 (February 14, 2014): 591–592.

Pfeiffer, James, and Rachel Chapman. "Anthropological Perspectives on Structural Adjustment and Public Health." *Annual Review of Anthropology* 39 (2010): 149–165.

Ponnou-Delaffon, Erin Tremblay. "In and Out of Place: Geographies of Revolt in Camus's *La Peste.*" *Studies in 20th & 21st Century Literature*, 39 no. 1 (2015): 1–13.

Rossella, Bonito Oliva, and Timothy Campbell. "From the Immune Community to the Communitarian Immunity: On the Recent Reflection of Roberto Esposito." *Diacritics* 36, no. 2 (Summer 2006): 70–82.

Rothstein, Mark A. "From SARS to Ebola: Legal and Ethical Considerations for Modern Quarantine." *Indiana Health Law Review* 12, no. 1 (2015): 227–280.

Saéz, Mari, et al. "Investigating the Zoonotic Origin of the West African Ebola Epidemic." *EMBO Molecular Medicine* 7, no. 1 (December 30, 2014): 17–23. doi: 10.15252/emmm.201404792.

Shuaib, Faisal, et al. "Ebola Virus Disease Outbreak—Nigeria, July–September 2014." *Morbidity and Mortality Weekly Report* 63, no. 39 (October 3, 2014): 867–872.

Stotesbury, John A. "Rudyard Kipling and His Imperial Verse: Critical Dilemmas." *Hungarian Journal of English and American Studies* 1, no. 2 (1995): 37–46.

Stoler, Ann Laura. "Colonial Archives and the Arts of Governance." *Archival Science* 2 (2002): 87–109.

Stuckler, David, Lawrence P. King, and Sanjay Basu. "International Monetary Fund Programs and Tuberculosis Outcome in Post-Communist Countries." *PLoS Medicine* 5 (July 2008): 1079–1090.

Tognotti, Eugenia. "Lessons from the History of Quarantine, From Plague to Influenza A." *Emerging Infectious Disease* 19, no. 2 (February, 2013): 254–259.

Toscano, Alberto. "The Tactics and Ethics of Humanitarianism." *Humanity* 5, no. 1. (Spring, 2014): 123–147.

Varpilah, Tornorlah, et al. "Rebuilding Human Resources for Health: A Case Study from Liberia." *Human Resources for Health* 9, no. 11 (2011): 1–9.

Wallis, Laura. "First U.S. Nurse to Contract Ebola Sues Texas Health Resources." *American Journal of Nursing* 115, no. 6 (June 2015): 16. doi: 10.1097/01. NAJ.0000466302.77895.c5.

Walters, William, and Anne-Marie D'Aoust. "Bringing Publics into Critical Security Studies: Notes for a Research Strategy." *Millennium: Journal of International Studies* 44, no. 1 (2015): 45–68, doi: 10.1177/0305829815594439.

Wander, Philip. "The Third Persona: An Ideological Turn in Rhetorical Theory." *Central States Speech Journal* 35 (1984): 197–216.

Watterson, Christopher, and Adam Kamradt-Scott. "Fighting Flu: Securitization and the Military Role in Combating Influenza." *Armed Forces & Society* (2015); 1–15. doi: 10.1177/0095327X14567364.

Weldon, Rebecca. "An 'Urban Legend' of Global Proportions: An Analysis of Nonfiction Accounts of Ebola Virus." *Journal of Health Communication: International Perspectives* 6, no. 3 (2001): 281–294. doi: 10.1080/108107301752384451.

Weldon, Rebecca A. "The Rhetorical Construction of the Predatorial Virus: A Burkian Analysis of Nonfiction Accounts of the Ebola Virus." *Qualitative Health Research* 11, no. 1 (2001): 5–25. doi: 10.1177/104973201129118902.

WHO Ebola Response Team. "Ebola Virus Disease in West Africa-The First 9 Months of the Epidemic and Forward Projects." *The New England Journal of Medicine* 371 (October 16, 2014): 1481–1495.

Wilkinson, Annie, and Melissa Leach. "Briefing: Ebola-Myths, Realities and Structural Violence." *African Affairs* 114, no. 454 (2014): 136–148.

MAGAZINE ARTICLES

Castner, Brian. "We Are Fighting an Enemy, and the Enemy Is Ebola." *Foreign Policy*, January 14, 2015. http://foreignpolicy.com/2015/01/14/us-army-general-volesky-fighting-ebola-outbreak-in-liberia/.

Cohen, Jon. "Exit Interview: CDC Epidemiologist Sees Hope for Controlling Ebola in Southeastern Liberia." *Science Magazine*, October 8, 2014. http://news.sciencemag.org/africa/2014/10/exit-interview-cdc-epidemiologist-sees-hope-controlling-ebola-southeastern-liberia.

Francis, David. "Ebola's Toll Was Horrific. It Could Have Been Much Worse." *Foreign Policy*, February 11, 2015. http://foreignpolicy.com/2015/02/11/epidemic-ebola-pentagon-obama-outbreak-africa/.

Fridriksdottir, Gudrun Sif. "The 'War' on Ebola." Mats Utas, October 27, 2014. https://matsutas.wordpress.com/2014/10/27/the-war-on-ebola-by-gudrun-sif-fridriksdottir/.

Frizell, Sam. "First Ebola Worker Quarantined under New Policy Tests Negative." *Time*, October 25, 2014. http://time.com/3538834/ebola-quarantine-new-york/.

Garrett, Laurie. "Ebola's Lesson." *Foreign Affairs*, September/October, 2015. https://www.foreignaffairs.com/articles/west-africa/2015-08-18/ebola-s-lessons?campaign=Garrett.

Garrett, Laurie. "Heartless but Effective: I've Seen 'Cordon Sanitaire' Work against Ebola." *The New Republic*, August 14, 2014. http://www.newrepublic.com/article/119085/ebola-cordon-sanitaire-when-it-worked-congo-1995.

Garrett, Laurie. "Liberia Is Stiffing Its Contact Tracers as Ebola Epidemic Continues." *Foreign Policy*, November 11, 2014. http://foreignpolicy.com/2014/11/11/liberia-is-stiffing-its-contact-tracers-as-ebola-epidemic-continues/.

Ghose, Tia. "Contagion: Science Fact?" *The Scientist*, September 16, 2011. http://www.the-scientist.com/?articles.view/articleNo/31179/title/Contagion—Science-Fact-/.

Greenberg, Karen. "America's Response to Ebola Looks Disturbingly Similar to the War on Terror." *Mother Jones*, November 12, 2014. http://www.motherjones.com/politics/2014/11/4-lessons-war-terror-apply-ebola-fight.

Kedmey, Dan. "Kaci Hickox: 'Stop Calling Me the 'Ebola Nurse'—Now!" *Time*, November 17, 2014. http://time.com/3588930/kaci-hickox-ebola-nurse/.

Latson, Jennifer. "Refusing Quarantine: Why Typhoid Mary Did It." *Time*, November 11, 2014. http://time.com/3563182/typhoid-mary/.

Lydersen, Kari. "Ebola Teams Need Better Cultural Understanding, Anthropologists Say." *Discover*, December 9, 2014. http://blogs.discovermagazine.com/crux/2014/12/09/ebola-cultural-anthropologists/#.VXHoY89VhBd.

Musabeyezu, Juliet, Yusuph Mkangara, and Hamma Amanuel. "The 'Africanization' of Ebola." *Harvard Political Review*, February 25, 2015. http://harvardpolitics.com/world/africanization-ebola/.

Preston, Richard. "The Ebola Wars." *The New Yorker*, October 27, 2014. http://www.newyorker.com/magazine/2014/10/27/ebola-wars.

Sherwood, Dave, and Colleen Jenkins. "Maine Settles Quarantine Lawsuit with Nurse Who Worked with Ebola Patients in West Africa." *Scientific American*, November 3, 2014. http://www.scientificamerican.com/article/nurse-kacihickox-and-state-of-maine-settle-quarantine-lawsuit/.

Weintraub, Karen. "From Senegal and Nigeria, 4 Lessons on How to Stop Ebola." *National Geographic*, October 25, 2014, http://news.nationalgeographic.com/news/2014/10/141024-ebola-nigeria-outbreak-lessons-virus-health/.

MISCELLANEOUS INTERNET SOURCES

Albertini, Bill. "The Geographies of Contagion." *Rhizomes: Cultural Studies in Emerging Knowledge* 19 (Summer 2009): Accessed October 7, 2015. http://www.rhizomes.net/issue19/albertini.html.

Anderson, Warwick. "Tolerance." Somatosphere, October 27, 2014. http://somatosphere.net/2014/10/tolerance.html.

Benton, Adia. "Race and the Immuno-Logics of Ebola Response in West Africa." Somatosphere, September 19, 2014, http://somatosphere.net/2014/09/raceand-the-immuno-logics-of-ebola-response-in-west-africa.html.

Bigon, Liora. "Bubonic Plague, Colonial Ideologies, and Urban Planning Policies: Dakar, Lagos, and Kumasi." *Planning Perspectives*, August, 2015. doi:10.1080/02665433.2015.1064779.

Bouchet-Saulnier, Françoise. "The Theory and Practice of Rebellious Humanitarianism." *Humanitarian Practice Network*, June 2003. http://odihpn.org/magazine/the-theory-and-practice-of-%C2%91rebellious-humanitarianism%C2%92/.

Brosseau, Lisa M., and Rachel Jones. "Commentary: Health Workers Need Optimal Respiratory Protection for Ebola." *Center for Infectious Disease Research and Policy*, September 17, 2014. http://www.cidrap.umn.edu/news-perspective/2014/09/commentary-health-workers-need-optimal-respiratory-protection-ebola.

De Waal, Alex. "Militarizing Global Health." *Boston Review*, November 11, 2014. http://bostonreview.net/world/alex-de-waal-militarizing-global-health-ebola.

Fearnley, Lyle. "The Disease That Emerged." *LIMN*, January, 2015. http://limn. it/the-disease-that-emerged/.

Gregory, Derek. "Fighting Ebola." *Geographical Imaginations*, November 15, 2014. http://geographicalimaginations.com/2014/11/15/fighting-ebola/.

Gregory, Derek. "Theory of the Drone 3: Killing Ground." Geographical Imaginations, July 29, 2013. http://geographicalimaginations.com/2013/07/29/theory-of-the-drone-3-killing-grounds/.

Grey, Thomas C. "The Holmesian Judge in Theory and Practice." *William and Mary Law Review* 37 (1995): 19–45.

Koch, Tom. "Ebola, Epidemics, Pandemics and the Mapping of their Containment." Remedianetwork.net, September 22, 2014. http://remedianetwork. net/2014/09/22/ebola-epidemics-pandemics-and-the-mapping-of-their-containment/.

Médecins Sans Frontières. "An Unprecedented Year: Médecins Sans Frontières' Response to the Largest Ever Outbreak." Médecins Sans Frontières, March, 2015. http://www.msf.org/sites/msf.org/files/ebola_accountability_report_final_july_low_res.pdf.

Médecins Sans Frontières. "Ebola in West Africa: Epidemic Requires Massive Deployment of Resources." Médecins Sans Frontières, June 21, 2014. http://www.msf.org/article/ebola-west-africa-epidemic-requires-massive-deployment-resources.

Médecins Sans Frontières. "Pushed to the Limit and Beyond: A Year into the Largest Ever Outbreak." Médecins Sans Frontières, March, 2015. https://www.doctorswithoutborders.org/sites/usa/files/msf143061.pdf.

Meyer, Michelle. N. "Will the Real Evidence-Based Ebola Policy Please Stand Up? Several Takeaways from *Maine DHHS v. Hickox*." November 6, 2014. http://www.thefacultylounge.org/2014/11/will-the-real-evidence-based-ebola-policy-please-stand-up-seven-take-aways-from-maine-dhhs-v-hickox.html.

Park, Sung-Joon, and René Umlauf. "Caring as Existential Insecurity: Quarantine, Care, and Human Insecurity in the Ebola Crisis." *Somatosphere*, November 24, 2014, http://somatosphere.net/2014/11/caring-as-existential-insecurity.html.

Sáez, Almudena Mari, Ann Kelly, and Hannah Brown. "Notes from Case Zero: Anthropology in the Time of Ebola." Somatosphere, September 16, 2014. http://somatosphere.net/2014/09/notes-from-case-zero-anthropology-in-the-time-of-ebola.html.

Steinhauer, Jason. "Ebola, Colonialism, and the History of International Aid Organizations." Library of Congress Blog. Last modified February 3, 2015. http://blogs.loc.gov/kluge/2015/02/ebola-colonialism-history-international-aid-organizations-in-africa/.

Wald, Priscilla. "Panic and Precaution: Ebola and the Outbreak Narrative." *The Conversation*, October 28, 2014. http://theconversation.com/panic-and-precaution-ebola-and-the-outbreak-narrative-32786.

World Health Organization. "Strengthening Health Security by Implementing the International Health Regulations, 2005." *World Health Organization*, August 6, 2014. http://www.who.int/ihr/procedures/emerg_comm_members_20140806/en/.

GOVERNMENT REPORTS AND PUBLICATIONS

Government of Liberia: Ministry of Health and Social Welfare and World Health Organization. *Liberia Health Situation Analysis, Final Report.* Geneva: World Health Organization, 2002.

Government of Liberia: Ministry of Health and Social Welfare. *Liberia Ebola Situation Report* no. 94, August 17, 2014. http://mohsw.gov.lr/documents/Liberia %20Ebola%20SitRep%2094%20Aug%2017,%202014.pdf.

U.S. Committee on Health, Education, Labor and Pensions Staff. *Joint Full Committee Hearing: Ebola in West Africa: A Global Challenge and Public Health Threat.* U.S. Committee on Health, Education, Labor & Pensions, September 16, 2014, http://www.help.senate.gov/hearings/ebola-in-west-africa-a-global-challenge-and-public-health-threat.

LEGAL CASES

Crayton v. Larabee, 110 N. Rep. 355, 220 N.Y. 493 (N.Y. Ct. of App. 1917).

Jacobson v. Massachusetts, 197 U.S. 11 (1905).

Selective Draft Law Cases, 245 U.S. 366 (1918).

U.S. ex rel. Siegel v. Shinnick, 219 F. Supp 789 (E.D. NY 1963).

Index

Abdullah, Ibrahim, 108, 111, 126
Adadevoh, Ameyo, 151, 178
Africanization, vii, 150–52, 220
Agamben, Gorgio, 12
Albertini, Bill, 143, 219
American exceptionalism, 3, 17 201–202, 207, 228
Anderson, Warwick, 180
Appadurai, Arjun, 22, 131–32, 157
Arendt, Hannah, 23
argumentative, 1, 9, 14, 16–17, 27, 36, 38, 54, 78, 85–86, 121, 124, 153
autoimmunization, 163, 167–72, 177, 180
Ayotte, Kevin, 17, 167, 173, 204

Bass, Jeff. 24, 166
Benton, Adia, 124, 166
Bergstresser, Sara M., 82
Biafra, 34–35
biocriticism, viii, 10, 20, 167, 180
Black Swan events, 221–22
Blattman, Chris, 107, 118–24
Brantly, Kent, 52–55, 62, 151, 193, 215
Brown, Donal, 213–14, 219
Brown, Hannah, 156, 177

Buck, Carrie, 77, 80, 97
bushmeat, 28, 34, 64, 205

Camus, Albert, 163, 178, 180
Carrilho, André, 152
Centers for Disease Control (CDC), 8, 12–13, 16–17, 20, 31, 39, 64–66, 70, 79, 82–83, 87, 89–93, 95–96, 98, 100, 102, 104–06, 133, 142–48, 166, 174, 178–79, 202, 215–17, 222
Chan, Kit Yee, 78
Chan, Margaret, 225, 230
Chapman, Rachel, 111–13
Chau, Arlene, 70
Chiappelli, Francesco, 1
cholera, 1, 11, 22, 25, 27, 43, 81, 211, 219
Christie, Chris, 80, 83, 87–88, 92–93, 97, 102
Cloud, Dana, 54–55
Collier, Stephen, 21, 132, 135, 201
communitas, 13, 168, 176–77, 180
Condé, Alpha, 31–33
Conteh-Morgan, Earl, 113–15
contract tracers, 4, 8–9, 16, 49, 52, 55–64, 66–71, 75, 176–77, 198, 213, 215, 220, 224, 228–229

cordons sanitaires, 4, 5, 7–8, 10, 17, 51, 67, 71, 78, 81, 88, 138, 147, 150, 156, 163–67, 170, 172–80, 200, 214
critical cultural studies, 18
critical rhetorical studies, 73

De Waal, Alex, 196–197
DeChaine, D. Robert, 30, 39
Delicath, John, 9, 21
Deloffre, Maryam Z., 194–95
DeLuca, Kevin, 9, 21
Democratic Republic of the Congo (DRC), (Zaire), 11, 38, 49, 65, 73, 133, 135, 138, 142, 165, 180
Derrida, Jacques, 10, 167–69, 171, 177, 180
Dhillon, Ranu, 56–58
Dionne, Kim Yi, 121, 124–25, 197
dispositifs, 4, 9–17, 21, 24, 27–28, 43, 50, 54, 56–58, 63, 70–71, 78–82, 92, 98, 107–09, 111, 119, 121, 132–35, 139, 142, 151, 153, 156, 164, 166, 168, 172, 177, 180, 189, 215, 218, 227, 230
Duncan, Thomas E., 11–12, 97, 134, 148, 154, 193

Ebola: apocalypse, 10, 17, 58, 63, 70, 121, 131–132, 137–38, 142, 144–45, 147, 152, 156, 163, 165, 175, 178, 199, 217–18, 231; denialism, 2–3, 15, 28, 32–33, 41, 43, 55, 61, 64, 155, 170, 174, 210, 215, 217; exceptionalism, 185–201; hunters, 4, 8; stigma, 5, 11, 57, 61, 65, 69, 77, 80–81, 96, 152, 168, 196, 210, 220–21, 224; transmission, 1–2, 7–8, 15–16, 20–22, 37, 47, 58, 62, 71, 80, 83, 92, 94–95, 98, 106, 132, 134, 140–42, 146, 149–50, 157, 159, 171, 174–75, 178, 210–11, 214–15, 217, 219–20, 222–23; Virus Disease (EVD), 1, 3–4, 6–8, 11–17, 20–21, 24–27, 35–40, 42, 46–47, 49–56, 58–62, 64, 68–79, 73, 75, 78, 85, 87, 96, 98–101, 104, 107, 109, 120, 132, 134–135, 137, 139, 141, 144, 151, 157, 164, 166, 170–71, 173–78, 180, 189–96, 200–03, 205, 209, 210, 213–

17, 220–25, 228–29, 231, 233; West African outbreak, 3, 5, 15–16, 22, 28, 36, 42, 51, 63, 65, 71, 107, 138, 151, 155, 165, 177, 209, 217–18, 220, 230, 234; Zaire, 1, 11, 22, 25, 69, 133, 138, 140–41, 143, 165, 180, 220.
Ebolaphobia, 216
Elbe, Stefan, 227
Esposito, Roberto, 10, 13, 22, 167–168, 177, 180–82
Evers, Claudia, 220

Farmer, Paul, 4, 113
Fauci, Anthony, 148, 177
Fins, Joseph, 6
Foucault, Michel, 4, 6, 10–11, 19–21, 55, 72, 83, 108, 152
Fox, Renée, 35–36
Frankel, Stephen, 110, 125

Garrett, Laurie, 27, 50, 67–68, 131, 133, 135–41, 150, 158, 165
Gatter, Robert, 93–95, 98, 102, 106
Gbanya, Miatta Z., 44, 49, 51
genealogical, 57, 83, 100, 108, 123
Ghana, 116
Gingrey, Phil, 216
global health security, 5, 9, 11, 28, 43, 210–11, 213–14, 223, 231
global North, 1–3, 7, 16, 25, 35, 56, 64, 71, 108, 112, 113–15, 118–19, 121, 124, 133, 135–36, 152, 157, 164, 174–75, 196, 212, 214–16, 220, 223, 226–27, 230–31
global South, 2–3, 108, 112, 121, 157, 164, 175, 196, 215, 220, 226–27, 231
Gostin, Lawrence, 100, 221–22
Greenberg, Karen, 196
Gregory, Derek, 171
Guild, Carissa, 59–61
Guinea, 1–2, 4, 8, 11, 13, 15–16, 20, 24–25, 30–33, 35–37, 40–43, 46, 52, 56–64, 68–75, 80, 83, 107–11, 118, 121, 123, 125, 133, 137, 150–51, 155, 157, 164–65, 167, 173–75, 179, 185, 188–89 194, 196, 200, 202, 209, 213, 219–221, 223–226, 229–230

H1N1 scare, 145
Heath, J. Benton, 2, 6
Henao-Restrepo, Ana Marie, 223–24
Heymann, David, 135, 210–13
Hickox, Kaci, 7, 16, 77–106, 207, 209, 217
Hodge, James, Jr., 51
Hoffman, Dustin, 143
Holmes, Oliver Wendell, Jr., 77
Hot Zone, 52, 93, 134, 142–43, 149, 218–19, 228, 231

ideograph, 9, 21, 112, 211, 213, 221
image events, 9, 20, 137, 152
immunitas, 13, 167–68, 177–78, 182
International Federation of the Red Cross and Red Crescent Societies (IFRC), 179
International Health Regulations (IHR), 2, 6, 18, 211–12, 230
International Monetary Fund (IMF), 9, 16, 42, 107–09, 111–25, 127–28, 141, 185, 229
Ivory Coast, 1, 175, 222

Jacobson v. Massachusetts (1905), 83, 101

Kekulé, Alexander, 64
Kelly, Ann, 156, 177
Kelly, Daniel, 56–58
Kenitkelenis, Alexander, 119–20, 124
Keränen, Lisa, 10, 167, 177, 180
Khan, Sheik Umar, 139
Ki-Moon, Ban, 87
Kontorovich, Eugene, 83–84, 99, 101
Koroma, Ernest B., 209

Lakoff, Andrew, 132, 135, 162, 201, 219
Lassa Fever, 11, 22, 25, 37, 45
LaVerdiere, Charles, 90–91, 94, 98–99
Leach, Melissa, 24, 234
Legters, Llewellyn, 142, 149
LePage, Paul R., 88, 90, 94, 104
Liberia, 1–2, 4, 7, 8, 11–13, 15–17, 20, 24, 26, 32, 35–37, 40, 49–53, 55, 56–58, 61–62, 64–71, 75, 80, 83, 107–11, 115–23, 125, 137, 147, 150–51, 154–56, 163–67, 170–75, 77–180, 183,

185, 189–94, 196–98, 200–03, 209, 213–14, 217, 219–23, 226, 229
Liu, Joanne, 28, 36, 43–44, 185, 188, 209–210
Liverpool School of Tropical Medicine, 109
Livingstone, David, 54
Livingstone, David N., 57
Lynch, Lisa, 136–37, 154

magic bullet, 145, 147, 223
malaria, 1, 11, 36, 39, 63, 109–10, 125, 164, 176, 196, 199
Mali, 1, 38, 150, 187, 226
Mallon, Mary (Typhoid Mary), 77, 80, 97, 99, 217
Mano River Union, 164–66
Mbembe, Achille, 210
McChrystal, Stanley, 153–55
McGee, Michael C., 21
McKerrow, Raymie, 175
Médecins Sans Frontières, (MSF), [Doctors Without Borders], 4, 8, 12, 14–15, 18, 22–46, 50, 58–59, 61–64, 69, 79, 85, 88, 108, 116, 133, 136, 138, 154, 174, 176, 179, 185–86, 188, 191, 194, 203–04, 209, 214, 220–21, 225, 229
medical humanitarianism, 3, 5, 23–24, 28, 34, 50, 53, 88, 108, 116, 120, 139, 143, 185–86, 189, 197–98, 227
Meyer, Michelle, N., 101, 106, 203
military humanitarianism, 3, 12, 17, 22, 27, 63, 136, 143, 154, 185–87, 195–96, 203–04, 227
Mitman, Gregg, 217
mobile rapid responses, 226
Moeller, Susan, 143
Murray, Clinton, 199
Musabeyezu, Juliet, 150–51
Mutsaers, Inge, 168, 177, 180
Muyembe, Jean-Jacques, 180

necropolitics, 40, 210
neo-colonial, 2, 28, 126
Nigeria 1, 11, 34–35, 38, 108, 151, 175, 178–80, 182, 216–18, 226
Nyenswah, Tolbert, 65, 170

Obama, Barack, 13, 17, 56, 64, 68, 98, 136, 138, 153, 185–86, 188–90, 193–202, 223, 228
Operation United Assistance (OUA), 8, 108, 187, 189–93, 195–98, 200, 204–207, 228
Osterholm, Michael, 221–22
outbreak narratives, 9, 13, 31, 36, 38, 132, 143, 175, 195, 199, 211, 216–18, 230

Parmet, Wendy, 98
Park, Sung-Joon, 7, 20
patient zero, 8, 15, 23–26, 30, 34, 36–38, 56, 64, 123–24, 133, 148, 151, 172, 191, 224
Personal Protective Equipment (PPE), 2, 12, 14, 37, 51–53, 60, 66, 70, 171, 173, 191, 203, 229
Pfeiffer, James, 111–13
Pham, Nina, vii, 7, 71, 95, 97–98, 105, 134, 148, 193, 209, 214, 216
Piot, Peter, 52, 135, 143, 223
precautionary principle, 8, 13, 78, 84, 92–93, 98, 106, 202
Preston, Richard, 52, 93, 133–135, 140, 142, 149, 156–57, 218–19, 231
Public Health Emergency of International Concern (PHEIC), 63

quarantines, vii, 4–5, 7, 10, 12–13, 17, 32, 35, 51, 56, 59, 66, 71, 78–92, 94–96, 98–101, 103, 106, 138, 140, 147, 150, 166–67, 171–77, 180, 182, 200, 202, 211, 214, 217, 222

Redfield, Peter, 35
Redipath, Daniel, 78
Responsibility to Protect (R2P), 9, 12 27, 229
rhetorical, 1, 4, 6, 8–12, 14, 15–20, 24–25, 28–29, 31, 37, 41, 52, 54, 58, 64, 70, 73, 79–81, 83, 87, 92, 94, 97, 100, 106, 108, 122, 132–34, 136–37, 142, 144, 166, 169–70, 193–94, 201, 215, 218, 220–21, 228, 230
Rosling, Hans, 63
rule of law, 6, 9, 11, 19, 21, 78, 86, 100

Sáez, Marí Almudena, 69, 156
savior complex, 43
Sawyer, Patrick, 178
Senegal, 38, 152, 175, 178–80, 222, 226
Shuaib, Faisalm, 179
Sierra Leone 1–2, 4, 11, 13, 15–16, 20, 24, 32, 35, 37, 40–42, 46, 52, 56, 58–60, 62–64, 66, 68–69, 79–80, 83, 85, 93, 96, 107, 109–11, 113–15, 118, 121–23, 125, 137, 150–51, 155, 157, 164–65, 167, 174–75, 179, 185, 188–89, 194, 196, 200, 202, 209, 213, 215, 219–20, 222–23, 226, 229
Sirleaf, Ellen Johnson, 49, 54, 115, 166, 170–71, 173–75, 190, 192, 196–97
Sloterdijk, Peter, 167–69, 171, 180–91
Soderbergh, Steven, 144–50
Spain, 11, 165, 226
Spanish flu, 131
Spencer, Craig, 85, 95, 97, 100, 105, 209, 216
Stoler, Ann, 108, 204
structural adjustment programs (SAPs), 111–17, 123, 202

Talbert-Slagle, Kristina, 153–56
Taleb, Nassim Nichols, 221–22
témoignage, 15, 29, 34–35, 42–44, 188
thanatopolitics, 10–11, 22, 25, 28, 42, 93, 121, 132, 137, 168–69, 177, 210, 218
Tognotti, Eugenia, 81, 101
Toscano, Alberto, 30, 189
traditional healers, 37, 69
tropical hermeneutics, 57

Uganda, 11, 62, 133, 138, 142
Umlauf, René, 7, 20
U.N. Mission for Ebola Emergency Response (UNMEER), 26, 50, 195
U.S. Agency for the International Development (USAID), 190–92, 198, 200–01

vaccines, 141, 143, 145–47, 149–50, 165, 169, 196, 202, 212–13, 216, 223–27
Varpilah, Tornorlah, 115–17

vernacular, 10, 26, 55, 57–58, 61, 70, 73, 147, 149, 154, 167, 170
Vinson, Amber, 71, 95, 97, 216
vital systems security, 132, 201
Volesky, Gary, 200–01

Wald, Priscilla, 9, 24
Waldon, Rebecca, 167
Wander, Philip, 55
Weizman, Eyal, 23, 28, 44
West Point, 17, 147, 163–79, 214

White Man's Burden, 53
White Man's Grave, 109–11, 123
Williams, Darryl, 194
World Bank, 9, 16, 26, 42, 50, 64, 107–25, 141, 185, 214, 229
World Health Organization (WHO), 2, 5, 8, 12, 14–15, 18, 25–28, 30–34, 37, 39, 42–43, 57, 63, 64, 70, 118, 126, 133, 136–37, 142, 151, 176, 179, 185, 187, 189, 209, 211, 214, 221–22, 224–25, 228, 230

About the Author

Marouf A. Hasian Jr. is professor of communication at the University of Utah.